Radiologic technology

Textbook of

Radiologic technology

CHARLES A. JACOBI

B.Sc., R.T.(A.R.R.T.)

Lecturer and Head, Department of Radiologic Technology,
College of General and Technical Studies,
Nevada Southern University, Las Vegas, Nevada;
formerly Assistant Professor, Medical Radiologic
Technology, and Member, Radioisotopes Committee, Oregon
Technical Institute, Klamath Falls, Oregon

DON Q PARIS

R.T.(A.R.R.T.)

Lecturer, Department of Radiologic Technology,
College of General and Technical Studies,
Nevada Southern University, Las Vegas, Nevada;
formerly Assistant Professor and Chairman, Medical Radiologic Technology,
Oregon Technical Institute, Klamath Falls, Oregon

Fourth edition

With 384 illustrations

The C. V. Mosby Company

Saint Louis   1968

Dedicated to students of

Radiologic technology

Foreword

This book should prove helpful to those who need help the most. It is a compilation of the instructional material that has been found by the authors to be the most effective in teaching students radiologic technology at Oregon Technical Institute.

It presents basic information and procedures. Frills have been intentionally omitted. Although this is a practical book to be used in basic instruction, it may also be used by the technologist of limited experience and the technologist "on his own" in the smaller hospitals and clinics.

The authors have made a valuable contribution to radiologic technology.

James M. Hilton, M.D.

Roentgenologist,
Associate Professor, Medical Radiologic
Technology, Oregon Technical Institute,
Klamath Falls, Oregon

Preface to fourth edition

To be current with changes in our profession and to be specific in the intent of this text, we have changed the title and the dedication. Other changes include the addition of a new chapter designed to assist in the orientation of students of radiologic technology. In conjunction with the new chapter there are corresponding additions in the illustrations. Also, there are many replacement illustrations throughout the text. We have rearranged several parts of existing chapters in order to present the technical information to the student in a better learning sequence. The chapter on special procedures has been expanded considerably to afford more specific information.

Acknowledgments of appreciation for permission to use certain illustrative material are gratefully extended to Machlett Laboratories Incorporated, General Electric Company, Standard X-ray Company, Picker X-ray Corporation, Tracerlab-Keleket Company, Victoreen Instrument Company, The W. B. Saunders Company, and Dr. Stanley Jacob and Mrs. C. A. Francone.

As in the previous editions, the assistance and encouragement of our wives and families have been a most welcome stimulus in our efforts.

Charles A. Jacobi
Don Q Paris

Preface to first edition

During our instruction of students in x-ray technology, we have felt the need for a text containing the areas of information necessary to our specialized field. We have tried, in developing the text, to include all the materials relevant to our field. We also have attempted to arrange the material in the sequence that will facilitate its use as a teaching tool.

A major problem in teaching a course in x-ray technology is the diversity of knowledge needed by a technician. This diversity is essential for operating x-ray equipment and obtaining the exact radiographs specified by the doctors. It would be impossible to teach each element in its entirety; therefore, we have explored thoroughly each individual area and have extracted the necessary principles and facts. To be expert in each field is unnecessary for a technician, but a good technician must have a rudimentary knowledge of allied areas.

It is not our belief that an x-ray technician should double as a repairman, but we do believe that he should understand the general principles of the working of the machine he operates. Therefore, he should have a knowledge of the principles of physics and electricity. Thus we feel that inclusion of the chapters on these subjects is justified.

However, a technician must know more than how to read a chart and to adjust the dials on a machine if he is to be of aid to the medical profession. Consequently, preceding each chapter on positioning, we have included a chapter on anatomy and physiology related to the particular area to be radiographed.

The development of this text has not been a haphazard or recent idea. While working as x-ray technicians, we began noting ideas which we thought would be helpful if we were to teach a course in the field or if we were ever to write a book based on knowledge gained by our experience. From an outline based on these notes, we were able to formulate the course in x-ray technology taught at Oregon Technical Institute. The course has been highly successful.

A more detailed contents than is usually found in books in the field of medicine and related sciences has been included to allow for quick and easy reference to various sections within this book.

We wish to express our sincere thanks and appreciation to the following for professional and technical advice, help, and illustrative material: Dr. James M. Hilton, our Radiologist and Course Supervisor; Dr. A. I. Thompson, our Medical Advisory Committee Chairman; Mrs. John Lake and Mr. Robert DeRosier, of our English Department, and Mrs. Robert DeRosier; Mr. Earl Bairey and Mr. William Finch, of our Graphic Arts Department; Mrs. Margaret Mansfield, R.T., who photographed the many radiographs loaned us by Dr. James M. Hilton and Dr. Earl Lawson; Miss Venita Merrill, Mrs. Catherine Parker Anthony, Dr. Carl C Francis and Dr. Gordon L. Farrell, and Dr. Barry J. Anson and Dr. Walter G. Maddock, for the use of illustrations from their publications*; and the General Electric X-Ray Department and Mrs. Catherine Parker Anthony, for the use of tabular material. Especially we wish to express our appreciation to our wives for their patience and to Mrs. Jacobi for her unselfish aid in typing the many manuscript copies.

Charles A. Jacobi
Donald E. Hagen

Klamath Falls, Oregon

*Merrill, Vinita: Atlas of roentgenographic positions, vols. I and II, St. Louis, 1949, The C. V. Mosby Co.

Anthony, Catherine Parker: Textbook of anatomy and physiology, ed. 4, St. Louis, 1955, The C. V. Mosby Co.

Francis, Carl C, and Farrell, Gordon L.: Integrated anatomy and physiology, St. Louis, 1957, The C. V. Mosby Co.

Anson, Barry J., and Maddock, Walter G.: Callander's surgical anatomy, ed. 3, Philadelphia, 1952, W. B. Saunders Co.

Contents

Chapter 5

Preventive maintenance, 68

Chapter 6

Radiographic principles, 73

Chapter 7

Film processing, 101

Chapter 8

Principles of radiographic quality, 108

Chapter 9

Bones of the extremities, 117

Chapter 13

Bones of the skull, 258

Chapter 14

Positioning for the skull, 273

Chapter 15

Anatomic physiology, 326

Chapter 16

Positioning for contrast studies, 351

Radiologic technology

Chapter 1

Introduction to radiography

U pon moving into a new neighborhood, we find that it is not only useful but necessary to become acquainted with the residents of the neighborhood and its customs; equally, entrance into a new professional field requires that we become acquainted with the persons and professions with whom we will be associated in our new endeavors. Entering into studies toward professional competence in the paramedical profession of radiologic technology, we need, first, to appreciate and understand the scope and sphere of radiologic technology, and then to become acquainted with the associated paramedical professions and medical specialties.

The practice of radiography is one of the several functions of radiologic technologists. Radiography, by definition, is the making of a record or photograph by means of the action of actinic rays (x-rays) on a sensitized surface, and a radiograph, or radiogram, is a film or other record so produced. Our professional society offers this definition: *a radiograph is a permanent photographic record of the structures through which a beam of ionizing radiation has passed.*

Paramedical professions and medical specialties

A radiologic technologist is a person trained to be expert in the performance of technical procedures that require the use of x-rays and/or radioisotopes and that are conducted under the supervision of medical doctors, dentists, osteopathic physicians, or veterinarians. He may be employed by any of these professional persons or by a hospital or clinic.

Another paramedical specialty is medical laboratory technology. A medical laboratory technologist is a person trained to be expert in the performance of technical procedures in the clinical laboratory that require the use of a variety of instruments and that are performed under the supervision of medical doctors, dentists, osteopathic physicians, or veterinarians. As a rule, the radiologic technologist works directly with radiologists and roentgenologists, and the medical laboratory technologist works directly with pathologists; however, this is not without exception.

Other paramedical professional personnel with whom radiologic technologists perform on the *medical team* include physical therapy technologists, nurses, and pharmacists.

Our discussion of purely professional persons will be restricted to medical doctors since the organizational structure of the paramedical profession of radiologic technology is so closely allied to the medical profession.

1

Medical doctors are graduates of medical schools. To enter medical school, one must possess, among many things, a baccalaureate degree in premedicine. Following graduation from medical school, the medical doctor must spend a period (usually 12 months) of *internship* in an AMA-approved hospital, i.e., a hospital approved by the Council on Medical Education of the American Medical Association (AMA) for medical internship. Upon satisfactory completion of the internship, the medical doctor must successfully write examinations required by the State Board of Medical Examiners in states in which he may wish to practice medicine.

If this new medical doctor, or one who has been in medical practice, desires to *specialize* in one field of medical practice, he will enter a *residency* for a specified number of years in a particular AMA-approved hospital. Upon the successful completion of his residency, the doctor will write a prescribed number of *medical specialty board examinations*. Successful performance with the board examinations entitles this doctor to practice his medical specialty in any state in which he holds a license.

Both roentgenologists and radiologists, then—with whom radiologic technologists often work closely—have completed a baccalaureate degree in premedicine, a graduate degree (M.D.) in medicine, a 1-year internship, and a 3-year residency: a total of 12 years of intensive study and practice (internship and residency) under strict supervision of skilled and experienced medical doctors.

Medical specialties differ in their requirements as to residency time period; otherwise, their requirements are very similar.

In alphabetical order the medical specialties are as follows:

A Allergy
ALR Otology, Laryngology and Rhinology
AM Aviation Medicine
Anes Anesthesiology
C Cardiology
CD Cardiovascular Diseases
CS Cardiovascular Surgery
CP Clinical Pathology
D Dermatology
FOP Forensic Pathology
GE Gastroenterology
GP General Practice
G Geriatrics
Gyn Gynecology
I Internal Medicine
Ind Industrial Practice
N Neurology
NS Neurological Surgery
OALR Ophthalmology, Otology, Laryngology and Rhinology

Ob Obstetrics
ObG Obstetrics and Gynecology
Oph Ophthalmology
Or Orthopedic Surgery
P Psychiatry
Path Pathology
Pd Pediatrics
PH Public Health
PL Plastic Surgery
PM Physical Medicine
PN Psychiatry and Neurology
Pr Proctology
Pul Pulmonary Diseases
R Roentgenology and Radiology
S Surgery
TS Thoracic Surgery
U Urology
VS Vascular Surgery

A radiologist is a physician with special experience in radiology. Radiology is the science of radiant energy and radiant substances, especially that branch of medical science that deals with the use of radiant energy in the diagnosis and treatment of disease.

Roentgenology is the branch of radiology that deals with the diagnostic and therapeutic use of roentgen rays. A roentgenologist is a physician who devotes himself to diagnosis and treatment by the roentgen rays (x-rays).

The other medical specialists and the general practitioners of medicine comprise the medical doctors for whom the radiologic technologists perform their skills and professional arts.

History of radiologic technology

Dr. W. C. Roentgen discovered x-rays on November 8, 1895, while experimenting with cathode rays generated in a Crooke's tube. Following release of the pertinent research and experimental data, these rays were produced in both Europe and North America. Dr. Roentgen's refusal of personal gain has permitted the origination and growth of many new branches of medical science and industrial technology.

One of the new medical science branches was that of radiologic technology. Near the turn of the century many physicians began to use these new rays in their medical practices. These men were forced either to operate their x-ray equipment personally or to train an assistant in these techniques. As a result, there was an increasing number of partially trained medical assistants operating the new x-ray equipment and using a variety of techniques.

In the same decade with Roentgen's discovery, there were numerous advances in knowledge of electricity and its application, in both diagnosis and therapy, to the practice of medicine. When Roentgen's discovery was made public, the application of electric currents in medical practice was receiving considerable attention. Ed C. Jerman, a talented electrician, was engaged with his father, a middle western physician, in this effort. With the release of information pertaining to the production of x-rays, Ed Jerman sought to assemble the necessary apparatus to produce x-rays. He became experienced in the operation of early x-ray machines and became well known in his own right to the medical profession and to the manufacturers of x-ray equipment; he is credited with starting the paramedical profession of x-ray technology in 1896.

Because of his knowledge of x-ray machines and the techniques of radiography, Ed Jerman received requests from equipment manufacturers to conduct schools for physicians' assistants; these were in the northern United States and in southern Canada around the Great Lakes. Thus, early in the twentieth century, Ed Jerman became the first professional teacher of *radiologic technology* in North America.

Mr. Jerman's driving enthusiasm, skill, and personality stimulated his students to want additional educational opportunities; their common desire caused these persons to gather for educational discussions. These meetings, conducted by Mr. Jerman, led to the formation of the American Association of Radiological Technicians on October 25, 1920. A second meeting was conducted by Mr. Jerman, as President, on June 27, 1921.

During its formative years this Association pressed for the setting of standards, and by joint committee action of the Radiological Society of North America and the American Roentgen Ray Society, a Registry for the purpose of certifying x-ray technicians was established on November 18, 1922. The original Registry Board was composed of both radiologists and technicians, representing their societies.

In 1925 membership in the American Association of Radiological Technicians was restricted to Registered Technicians.

The Second Annual Meeting was conducted in Chicago in April, 1927, after a reorganizational meeting in 1926. During the next several meetings, emphasis was given to improving educational standards and to the establishment of an official journal, *The X-ray Technician*. Annual meetings, now called Conventions, have been conducted each year since 1927.

Current educational patterns

Presently three distinct patterns (methods) of education and training are acceptable to the American Medical Association's Council on Medical Education, the American College of Radiology, and The American Society of Radiologic Technologists. In each method the hospital experience is the approved training period and is so stipulated by certain governing bodies.

Hospital school

The traditionally accepted method is the approved 24-month hospital school. In these schools the students spend a required minimum time in classroom lecture, followed by observation and practical experience under the direct supervision of Registered Technologists and/or Radiologists. Upon completion of the 24-month period of training in the hospital school the graduates apply to The American Registry of Radiologic Technologists for examination.

The national Registry examinations are conducted in specified cities in the United States.*

College–hospital school

The combined college curriculum and hospital experience is an increasingly popular method of training for the profession of radiologic technology. In this method the students are accepted in approved hospital schools prior to their initial enrollment in the affiliated college. The college curriculum follows the basic science and humanities offerings suggested as preparation for the hospital "externship (practicum)."†

In these situations there is considerable variation between schools. However, a minimum of four semesters in college and 2,400 clock hours of practical experience in the hospital is a distinct requirement of the program. Depending upon a variety of circumstances, the students may complete predetermined parts of the hospital experience in the summer months and during the second school year.

The application for Registry examination is made in the same manner as from the hospital school.

Technical college–hospital school

A more technologically oriented method is that of certain universities that include a college of technical studies.

This more advanced method provides instruction and laboratory practice using a variety of "live" radiographic and x-ray therapy units in the university. The uni-

---

*Information about when and where the examinations are conducted may be obtained from The American Registry of Radiologic Technologists, 2600 Wayzata Blvd., Minneapolis, Minnesota 55405.

†Externship implies that the student is "externing" from the college, since his graduation from the college requires successful completion of the specified period of practical experience.

versity experience is integrated with the required 2,400 clock-hour practicum in affiliated, approved hospitals.

This method provides for both Associate and Baccalaureate degrees in Radiologic Technology. Application for the examination of The American Registry of Radiologic Technologists is made as in the preceding methods.

Professionalism

In 1932 it was decided to change the name of the Association to The American Society of X-ray Technicians; this change went into effect in 1934. Also in 1932, the Registry was first called The American Registry of X-ray Technicians.

The American College of Radiology and The American Society of X-ray Technicians became the official co-sponsors of The American Registry of X-ray Technicians on May 6, 1943. In 1945 the Council on Medical Education and Hospitals of the American Medical Association accepted the responsibility of inspecting and approving training schools for x-ray technicians.

Continuous *upgrading* of the profession of radiologic technology through increased and expanded educational requirements is a mark of our progress. The inclusion of academic courses is now an integral part of most training programs. The general trend in the next few years is to include more academic courses in the curriculum; many of our training programs are now the final part (externship) of an academic program.

Continuous progress and expansion is seen in other facets of our paramedical profession. During the Annual Convention in 1962 certain name changes were approved and adopted. The American Registry of X-ray Technicians is now The American Registry of Radiologic Technologists (ARRT), and The American Society of X-ray Technicians is now The American Society of Radiologic Technologists (ASRT). The journal, *The X-ray Technician*, is now called *Radiologic Technology*. These changes in nomenclature indicate the expansion of our knowledge and performance to include the uses of radioactive isotopes.

Upon becoming registered with the ARRT, it is possible to pursue additional studies and training in either of two *specialty fields* and to write the examinations to be certified as either a *Nuclear Medicine Technologist* or a *Radiation Therapy Technologist*.

The increasing responsibilities of radiologic technology convey corresponding responsibilities of ethical conduct and activities.

Ethics
Ethical inclusions

Ethics relates to the mode of conduct and behavior. A pattern of proper and ethical conduct *at all times* is essential in those who intend to practice any profession. The ethical practices of the profession of radiologic technology are of such broad scope as to make it necessary for those persons engaged in this profession to consider carefully all of their actions and performances both on and off duty.

Some of the more important ethical considerations are explained in the following paragraphs. These are (1) respect for the medical profession; (2) loyalty to the employer, whether radiologist, other specialist, or general practitioner; (3) clear conversational English and correct grammar; (4) personal appearance;

(5) punctuality; (6) personality; (7) respect and care for the patient; (8) obligations to community and profession; (9) respect for paramedical profession; (10) discretion with professional information; and (11) a general knowledge of the economics of the practice of radiology and of hospital operation.

Respect for the medical profession must be considered as an inherent attitude of all the paramedical groups. The technologist must consider the many years of highly complex and specialized training through which all physicians have progressed. Such consideration will develop an appreciation of the professional skill and achievement of the medical profession. In the various demonstrations of respect, actual respect is given to the profession of medicine rather than to the individual physician.

Each physician should be treated with courtesy and his requests acknowledged with courteous reply and efficient response. Individual preference must be avoided; except for emergency cases, which always have priority, all requests must be followed in the sequence given.

If department routine is such that the radiologic technologist is present during the radiograph reading period, he should address the radiologist in charge unless addressed by other physicians.

Loyalty is an important obligation. Because a technologist is efficient and loyal to his employer, he is permitted to apply his abilities to better advantage with the patients. Disloyalty usually precludes the assumption of any degree of responsibility; therefore, it is likely that the employer cannot consider such a person worthy of consideration.

When a young radiologic technologist, just graduated and registered, applies for and receives his first position, he begins to establish his professional reputation. The technologist should build a reputation for loyalty and reliability. His registration does not guarantee that he will become a useful employee in a particular organization. The technologist must prove by deed that he is responsible and altogether useful and efficient. Once this is accomplished, he can expect high recommendation if it becomes necessary to change employers.

Regardless of the technologist's expertness and capabilities, a new position usually places him at a loss for a period of several weeks, until he has learned to adapt himself to the new methods and routine.

Clarity in conversational English and correct grammar are important because of the requirements for intelligent communication with professional people and with the patients, who normally represent a cross section of the entire populace. If instructions are not lucid and correct, understanding may be lost. Correct English usage is, of course, also highly important in the art of writing. Many radiologic technologists, as a part of their duties, are required to type the radiologic reports, and correct spelling and good grammar are therefore necessary.

Personal appearance is equally important since the continuous exhibition of neatness, cleanliness, and alertness tends to instill in the patients a sense of confidence in the efficiency of the technologist. A patient is quite naturally in a state of some anxiety during radiographic procedures. Although these procedures are commonplace to the technologist, they are usually quite strange to the patient. The exhibition of self-confidence and assurance tends to establish a feeling of trust within the patient. Such establishment of trust is highly contributory to the patient's progress and recovery and to his contentment while in the department or hospital.

Punctuality in professional capacity is, of course, mandatory. Punctuality in social obligations is of almost equal importance, for many people will compare attitudes of professional persons while off duty with anticipated attitudes while on duty.

Personality may be defined as that set of innate characteristics that distinguishes one person from another, or that which causes a person to maintain individual identity. Good personality may be developed, and such development is actually necessary for those who are not gifted with an innately attractive personality if they intend to pursue their chosen profession.

An attractive personality usually includes such attributes as a willingness to cooperate and accept, without complaint, additional responsibilities and extended work hours.

Respect and care for the patient must be evidenced in all of the contacts with patients necessary in fulfillment of duties. The modesty and comfort of all patients must be respected by the technologist.

Many radiographic positions will necessitate some lack of comfort for the patient; such requirements need explanation. Patients who are debilitated from any cause require special handling. Elderly patients require additional explanation of orders, as do children and deaf persons.

The use of fresh linens and proper cleansing of the radiographic table and the cassettes are obvious requirements. When permitted, additional cover for warmth should be applied on both the radiographic table and the stretcher. Constant observation for and preventive measures against shock are required.

The obligations to the community and the profession are quite numerous. As a member of one of the paramedical professions, a radiologic technologist is obligated to uphold the ideals of his profession in his community.

In small communities, it is expected that professional persons will actively participate in community enterprises and in some of the service organizations. In any community, active participation in professional society efforts is highly desirable. A professional society is the *only ethical medium* through which expression of personal ideals of a professional nature may be communicated. It is through participation in the professional radiologic technologist societies, state and national, that continued growth and advancement of professional standards will be achieved. No single individual is sufficiently strong to promulgate particular ideals. Through effort of the group in the society, such ideals, if desirable, are usually achieved.

Respect for paramedical professions is as necessary as respect for the medical profession. The radiologic technologist is in almost continuous contact with groups similar in function and ideals to his own. Interprofessional cooperation is vital to the fulfillment of duty in each profession.

Discretion with professional information is an absolute must. Information regarding any patient must never be divulged in any manner. Tact and studied statements are an attribute of each successful technologist.

Refusal of radiographic information to both patient and family must be achieved in a manner that precludes antagonism. Divulging any information regarding radiographic interpretation or results is a distinct violation of professional ethics and subjects the violator to severe reprimand.

Knowledge of the economics of the practice of radiology and hospital operation is important to both the employee and the employer. It is of the utmost importance to the employee since this knowledge will serve to enlighten him about the many facets contributing to the successful operation of the establishment. One cannot evaluate profit by the expedient of comparing film and solution cost with salary. The responsible technologist will investigate new methods that may make the total operation economically more sound. Reasonable suggestions for improvement are always in order.

Hospitals are, statistically, one of the larger businesses in the United States. A radiologic department is one of the major expenditures in a hospital; properly operated, it is one of the major contributors toward successful operation of the organization.

Courtesy, cooperation, and communication, the three C's of modern medical precept, are the summation of effort in all departments. When each of these items becomes an integral part of the routine of the technologist, he will begin to practice professional ethics.

Ethical activities
The technologist's obligations in his work

The work of the radiologic technologist and of his department is indispensable to the practice of medicine in all its branches. A well-produced radiograph is necessary to the establishment or ruling out of a diagnosis of pathology. In these days of modern lawsuits there are many situations in which a radiograph is not only standard but imperative. For example, any physician who undertakes to treat the "sprained ankle" without benefit of radiologic diagnosis is quite liable for a malpractice suit, since many radiographs of "sprained ankles" demonstrate fractures of the lateral malleolus, or the like.

The importance of good and complete radiographs in the diagnosis of chest pathology and of abdominal pathology cannot be overstated; a negative radiograph (one without demonstration of pathology) is by no means time and effort wasted! A negative radiograph serves to rule out the presence of many suspected conditions of pathology—tuberculosis, cancer, fracture, or the like, and the existence of a well-exposed *negative* radiograph is one step nearer to the diagnosis.

In obtaining radiographs of any part of the body, there is a minimum number of views that must be made, and these views should be supplemented by the technologist (with routine consent of the department head) on his own volition upon recognizing the need. In the past a posterior (A-P) and a lateral view were usually sufficient, but in modern radiological practice many diagnoses can be missed without further radiographic views. For example, ulnar flexion (radial deviation) of the wrist is, probably, the *single* view that may demonstrate a fracture of the scaphoid. This view is presently a standard (routine) view, and to omit it may be the cause of a missed diagnosis of fractured scaphoid—which may result in a lawsuit. Many orthopedic surgeons, in addition to the routine views of the wrist, will request three lateral views, at different densities (penetrations); it is significant that, more often than not, one of the three lateral views may demonstrate a fracture of the scaphoid. Therefore, do not hesitate to make additional radiographs when they are deemed necessary and when authority is granted. It is better to make one or two additional radiographs than to make the minimum number and have the diagnosis missed.

An x-ray machine must have a control panel (Fig. 1-3) upon which the determinations of kilovoltage, milliamperage, and time are made. Kilovoltage, milliamperage, and time (in seconds or parts thereof) are the *three prime factors* of x-ray production. This panel may have numerous auxiliary meters and selector switches, such as line amperage, line voltage, etc.

The control panel will always present (1) an *on-off* (line) switch, which activates most of the circuits of the x-ray machine; (2) a device by which the milliamperage is selected; (3) a device to select the kilovoltage; and (4) a device to select the exposure time. The exposure switch usually extends from the control panel on a short cord (except on mobile units). The kilovoltage (kvp) is the voltage (force and penetrating ability) of x-ray production and is the *tube voltage*; the milliamperage times the exposure time is the milliampere-seconds (mas) and is the *tube current*. The milliampere-seconds is the quantity and intensity of x-ray production. The usual sequence of selection for operation is as follows:

1. Turn line switch to *on* position.
2. Check (and adjust if necessary) the line voltage.
3. Select milliamperage.
4. Select time (and determine that ma × time gives the correct mas).
5. Select kilovoltage.
6. Check all selections against the tube-rating chart (see Fig. 1-4, a sample tube-rating chart).

An x-ray machine has a number of transformers and other electrical items usu-

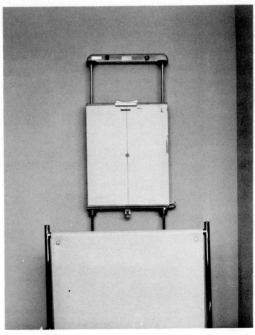

Fig. 1-2. Wall rack for cassette in chest radiography. An aligned grid with a 72-inch focal-film distance is in the cassette slot. The lead curtain is in place on the curtain stand.

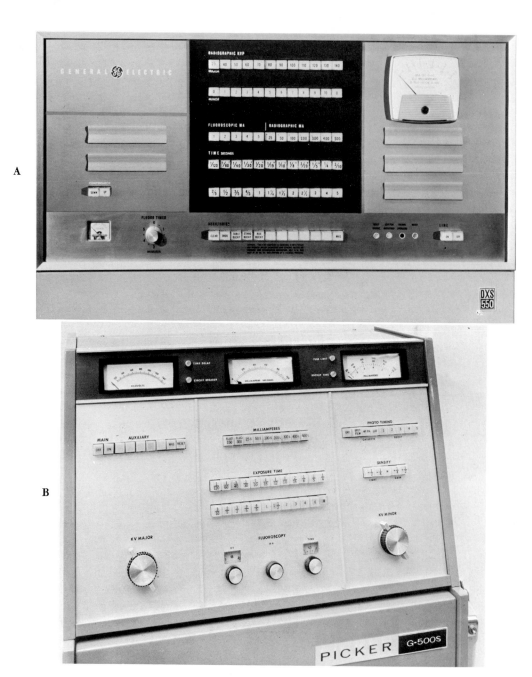

Fig. 1-3. Control panels of four x-ray machines in current use. **A,** General Electric Model DXS 550 (courtesy General Electric Co.). **B,** Picker Model G-500S (courtesy Picker X-ray Corp.). **C,** Keleket 500 MA (courtesy Tracerlab-Keleket). **D,** Standard Model Ultima 600 (courtesy Standard X-Ray Co.).

ally immersed in an oil bath and situated at some distance from both the table and control panel. From the upper surface of the transformer extend the *high-voltage* (high-tension) cables to the various x-ray tubes.

A most important part of the x-ray machine is the x-ray tube (Figs. 1-5 and 1-6). X-rays are generated in the tube and pass from the tube through the *port* (window) in the metal case that surrounds the x-ray tube.

The three principal items necessary in a modern, hot-cathode x-ray tube are the cathode, anode, and an evacuated glass envelope to contain the cathode and anode.

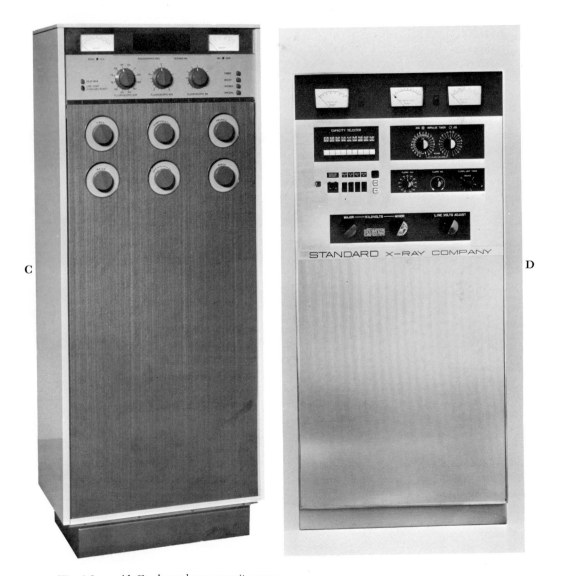

C   D

Fig. 1-3, cont'd. For legend see opposite page.

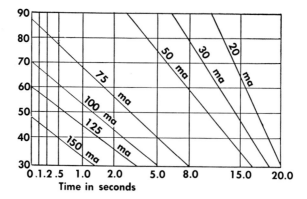

Fig. 1-4. Tube-rating chart. This is a diagram of a tube-rating chart and has no reference to any specific tube. Any combination of values found to the left of the sloping milliamperage line is acceptable, whereas those on the line and to the right are too high for the tube. Example: 200 mas at 70 kvp cannot be obtained safely using either 125 or 100 ma, but can safely be obtained when using 50 ma for 4 sec.

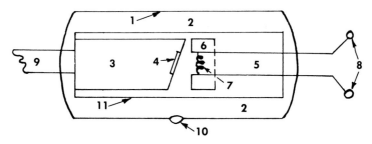

Fig. 1-5. X-ray tube, stationary anode.

1. Metal shielding
2. Insulating oil
3. Anode
4. Tungsten target
5. Cathode
6. Focusing cup

7. Cathode filament
8. Wire connections to secondary side of filament transformer
9. Anode connection to secondary circuit
10. Port (window) in metal shield
11. Evacuated glass envelope

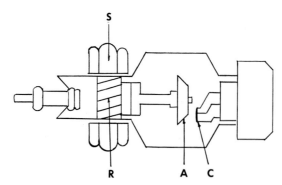

Fig. 1-6. X-ray tube, rotating anode. The anode disk rotates at approximately 3,000 rpm, thus permitting a constantly changing area of bombardment by the cathode electron stream.

A Anode   C Cathode   R Rotor   S Stator

X-rays

Radiologic technologists must, of course, have knowledge of the nature of x-rays and of x-ray production; however, in this introductory chapter no attempt is made to discuss the subject in depth. A few summary paragraphs at this time will suffice; later chapters will set out the subject in greater detail.

X-rays are any of the radiations (electromagnetic waves) of the same nature as light radiation but of an extremely short wavelength, about one angstrom (1Å) unit,* emitted primarily as the result of a sudden change in the velocity of a moving electron (electric charge), as when rapidly moving cathode rays strike a solid obstacle, or target, in a vacuum tube, and as the result of changes in the atoms in the target (anode) due to this impact.

The most notable properties of these rays are (1) ionization of a gas through which they pass, (2) penetration through various thicknesses of all solids, (3) production of secondary rays, and (4) action on photographic plates, fluorescent screens, etc., like that of light.

These radiations were first discovered by W. C. Roentgen, a German physicist, on November 8, 1895, while he was working with highly exhausted vacuum tubes. Because of their unknown nature he called them x-rays; however, they are frequently called roentgen rays in honor of the discoverer.

X-rays are one of the forms of energy existing as electromagnetic waves. Collectively, these several waves comprise the electromagnetic wave spectrum. A spectrum is the series of images formed when a beam of radiant energy is subjected to dispersion and then brought to focus so that the component waves are arranged in the order of their wavelengths.

X-rays and the electromagnetic wave spectrum

The longer wavelengths in the electromagnetic wave spectrum are the radio waves; the shorter wavelengths are the cosmic† waves or rays. *Cosmic rays con-*

---

*An angstrom unit is a unit of measure of wavelength and is equal to one one-hundred millionth of a centimeter. It is written also 1×10^{-8} cm.

†The electromagnetic portion of cosmic rays is usually referred to as high-energy gamma rays.

Table 1-1. Approximate wavelength range in angstrom units of electromagnetic waves

Radiations	*Wavelengths in Å units*
Radio waves	10^{14} to 10^{11}
Hertzian waves	10^{10} to 10^{9}
Short electric waves	10^{8}
Infrared rays	10^{7} to 10^{5}
Visible light rays	10^{4}
Ultraviolet light rays	10^{3}
X-rays	10^{2} to 10^{-1}
Gamma rays	10^{-2}
Cosmic rays	10^{-4}

sist of high-energy electromagnetic waves, gamma rays, and assorted electrons, protons, neutrons, positrons, etc.

Table 1-1 lists the electromagnetic waves in their respective positions in the electromagnetic wave spectrum.

X-rays are sometimes compared with visible light, and indeed they differ from visible light in but few qualities. Just as light rays strike a film emulsion and cause certain physical reactions within the crystalline structure of the emulsion, in the shape of the source of the reflected light rays (latent image), so do x-rays pass through an object or structure and strike the film emulsion to cause a similar sequence of events.

It is the nature of x-rays that each travels in a straight line from its source to the object it strikes, including the film. Since the source of x-rays in diagnostic x-ray tubes is very small (1 or 2 square millimeters), the x-rays diverge from this "point," travel to the structure and through it to the film, and cause an image (shadow) somewhat larger than the actual size of the structure (Fig. 1-7).

The image so formed is *latent;* i.e., the image is not visible and must be rendered *manifest* (visible) by a sequence of chemical events in the processing (dark) room.

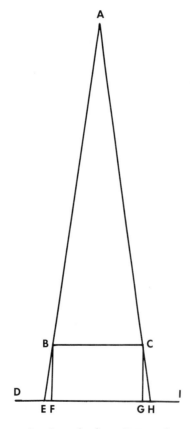

Fig. 1-7. A vertical line from point **A** to the base, **D-I**, is drawn to represent a 40-inch ffd (focal-film distance). The object x-rayed, **BFGC**, is 6 inches thick (vertical) by 10 inches wide. The projected size of **E-H** over **BC** (or **FG**) is an increase of 0.118, or 11.8%.

Film holders

Since light rays affect film emulsions much as do x-rays, it is necessary to contain the x-ray films in lightproof holders. These may be cardboard holders or metal and plastic cassettes.

Cardboard holders are simply constructed and may be either stiff or flexible. These holders (see Fig. 1-8, *C*) consist of two pieces of cardboard connected either at one end or at one side by some flexible material. The holders are made in the various film sizes. There is a tube side and a back side in each holder. The

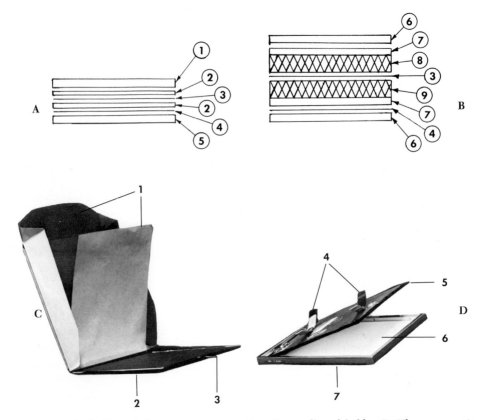

Fig. 1-8. Film holders. **A** diagrams a cross section of a cardboard holder. **B,** The cross section of a cassette.

1. Cardboard front (tube side)
2. Paper envelope
3. Film
4. Lead foil
5. Cardboard back
6 (**upper**). Radiolucent front (tube side)
6 (**lower**). Metal frame
7. Cardboard
8. Emulsion of phosphors
9. Emulsion of phosphors

C, Cardboard holder. **D,** Intensifying screen cassette.

1. Opened paper envelope for x-ray film
2. Tube side of cardboard film-holder
3. Locking clip
4. Spring locks on cassette back
5. Cassette back
6. Upper (tube-side) intensifying screen
7. Tube side of cassette

back side contains a thin lead foil sheet to absorb the back scatter and to prevent the fogging of film by secondary rays. An envelope to encase the film is glued to the inside of the back. (Note: When loading or closing the envelope, place the larger flap directly over the film.) A clamping devise is placed at the end or side opposite the flexible connection between the two cardboards. Since the paper that usually encases the film has no effect on the film in a cardboard holder, this paper may be left around the film as additional light prevention. *The total radiographic effect upon the film exposed in a cardboard holder is from the x-ray energy.*

Cassettes are usually made of aluminum or some other equally radiolucent substance supported within a strong metal framework. A cassette has an aluminum front (tube) side and raised metal sides and ends into which the back fits. The back is hinged to the front on one end (or side). Spring locks are so fitted into the back that when they are locked, the cassette is tightly closed. In order to seal out light, the sides and ends have felt padding on the inner surfaces. A thin lead foil sheet is contained in the back to prevent back scatter. The cassettes contain one pair of *intensifying screens* between which the film is sandwiched. The intensifying screens function to augment the x-ray energy by adding light energy to the total energy quantity striking the film emulsion. Intensifying screens are attached to both the front and back sides of the cassette. These screens sandwich the film. Fig. 1-8, *B,* is a cross-section diagram of a cassette.

Like the cardboard holders, the cassettes are made the same sizes as the films. The sizes are 5″ × 7″, 6½″ × 8½″, 8″ × 10″, 9″ × 9″, 10″ × 12″, 11″ × 14″, 7″ × 17″, 14″ × 17″, and 14″ × 36″. Cassettes are either flat or curved. Special cassettes for use with phototimers contain no lead so the remnant rays pass through the cassette to the fluorescent screen in the phototiming device (see pp. 95 and 96).

Cassette screen cleaning

Successful radiograph production depends upon a variety of conditions, including the maintenance of clean and lint-free intensifying screens in the cassettes.

Depending upon the frequency of use and upon other routine conditions, the cassettes should be inspected at periodic intervals. When lint is found on an intensifying screen, it can usually be removed with a special "antistatic" brush.

Other contaminating foreign objects on the screen surface should be removed as soon as possible with one of the following liquid cleaners:

1. Commercial screen cleaner and/or antistatic solution
2. Anesthetic ether
3. Pure grain alcohol
4. Warm water and very mild soap

Screens should be cleaned as often as is necessary and usually on a scheduled rotating basis. Monthly cleaning of all cassettes in small radiological departments should be considered routine.

To clean screens, moisten a small piece of clean cotton with the liquid cleaner and lightly rub the screen surface in a crosswise motion; then quickly remove any excess cleaner with a dry piece of cotton and place the cassette on its edge like an open book to allow thorough drying before reloading.

A simple card-file index for cassette maintenance should be arranged with corresponding screen-cassette numbers for each series of cassette sizes. Screen installation and cleaning dates should be recorded on a routine basis.

Film processing

In this section only the simplest aspects of the rather complicated chemical reactions will be explained in conjunction with the basic mechanical steps of film processing.

In order to make the latent image manifest, it is necessary to change the chemical and physical natures of certain parts of the film emulsion, especially the silver.

Explained simply, the exposed x-ray films are suspended in suitable hangers and immersed for an exact period of time in the developing solution, where the latent image is made manifest. Next the film (in its hanger) is removed from the developing solution, permitting none of the developing solution to drip back into the developing tank. The film is then immersed in the water bath for a few seconds and is next immersed in the acid stop bath for an exact interval of 30 seconds. Following the acid stop bath, the film is immersed in the fixing solution for a period of time at least twice as long as the time in the developing solution.* In the fixing bath the film surface is hardened, and the manifest image is fixed. Following the fixing bath, the film is again washed, then rinsed in a photoflow (detergent) solution, and then dried. The total process may take as much as 45 minutes to an hour in manual processing rooms. Use of automatic processing machines reduces the total time to as little as from 90 seconds to 15 minutes.

To obtain satisfactory results, it is necessary that certain routine procedures be developed and followed. *The proper processing of x-ray film is just as important as the original exposure of the film.* The very best exposure is easily rendered useless or nearly so by careless or improper darkroom technique. In order to develop good habits in any procedure, a strict routine is necessary. The following routine is suggested for a manually operated processing room.

1. Close and lock doors tightly.
2. Be sure that solutions are well stirred and that the amount of solution fully covers the film.
3. Check temperatures of the solutions and water carefully.
4. Set the timer clock accurately.
5. Be sure that all lights except the safelight are out.
6. Hold the cassette with the tube side down and the hinges away from you and place it on the loading bench.
7. Grasp the corners nearest you and remove the film. Be sure to refrain from touching the rest of the film. Avoid dragging the film across the cassette.
8. Place the end of the film that you are holding in the bottom of the hanger, being certain that you have closed the cassette before bringing a hanger across its face.
9. Clamp the corners you hold into the hanger, then turn the hanger over and

---

*Fixing time is twice as long as "clearing" time; sometimes as little as 3 minutes in fresh fixer.

secure the other two corners. Never allow the film to override on the sides of the hanger or on the ends.

10. Agitate the suspended film as it is immersed into the developer and simultaneously start the timer clock.*

11. Dry your hands and reload the cassette.

12. After the proper time interval has elapsed, remove the suspended film from the developer and rinse it in a running water bath for a minimum of 30 seconds, agitating it *vigorously.* Allow the excess water to drain off the film. No-screen film requires 45 seconds to wash.

13. Immerse the film in an acid stop bath for 30 seconds.

14. Place the suspended film in the fixer and start the timer clock.

15. After the proper time interval has elapsed, remove the suspended film (now the radiograph) and rinse it at least 30 minutes in a running water bath before immersing it in the photoflow.

16. Place the film in a drier.

The solution on the film should never be allowed to drip into the developer tank because the solution that adheres to the film is partially exhausted and will tend to weaken the developing solution earlier than necessary. The fixer is not so weakened. The developer and fixer baths should be maintained at their required levels by frequent additions of specific replenishing solution throughout the day. Following each addition of new replenisher, the solutions should be well stirred. *Remember that there are three equally important solutions in the darkroom: developer, water bath, and fixer.*

Equipment

In most darkrooms the developer will be in the left-hand tank as the technologist faces it, the water bath in the center, and the fixer in the right-hand tank. In a strange darkroom, the developing solution can be identified by its *slippery* feeling. The fixer will have a *vinegary* odor when fresh.

Through-the-wall water baths are highly advantageous in that they enable the physicians to view wet radiographs without disturbing the processing routine.

The darkroom illuminator should be equipped with a light source that has no afterglow.†

The well-designed darkroom should be completely light-proof. There should be a clean and dry loading bench away from the solution tanks to eliminate the danger of moisture and chemicals splashing upon the bench. The hangers should be so placed upon the wall over the loading bench that they will not hang over the cassette-loading area, yet will be within easy reach of the technologist.

If the darkroom is equipped with an overhead safelight, this light (if indirect) should be located a minimum of 4 feet from the loading bench. The illumination from the safelight should be filtered with a *Wratten 6B* filter and contain a globe no stronger than 25 watts. A direct overhead safelight requires the same

---

*Agitation in the developing solution should be continued throughout development (or sufficiently long to prevent the formation of *air bells*).

†In this particular use, afterglow refers to a glow of refulgence remaining after a light has disappeared. The radiographic use refers to a condition in an intensifying screen wherein the screen continues to emit light after the x-ray energy has ceased to strike the screen.

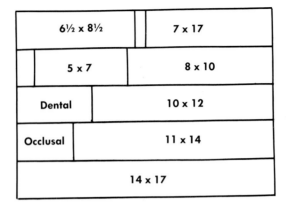

Fig. 1-9. The diagram demonstrates one method of placing films of different sizes in the film bin.

filter, a 15-watt globe, and should be a minimum of 6 feet from the loading bench.

The *safeness* of the safelight may be tested in the following manner. With only the safelights on, place an exposed film on the loading bench. Place some opaque object, such as a coin, on the film and expose the film to the safelights for *15 seconds exactly*. Process the film. The visible outline of the coin indicates that the lights are too strong and that some exposure of the film has occurred. Exposed films are seven to eight times more sensitive to safelight fogging than are unexposed films. If unexposed films are used for this purpose, the required time is *2 minutes*.

A film bin should be placed in the loading bench so that films may be obtained from it without disturbing the loading surface. A diagram of such a bin is shown in Fig. 1-9. It is desirable to establish a routine in loading the bin so that the technologist may always be certain of the kind of film located in designated places.

It is advisable to have the film bin wired so that the lights will be turned off when the bin is opened. The safelights need not be in this circuit.

The darkroom should have adequate ventilation or an air-exhaust system. Careful installation of an air-exhaust fan will prevent entrance of light and moisture.

Pass boxes between the darkroom and adjacent radiographic rooms and halls are a great convenience and tend to prevent accidental entrance of light.

Entrance into the darkroom may be achieved through a variety of methods, each of which precludes the entrance of light. Probably the best method is to use a *light maze* (an arrangement of joined pathways into the darkroom). However, there are conditions under which the required space for a maze is unavailable. A second method is that of spacing two doors at either end of a short and darkened cubicle or hall. In this method, one of the doors leads directly into the darkroom from the darkened hall and the other door leads from the hall into the outer areas. These doors are then equipped with locks that prevent both doors from being opened at the same time.

Chapter 2

Fundamental electricity and magnetism

In a text of this academic level, one must assume that the student has a knowledge of basic physics and chemistry. In general, it is our intent to review briefly some facts and theories of physics and chemistry that have a direct application in our profession. Theories and postulates are accepted as they are presented in texts on these subjects.

Fundamental concepts of matter

Matter is defined as anything that has mass or weight and occupies space. Matter represents a given quantity of energy. *Energy is the ability to do work.* Energy is *kinetic* when performing a task and *potential* when available but not operational. *By the laws of conservation of mass and energy, the total quantity of mass and energy is constant, although mass and energy may be converted one into the other.*

Matter always exists in one of three states: solid, liquid, or gas. Ninety-two simple forms of matter that cannot be further subdivided make up the structure of the universe. These forms are elements.* All matter, then, consists of one or more of these elements in combination. Any one element in its pure state consists of many atoms, which exist either as single entities or in combination as molecules. A *molecule is an aggregation of atoms, that is, a chemical combination of two or more atoms that form a specific chemical substance. An atom is the smallest quantity of an element that can exist and still retain the chemical properties of that element.*

However, atoms are not the smallest particles found in nature; within the atom are contained several much smaller particles such as protons, neutrons, and electrons. The protons and neutrons are contained within the nucleus of the atom, and the electrons are considered to orbit about the nucleus. *The proton is a positively charged particle of matter with a mass approximately that of the nucleus of the hydrogen atom. The neutron, which is slightly larger in mass than the proton, is electrically neutral. The electron, which is a negatively charged particle of matter, has a mass approximately 1/1840 of that of the proton.*

---

*At least eleven additional elements have been produced artificially.

The radius of the nucleus of an atom has been estimated as approximately 10^{-12} cm* and the radius of the electron orbits about the nucleus as approximately 10^{-8} cm. The proton mass has been estimated as approximately 1.00758 AMU (atomic mass unit), the neutron mass as approximately 1.00894 AMU, and the electron mass as approximately 0.00055 AMU.

The minuteness of each particle (nucleon) in the atomic nucleus is no measure of the energy required to remove a single nucleon from the nucleus of that atom. The energy required to remove a neutron or proton from an atomic nucleus is called the *binding energy*. If an atomic nucleus were to be assembled from individual neutrons and protons, the energy that would be released would be the total binding energy of the nucleus. The binding energy of a particular nuclear particle is measured in millions of electron volts. The symbol for one million electron volts is 1 mev.

The binding energy varies from one element to another; the greatest variations occur between hydrogen and neon. Following are some of the elements and their corresponding binding energies.

H (hydrogen)	1.0 mev	Ne^{20} (neon-20)	8.0 mev
He (helium)	2.6 mev	Ga^{70} (gallium-70)	8.7 mev
He^4 (helium-4)	7.1 mev	U^{240} (uranium-240)	7.6 mev
Li^6 (lithium-6)	5.2 mev		

The energy increases gradually from elements with atomic weight 20 to those with atomic weight 70, and decreases gradually from elements with atomic weight 70 to those with atomic weight 240. The binding energy must not be confused with the electrical charges of atoms.

Under normal conditions, the atom is electrically neutral. There is normally one electron in orbit for each proton in the nucleus. Circumstances often alter the structure and stability of atoms. A deficiency of one or more electrons will render the atom electrically positive, due to the excess of positive charges in the nucleus. A surplus of orbital electrons renders the atom electrically negative because more negative charges exist in the orbits than positive charges in the nucleus. *When an atom either gains or loses one or more electrons, the atom becomes ionized and is either a negative ion or a positive ion.*

The periodic table[†] is an orderly arrangement of the elements according to increasing number of protons within the nucleus. In this table the elements are in eight vertical *groups* according to family and seven horizontal *periods* according to the increasing atomic number. *The atomic number[‡] is the number of protons within the nucleus. The atomic weight is the sum of the number of protons plus the number of neutrons.* In the periodic table, hydrogen is the first element. Hydrogen, a gas, has one proton as its nucleus and one electron in orbit. Since a single proton comprises the entire nucleus of the hydrogen atom, both the atomic number and the atomic weight are 1.

From inside to outside, the labels of the orbits are K, L, M, N, O, P, and Q. Compared to the size of the nucleus, there is an enormous distance between the K orbit and the nucleus and between each two orbits. The orbits are frequently

---

*The expression 10^{-12} cm is a simplified method of writing the number 0.000000000001 cm. The expression 10^{10} is a shortened method of writing the number 10,000,000,000.

†See Appendix for list of elements.

‡This is the number that determines the chemical nature of the atom.

referred to as energy levels since certain measurable quantities of energy are required to move an electron from an orbit near the nucleus to one farther away or to remove an electron entirely from the atom. The electron of the hydrogen atom orbits in the K energy level.

Helium, a gas and the second element in the periodic table, has atomic number 2 and atomic weight 4. This indicates the presence of two protons and two neutrons in the helium nucleus. The two electrons of the helium atom orbit in the K energy level. (See Fig. 2-1.)

A major consideration in radiologic technology is the physical nature of

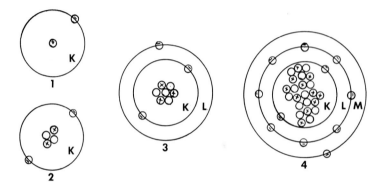

Fig. 2-1. Diagrams of atomic structure. **1** Represents hydrogen, with one proton in the nucleus and one electron in the *K* orbit. **2** Represents helium, with two protons and two neutrons in the nucleus and two electrons in the *K* orbit. **3** Represents lithium, with three protons and four neutrons in the nucleus, two electrons in the *K* orbit, and one electron in the *L* orbit. **4** Represents sodium, with eleven protons and twelve neutrons in the nucleus, two electrons in the *K* orbit, eight electrons in the *L* orbit, and one electron in the *M* orbit.

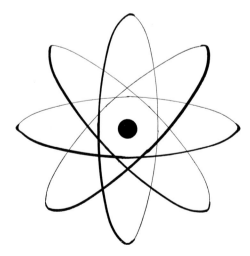

Fig. 2-2. Diagram of one of the modern concepts of atomic structure. Each electron radius is approximately equal in length to all other electron radii in the atom.

tungsten. Tungsten has atomic number 74 and atomic weight 184. It therefore has 74 protons and 110 neutrons in its nucleus. The orbits require varying numbers of electrons. The arrangement of the 74 electrons in their respective orbits, from inside to outside, is as follows: K-2, L-8, M-18, N-32, O-12, and P-2. (See footnote on p. 41 for further discussion of tungsten.)

Electricity

Electricity can be produced in many ways. Hydroelectric and steam generators are the major sources of alternating current (A.C.) However, electricity can be produced through *magnetism, chemical reaction,* or *friction.* All electrons are exactly alike, each bearing the same negative electric charge. The negative charge on one electron exactly neutralizes the positive charge on one proton.

The outer orbital electrons are rather loosely attached; some of these may be removed from their atoms by friction or other strong, positive attractions. When a silk cloth is rubbed on a glass rod, the silk becomes negatively charged and the glass rod takes on a positive charge. This is the result of electrons being removed from the glass rod by friction and collected in excess on the silk cloth. A deficiency of electrons exists on the glass rod following this procedure. The negative electric charge on the silk cloth can be neutralized by again placing the glass rod in contact with the silk cloth. In fact, the negative charge (excess of electrons) causes the silk to be attracted by the positively charged glass rod, and when it is pulled back to the rod, a neutral condition is produced.

If electrons are caused or permitted to flow along a conductor, a current of electricity is said to move along the conductor. If a bar of copper and a bar of zinc are placed vertically in a glass or rubber cylinder, the lower halves of each are immersed in sulfuric acid, copper wires are attached to the exposed end of each bar, and a galvanometer, which is an instrument for measuring electric current, is attached to the free ends of the two wires, all the conditions necessary for the production of a flow of electric current and its measurement are present. (See Fig. 2-3.) It will be noted that the galvanometer needle is always deflected in the same direction because the flow of current is always in this same direction. This type of electricity is *direct current* (D.C.). In this example, a current of elec-

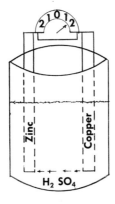

Fig. 2-3. Wet-cell battery. The electron flow is from the negative zinc to the positive copper, making direct current with a positive (right) deflection of the galvanometer needle.

tricity flows because the sulfuric acid attacks the zinc and releases negative electrons, zinc sulfate, and hydrogen ions. The electrons move along the zinc to the conductor through the galvanometer and to the copper, where they combine with the hydrogen ions to form hydrogen gas. Note that the number of electrons remains constant in this system but that the chemical reaction releases energy.

An electric current will flow along a conductor whenever there exists a difference in potential or voltage between two connected points. *Electric current may be defined as electrons in motion or the rate of flow of electrons along a conductor. The potential difference across or between two points or terminals is known as electromotive force (emf) and is measured in volts.* A difference in potential exists if there is a difference in electron pressure at any two points in the conductor; *emf is also measured in volts and is defined as that which causes a flow of current.*

The emf of a circuit is considered to be the total voltage of the circuit—also, the potential drop across the entire circuit. Electrons will leave a point of low positive charge and travel to a point of high positive charge.

Because the quantity of charge on an electron is very small, it is impossible to detect it by ordinary current-detecting meters. For this reason a larger unit of electric charge is generally used. *This larger unit is called a coulomb and equals the charge on 63×10^{18} electrons.* The ampere is the unit used to measure the rate of flow of electricity. *An ampere is a flow of one coulomb per second.* The unit of current is the ampere. Alternatively, *a coulomb is the total quantity of electricity that moves when a current of one ampere flows for exactly one second.* The term ampere-seconds is often used to describe the amount and duration of electric flow.

Just as water flowing through a pipe must overcome the frictional resistance offered by the walls of the pipe, electricity must overcome an electric resistance tending to restrict the passage of electrons along a conductor. *The unit of electric resistance is the ohm. An ohm is the resistance equal to the resistance of a column of mercury having a mass of 14.4521 grams, a uniform cross section of approximately one square millimeter, and a length of 106.3 cm at 0° C.* Ohm's law states: *the current strength in any conductor varies directly as the electromotive force and inversely as the resistance.*

The previous paragraphs have presented some of the fundamental units of electricity; the volt is the unit of pressure, the ampere is the unit of current, the ohm is the unit of resistance, and the coulomb is the unit of electric charge. A given current will be caused to move along a wire through a given resistance as a result of the pressure of a given voltage. The formula $E = IR$, where E is the electromotive force in volts, I is the current in amperes, and R is the resistance in ohms, expresses this condition. Electric power (rate of doing work) is rated in units called watts. *Watts are the product of volts and amperes.* Electric work is stated in units such as watt-seconds, watt-hours, or kilowatt-hours, which are obtained by multiplying the power in watts by a convenient unit of time.

Alternating current

There are two kinds of current electricity, direct current (D.C.), which we have discussed, and alternating current (A.C.). The basic laws and units that relate to direct current also hold for alternating current.

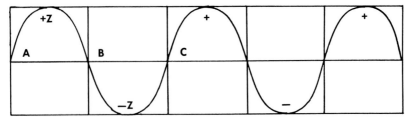

Fig. 2-4. Sine wave diagram. Between *A* and *C* there is one complete cycle. From *A* to *B* the current flows in a positive direction; from *B* to *C* the current flows in a negative direction. In 1 second there are 60 complete cycles, as from *A* to *C*, which contain a total of 60 positive half cycles and 60 negative half cycles. This diagram also represents the flow of an alternating current. The current rises from zero voltage at *A* to its maximum positive peak (the positive zenith) at +Z, falls back to zero at *B,* rises to the negative peak at −Z, and falls back to zero at *C.*

Direct current is a flow of electrons in a single direction. Alternating current is a flow of electrons in one direction immediately followed by a flow in the opposite direction. Alternating current has proved more efficient than direct current in transmission over great distances, and more easily distributed where used.*
Most of the electricity used in modern industry and homes is transmitted as alternating current and converted locally to direct current if required.

If current is plotted against time, alternating current exhibits a characteristic rising and falling curve that, when projected as a graph, approximates a *sine wave. The number of complete cycles that occur each second is the frequency of the current.* A complete cycle includes the half cycle flowing in the positive direction and the half cycle flowing in the negative direction. (See Fig. 2-4.) The usual current supply in American cities is 60 cycles a second.

It is necessary to use high voltage to conduct an alternating current efficiently over long distances. High voltage results when the alternating current passes through a step-up transformer. At distribution points, which supply houses and industrial establishments where voltage requirements are usually much lower, the alternating current passes through a step-down transformer; the result is reduced voltage and increased available amperage.

X-ray machine circuits require several voltages, which are furnished from the supply line. The supply line voltage is transformed in the x-ray machine according to requirements. In order to understand the principles involved in transforming alternating current, some knowledge of magnetism is necessary.

Magnets and magnetism

A *magnet is a body capable of exerting and being acted upon by magnetic force and attracting to itself magnetizable substances such as iron and steel.*

A piece of soft iron may become a magnet under certain conditions. If the iron is in bar form, the magnetic properties will be demonstrated as in Fig. 2-5. If a bar magnet is placed beneath a sheet of paper and iron filings are sprinkled

---

*Recent advances in the processes of electrical transmission and distribution indicate a probable increase in the use of direct current.

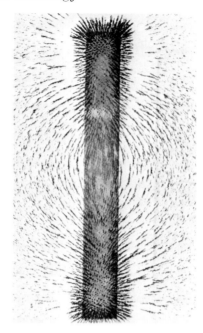

Fig. 2-5. Photograph of iron filings sprinkled on a clear surface and falling in the magnetic lines of force surrounding the magnet.

on top of the paper, the iron filings will fall on the paper in the pattern of the "lines of force" exerted by the magnet.

If two magnetized bars are suspended so that each may move freely and the magnets are brought close to each other, it will be noticed that one or both magnets will always swing about so that a particular end of one magnet seeks a particular end of the other. This is because the magnetic lines have direction that gives the magnets north-seeking and south-seeking poles. *Like poles repel and unlike poles attract.* This experimental evidence demonstrates that there are actually lines of force in a particular pattern about any magnet.

Flux lines (lines of force) also form around a wire when a current of electricity flows along the wire. The direction of the flux lines is counterclockwise; when the thumb of the left hand is extended in the direction of the electron flow, the fingers (of the left hand) point in the direction of the flux lines.

The preceding information is easily demonstrated by passing a bare copper wire through the center of a piece of thin paper and connecting the two ends of the copper wire to the terminals of a flashlight battery. After the connections are made and the current is flowing, sprinkle some iron filings on the paper near the copper wire; the iron filings will fall in the pattern of the flux lines. If the battery terminals are reversed, new iron filings sprinkled on the paper will assume a somewhat different pattern.

Transformers

A transformer is an electric device that either steps up (increases) or steps down (decreases) the incoming voltage.

If a copper wire, the free ends of which are attached to a galvanometer, is moved through a magnetic field so that the lines of force are cut by the wire, a deflection of the hand of the galvanometer will occur. If the movement of the wire is in the opposite direction, the deflection of the galvanometer hand will also be in the opposite direction. This process is one of inducing a current of electricity to flow along a conductor—the process of *electromagnetic induction.*

As stated earlier, magnetic lines of force exist around any wire along which an electric current is flowing. If a second wire is placed parallel to and near a wire conducting an alternating current, an alternating current of electricity will be caused to flow along the second wire; the alternations will be of equal duration but opposite in direction to the inducing current. *This is the principle of mutual induction* and is the process used in most transformers to change or alter the incoming alternating current.

Experimental evidence demonstrates that alternating current flowing in a coil will induce a second alternating current to flow in the opposite direction in a second coil placed within the field of the first coil. This induced current is even stronger when the two coils surround a soft iron core. When such magnetic cores are placed in a magnetic field, they increase the number of magnetic lines and thereby improve transformer efficiency. Fig. 2-6 is a diagram of a two-winding transformer.

Transformers and transformer capacities and types may be classified according to ratio. The ratio of a transformer reveals whether the transformer is a step-up or a step-down type and how much it changes the incoming voltage. *The ratio is determined by dividing the number of windings in the incoming (primary) coil by the number of windings in the outgoing (secondary) coil.* Thus, if a transformer has one winding in the incoming coil and two windings in the outgoing coil, the transformer ratio is 1:2 and the transformer is a step-up type. This transformer will deliver *approximately* twice as much voltage as was delivered to it. If the windings were reversed, the transformer would be a step-down type and would deliver *approximately* one half the voltage delivered to it. Voltage is delivered *to* the incoming coil and delivered *from* the outgoing coil of a transformer.

The outgoing power (watts) cannot exceed the incoming power (watts) and is actually less in quantity due to hysteresis,* eddy current losses,† resistance, and other factors. In ordinary loads the transformer loss usually will not exceed 5%, but in high-voltage transformers, such as those used in x-ray machines, the loss is much greater.

In an x-ray machine, the *autotransformer* is the *kilovoltage selector;* it supplies the primary side of the high-voltage transformer with the predetermined voltage. The autotransformer consists of a single wire wrapped around a soft iron core. The free ends of the single wire connect to the incoming supply line. A series of taps, for selection of output voltages, is on the side opposite to the primary source. The single wire serves as both the incoming and outgoing coils of the transformer. The output may be determined from the following: *The voltage*

---

*Hysteresis is a lagging or retardation of the effect.

†An eddy current is an induced electric current circulating wholly within a mass of metal. Such currents are converted into heat, thus causing serious waste.

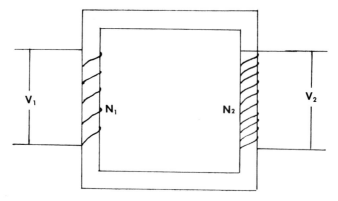

Fig. 2-6. A two-winding transformer. This is a step-up transformer with a 1:2 ratio. (The electrical symbols used throughout the text are copied with kind permission from the American standard graphical symbols for electrical diagrams, approved March 29, 1954, courtesy Institute of Radio Engineers, Inc.)

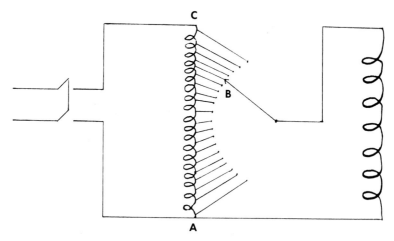

Fig. 2-7. Autotransformer. The supply line furnishes 110 volts. There are 20 windings between *A* and *C* and 16 windings between *A* and *B*. Eighty-eight volts will be delivered to the primary side (incoming side) of the high-voltage transformer from the autotransformer.

maintained between the minimum side of the transformer and the outgoing tap selected is in the same ratio to the total incoming voltage as the number of windings between the minimum side and the selected outgoing tap is to the total number of windings. This statement is expressed in the following proportion: $x{:}I$: : $w{:}W;$ where x is the voltage delivered from the autotransformer. I is the supply line voltage, w is the number of windings between the minimum side (A) and the selected output tap (B), and W is the total number of windings between the minimum side (A) and the maximum side (C) (see Fig. 2-7). That is, $x{:}110$: : $16{:}20; 20x = 1760; x = 88$ volts delivered at B.

The autotransformer may be designed as a step-down transformer or a step-down-step-up transformer by extending the number of windings beyond the maximum side. Fig. 2-7 is a diagram of the step-down type of autotransformer.

REFERENCES

Boast, Warren B.: Principles of electric and magnetic circuits, New York, 1950, Harper & Brothers.

Delario, A. J.: Roentgen, radium, and radioisotope therapy, Philadelphia, 1953, Lea & Febiger.

Miller, Franklin, Jr.: College physics, ed. 2, New York, 1959, Harcourt, Brace & World, Inc.

Robertson, John Kellock: Radiology physics, ed. 3, Princeton, N. J., 1955, D. Van Nostrand Co., Inc.

Weyl, Charles, and Warren, S. Reid, Jr.: Radiologic physics, ed. 2, Springfield, Ill., 1951, Charles C Thomas, Publisher.

White, Harvey E.: Modern college physics, Princeton, N. J., 1962, D. Van Nostrand Co., Inc.

Chapter 3

X-ray machine circuitry

Power supply

The electric power supply to most American installations is either 110-120 or 220 240 volts, 60-cycle, single-phase A.C. Most portable x-ray equipment requires 110-120 volts whereas most stationary equipment requires 220-240 volts.* In electricity a single alternating current is termed a single-phase current (Fig. 2-4). In a three-phase system, three currents flow, differing in phase from each other by 120 degrees (Fig. 3-1).

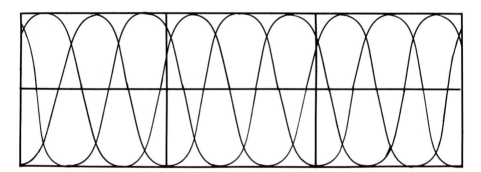

Fig. 3-1. Diagram of three-phase system. Above the center line, or the positive pulse side, there are three peaks; the center peak can represent the single peak in a single-phase diagram.

The supply line consists of either two or three wires; in either case, the voltage may be either 110 or 220. If there are three wires, the middle wire is neutral, and there are 110 volts between it and either of the other two wires, or 220 volts between the two outside wires.

X-ray machines employ many circuits for operation. Three of these circuits form the basis of all operation: the *primary*, or low-voltage, circuit; the *secondary*, or high-voltage, circuit; and the *filament*, or heating, circuit. However, all of the electricity used in operating the x-ray equipment is obtained from a single source, the supply line.

---

*Greater power economy can be effected by the use of three-phase power distribution systems. A common potential between any two of the three principal conductors in a three-phase system for office buildings is 208 volts.

Primary circuit

The primary circuit supplies the autotransformer, the primary side of the high-voltage transformer, the timing circuit, and the many other low-voltage circuits necessary for the operation of modern equipment.

A voltage load of 110-120 or 220-240 volts and an amperage load varying from 10 to 100 amperes, according to requirements, flow along the primary circuit. Further requirements of the primary supply are for alternating current, which is usually 60 cycles each second, i.e., 60 positive half cycles and 60 negative half cycles. (See Fig. 2-4.)

Upon entering the x-ray machine, the primary current passes through the following: primary switch, line-voltage regulator and meter, autotransformer, circuit breaker, oil-immersed magnetic contactor, timer, x-ray exposure switch, ammeter, milliampere selector, and filament transformer. Following manual selection of the eventual secondary kilovoltage, by means of the autotransformer, the primary current enters the primary side of the high-voltage transformer. (See Fig. 3-2.)

The supply line voltage is fused at the primary switch. The *primary switch* permits the supply line voltage to enter the primary circuit when the switch is closed. This switch is usually mounted on the control panel and labeled the *line switch*.

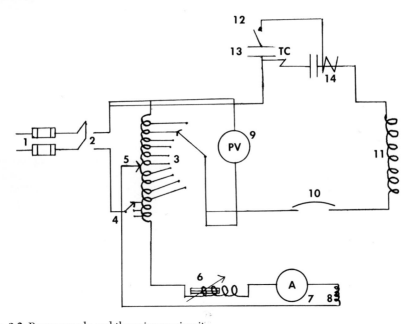

Fig. 3-2. Power supply and the primary circuit.

1. Fuses
2. Primary switch
3. Autotransformer
4. Line voltage compensator
5. Circuit connector for filament transformer
6. Choke coil
7. Filament ammeter
8. Primary of filament transformer
9. Prereading voltmeter
10. Circuit breaker
11. Primary of high-voltage transformer
12. Hand or foot switch
13. Timer to close circuit
14. Magnetic contactor (oil immersed)

The *line voltage regulator* is a part of the primary side of the autotransformer and regulates the incoming voltage. The *line voltage meter* is in parallel with the supply line and shows the voltage delivered to the autotransformer. In some equipment there is a *prereading kilovolt meter* in parallel with the autotransformer between it and the primary side of the high-voltage transformer. The purpose of this meter is to register, prior to exposure, what kilovoltage will be delivered during the exposure. Such a meter requires factory precalibration.

The *circuit breaker* is in series with the exposure switch and magnetic contactor. The timer circuit includes the timer, magnetic contactor, and hand or foot (exposure) switch. The circuit breaker functions to ensure against overload of the delicate equipment of the x-ray machine (see p. 69) since it may be set to *break* at any desired load; it is quite easily reset.

The *autotransformer* was discussed on pp. 29 and 30.

The *oil-immersed magnetic contactor* acts as a heavy current relay and is actuated by the small current flowing through the hand switch and timer. This condition reduces the danger of shock to the operator and the electrolysis at the contact points, which regulate the heavy current. Closure of the *exposure*

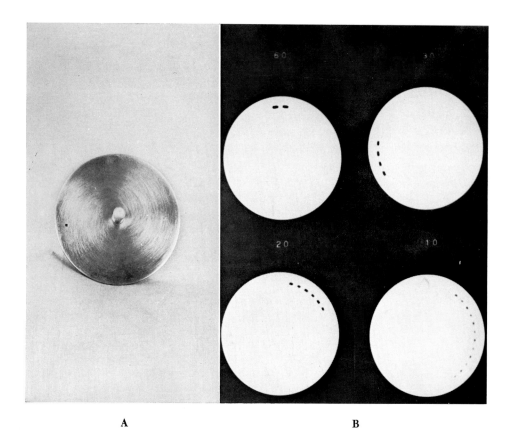

A   B

Fig. 3-3. A spinning top is shown in **A.** The photographs of the spinning top in **B** show the following numbers of dots for corresponding times on a full-wave rectified unit: two dots, 1/60 sec; four dots, 1/30 sec; six dots, 1/20 sec; and twelve dots, 1/10 sec.

switch causes the magnetic contactor to close and complete the circuit to the primary side of the high-voltage transformer.

Timers are incorporated into the x-ray machine to initiate timing and to terminate the exposure. Timers connect, in the primary circuit, to the primary side of the high-voltage transformer. At least three types of timers are commonly used: synchronous, impulse, and electronic. Some manufacturers incorporate a synchronous timer and an impulse timer into the same x-ray machine to permit

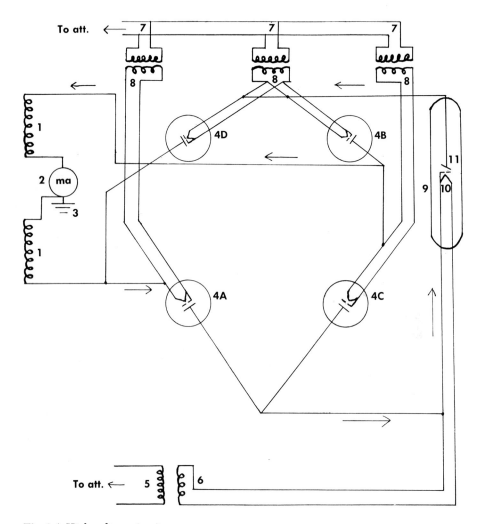

Fig. 3-4. High-voltage circuit.

1. Secondary side of high-voltage transformer
2. Milliammeter
3. Ground
4. Valve tubes
5. Primary side of filament transformer
6. Secondary side of filament transformer
7. Primary side of valve-tube transformer
8. Secondary side of valve-tube transformer
9. X-ray tube
10. X-ray tube filament (cathode)
11. X-ray tube anode

a wider range of accuracy in exposure time. Others combine an electronic timer and an impulse timer for this purpose. A *synchronous timer* is operated by a synchronous motor. The usual range of exposure time for this type is $\frac{1}{20}$ second to 20 seconds. An *impulse timer* is operated by impulses of current passing through the timing circuit; there are 60 current impulses each second in half-wave rectified equipment and 120 current impulses each second in full-wave rectified equipment. The usual range of exposure time for this type is $\frac{1}{120}$ or $\frac{1}{60}$ second to $\frac{1}{5}$ second. The impulse timer is quite accurate because the exposure is initiated and terminated at, or very close to, the zero point of the alternating current cycle. The *electronic timer* is operated by means of a series of electronic tubes and relays and is useful over a range of exposures. The minimum exposure time is $\frac{1}{30}$ second. Fourteen seconds is a common maximum exposure time. Another method of controlling exposure time uses the *triode valve tube.* This method of timing exposures involves withholding current between the outside (end) plates of the tube until the negative bias* of the middle (third) plate has been overcome by a predetermined voltage stored in a condenser. As a timer, the triode tube is useful in rapid-fire exposures in angiocardiography and other highly specialized radiographic procedures where many exposures are required each minute.

There are several conditions under which the timer may either fail completely or function improperly. If the timer accuracy is in question, a spinning top (see Fig. 3-3) should be used to check the actual length of exposure with that of the selected time. The factors to use for spinning top radiographs are 60 to 65 kvp, 50 or 100 ma, 0.1 second, and a 30- or 40-inch ffd. No less than five exposures should be averaged for final evaluation. Since there are 120 current impulses in full-wave rectified current, there should be 12 exposure dots on the radiograph in 0.1 second; with 60 impulses in half-wave rectified current, there should be six exposure dots on the radiograph in 0.1 second.

The radiographic density of the dots should be equal in degree. In full-wave rectified units, alternate light and dark dots may indicate either of two conditions: faulty valve tubes or faulty Thyrx timer tubes.

If the filament of valve tube 4-A or 4-B (Fig. 3-4) emits a quantity of electrons remarkably different from the quantity emitted by valve tube 4-C or 4-D, correspondingly different valve tube currents will occur in the alternate half-cycles of a given exposure; variations in valve tube current in this instance will cause corresponding variations in the emf of the secondary current.

A Thyrx timer requires a lead power thyratron tube and a trail power thyratron tube. If the valve tubes function correctly, it is logical to suspect the efficiency of the thyratron power tubes. If the lead tube of this timer is faulty, the first, third, and all alternate dots will be light; if the trail tube is faulty, the second, fourth, and all alternate dots will be light. (See item 4, p. 68, and item 8, p. 69.)

Phototiming, discussed on pp. 95 and 96, is used to obtain the same degree of radiographic density in sequence radiographs as in spot-film fluoroscopy and radiography and other procedures.

The *ammeter* is in series with the primary circuit to register the amperage load of the filament current. In older equipment and in some modern equipment,

---

*Bias is the direct voltage in the grid circuit of an electron tube.

a certain selection of amperage prior to actual exposure will determine the value of the milliamperage (tube current). Most modern x-ray machines provide an automatic control of the tube current for different kilovoltage values, accomplished through the use of a space-charge compensator (see pp. 48 and 49).

The *milliampere selector*, often called the *technique selector*, is in series with a *choke coil*, or rheostat, and the oil-immersed *filament transformer*. This transformer is a step-down transformer and supplies the filament of the x-ray tube with sufficient amperage to heat the filament. The filament transformer supplies a current that does not exceed 5 amperes at no more than 15 volts.

Secondary circuit

The secondary circuit begins and ends at the secondary side of the high-voltage transformer and conducts the high voltage used in the production of x-rays.

The high voltage is induced in the secondary side of the high-voltage transformer by mutual induction from the primary voltage in the primary side of this same transformer (see pp. 28 and 29). Since the primary voltage source is alternating current, it is obvious that the secondary voltage will be produced as an alternating current. Because the secondary voltage is alternating, this power supply must be rectified prior to entering the x-ray tube, since the production of x-rays in the hot cathode tube requires that the high voltage be *unidirectional*, i.e., flowing from the cathode to the anode of the x-ray tube. (See pp. 38 to 40.)

The secondary voltage flows through the following: secondary side of the high-voltage transformer, valve tubes, x-ray tube, and milliammeter. The exposure switch, located in the primary circuit, automatically controls the secondary voltage and current since they are obtained by mutual induction. (See Fig. 3-4.)

The entire high-voltage transformer is oil-immersed to prevent shock.

The *milliammeter* in modern, shockproof equipment is in series in the high-voltage circuit, mounted in the control panel, and grounded at the midpoint of the secondary side of the high-voltage transformer. The milliammeter measures tube current averages, not the peak values. *One milliampere is 1/1000 of an ampere.*

In some modern equipment using tube currents in excess of 300 ma, a *milliampere-second* meter is in series with the milliammeter. This meter registers the total milliampere-seconds used in any one exposure. A red signal warning light is usually in series with the milliampere-second meter. The warning light flashes on when the exposure is made, to call attention to the number of milliampere-seconds employed, so that if the selection is great enough to overload the x-ray tube, the operator can terminate the exposure.

The milliampere-second meter also provides a more accurate registration of the true value of the milliamperage during very short exposures.

Filament circuit

The primary circuit supplies current to the filament circuit, which is frequently called the *heating circuit*. The filament transformer induces the heating current, which flows through the cathode of the x-ray tube. The heating current for the valve-tube cathodes originates from a fixed position on the autotransformer. The current functions to produce sufficient heat in the cathode filaments

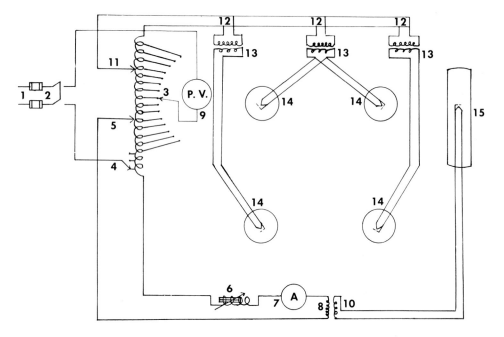

Fig. 3-5. Filament (heating) circuit.

1. Fuses
2. Primary switch
3. Autotransformer
4. Line-voltage regulator
5. Circuit connector for filament transformer
6. Choke coil
7. Filament ammeter
8. Primary side of filament transformer
9. Prereading voltmeter
10. Secondary side of filament transformer
11. Valve-tube filament transformer connection
12. Primary side of valve-tube transformer
13. Secondary side of valve-tube transformer
14. Valve-tube filaments
15. X-ray tube cathode filament

to conduct the secondary voltage, through thermionic emission (see pp. 46 and 47 and Fig. 4-7), across the terminals of the valve and x-ray tubes. (See Fig. 3-5.)

Rectification

Rectification is the restriction of the flow of current to a particular direction; i.e., the flow of current in each half cycle is in a direction useful in the production of x-rays.

Rectification may be achieved by use of the x-ray tube alone. In such an instance, the rectification is called *self-rectification.* This type is satisfactory in limited circumstances and is a form of half-wave rectification. In general, rectification is classified as either *half-wave* or *full-wave.* Fig. 3-6 presents diagrams of the current flow in a self-rectified circuit and of the current flow in a half-wave rectified circuit.

In the operation of self-rectified or half-wave rectified equipment, *only half the current impulses* produce x-rays. Current can flow only from the cathode to the anode. Consequently, current flowing in the opposite direction is blocked.

The cathode in full-wave rectified equipment receives *all the current im-*

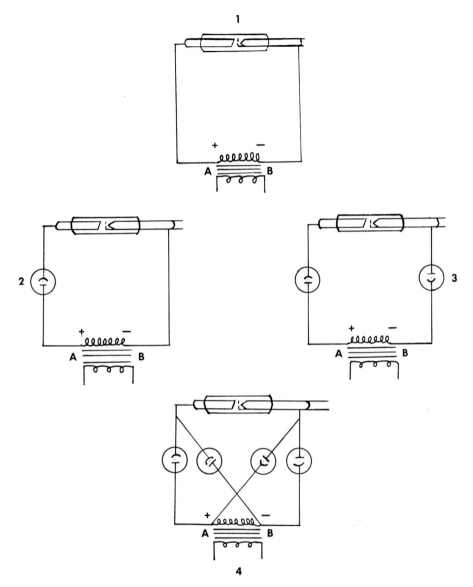

Fig. 3-6. Diagrams of rectification circuitry. **1,** Self-rectification. **2,** Half-wave rectification, one valve tube. **3,** Half-wave rectification, two valve tubes. **4,** Full-wave rectification, four valve tubes.

pulses from the same direction, thus permitting full current flow. Fig. 3-6 also diagrams the current flow in a full-wave rectified circuit.

The valve tubes are in series with the rectifier circuit. There is a slight loss in the kilovoltage during travel from cathode to anode in a valve tube, primarily because the valve tube operates at less than saturation current. (See pp. 48 and 49.) This loss seldom exceeds 3 kilovolts. Valve tubes are discussed on pp. 43 and 44.

Fig. 3-7 is a diagram of the basic circuits of a full-wave rectified x-ray machine.

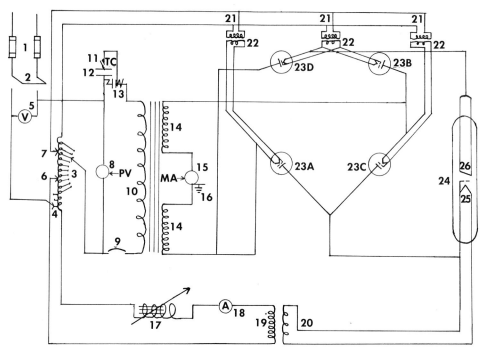

Fig. 3-7. X-ray machine circuitry with full-wave rectification.

1. Fuses
2. Primary switch
3. Autotransformer
4. Line-voltage regulator
5. Line-voltage meter
6. Fixed position for x-ray tube filament transformer
7. Fixed position for valve-tube filament transformers
8. Prereading voltmeter
9. Circuit breaker
10. Primary side of high-voltage transformer
11. Exposure switch
12. Timer to close circuit
13. Magnetic contactor
14. Secondary side of high-voltage transformer
15. Milliammeter
16. Ground
17. Choke coil
18. Filament ammeter
19. Primary side of filament transformer
20. Secondary side of filament transformer
21. Primary side of valve-tube transformers
22. Secondary side of valve-tube transformers
23. Valve tubes (*A* and *B* in first half cycle, *C* and *D* in inverse half cycle)
24. X-ray tube
25. X-ray tube filament
26. X-ray tube anode

REFERENCES

Boast, Warren B.: Principles of electric and magnetic circuits, New York, 1950, Harper & Brothers.

Robertson, John Kellock: Radiology physics, ed. 3, Princeton, N. J., 1955, D. Van Nostrand Co., Inc.

Selman, Joseph: The fundamentals of x-ray and radium physics, Springfield, Ill., 1954, Charles C Thomas, Publisher.

Weyl, Charles, and Warren, S. Reid, Jr.: Radiologic physics, ed. 2, Springfield, Ill., 1951, Charles C Thomas, Publisher.

Chapter 4

X-rays and other radiations

X-ray tubes

Modern x-ray tubes consist of three essential parts: *an evacuated glass envelope, a hot-filament cathode, and an anode with a suitable target.* The hermetically sealed glass envelope contains the cathode and anode. Electric current flows to and from the cathode and anode without destroying the vacuum. A shielding material, which contains a port (window) to permit the passage of x-rays through a limited aperture, encases the evacuated tube. The port material must be radiolucent. The anode contains a small tungsten* block (button) in its face nearest the cathode. The tungsten block, approximately 2 mm thick, is the target for the cathode electrons. (See Figs. 4-1 and 4-2.)

A molybdenum focusing cup surrounds the cathode filament. The focusing cup concentrates the electrons emitted from the filament onto a small area of the anode target. Since the filament is linear in shape, the electrons impinge upon the target in a line. The anode angles slightly away from the cathode so that the x-rays emitted at right angles to the electron beam appear to be coming from a point instead of a line (see pp. 45 and 46 and Figs. 4-5 and 4-6).

The anodes of diagnostic x-ray tubes may be either stationary or rotating. In most rotating anode tubes, the beveled (angled) edge of the *disk* circumference forms a 15-degree angle with the transverse plane of the x-ray tube. The beveled edge slopes away from the cathode. The cup focuses the electrons at the lower edge of this bevel. (See Fig. 4-2.)

The metal shielding that surrounds the glass tube serves to prevent the escape of nonuseful rays. Specifically refined oil occupies the space between the glass tube and the shielding. Between the x-ray tube and the port, the oil serves as the *inherent filter* (built-in filter) of the x-ray tube. The filtering effect of the inherent filter should be equivalent to that of a minimum of 0.5 mm of aluminium. Included in the structure of the metal shielding is a slot for additional filters; im-

---

*Because of the following six physical characteristics, tungsten is the element chosen as the target of an x-ray tube:

Z number (atomic number)	74
Density	19.3
Melting point	3370° C.
Temperature of volatilization	high (evident at 1800° C.)
Thermal conductivity	0.35
Specific heat	0.03

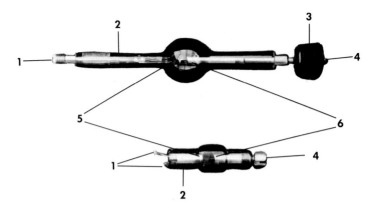

Fig. 4-1. Stationary anode x-ray tubes. Upper photograph is of an early Coolidge, nonshockproof tube; lower one is of a tube encased in metal and surrounded with oil.

1. Cathode connections
2. Evacuated glass envelope
3. Metal fins for air cooling
4. Anode connection
5. Cathode
6. Anode

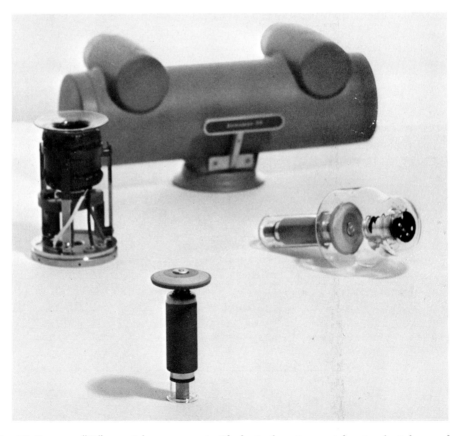

Fig. 4-2. Dynamax "50" x-ray tube components. Clockwise from top: metal casing for tube, anode and cathode in evacuated glass envelope, rotor and target, and stator windings. (Courtesy The Machlett Laboratories, Inc.)

mediately beneath this is a second slot for attachment of various cones (see pp. 84 to 88).

Tubes designed for use in x-ray therapy are similar to radiographic tubes; the chief differences are that the anodes and targets of therapy tubes are larger and the electrons do not impinge on as small a spot.

Valve tubes

Valve tubes differ somewhat in construction from x-ray tubes. The valve tube anode face is at right angles to the cathode stream. The electron stream strikes the entire anode face. There is no tungsten block in the valve tube anode. (See Figs. 4-3 and 4-4.)

It has been stated (pp. 38 to 40) that the valve tube's function is to conduct the secondary current along a predetermined circuit.

A good valve tube will *not* produce x-rays because the electrons cannot cross the valve at high speed. The design of a good valve tube is such that the tube current is maintained well below saturation. Consequently, the voltage drop is very small (see pp. 48 and 49).

Two types of valve tube filaments are available, and each type performs satisfactorily. The principal difference between the two types permits considerable difference in operation. The *tungsten filament* valve tube requires approximately 12 volts to operate the filament current. The *thoriated tungsten filament*

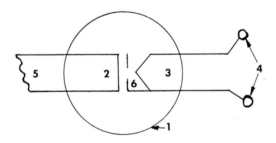

Fig. 4-3. Valve tube diagram. (See also Fig. 4-4.)

1. Evacuated glass envelope
2. Anode
3. Cathode

4. Cathode connections to secondary side of valve-tube transformer
5. Anode connection to high-voltage circuit
6. Cathode filament

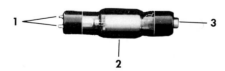

Fig. 4-4. Valve tube photograph. Cathode and anode are hidden from view by the metal sleeve surrounding them.

1. Cathode connections
2. Evacuated glass envelope
3. Anode connection

valve tube requires approximately 6 volts to operate the filament current; the thorium coating becomes the source of electrons and permits the lower operating voltage, thereby prolonging tube life.

Cathodes

The cathode has a negative charge in relation to the anode. The filament circuit of the x-ray machine supplies the cathode filament with the necessary heat. Also, one side of the cathode filament connects to the secondary side of the high-voltage transformer to conduct the secondary current across the x-ray tube.

The construction of the focusing cup, the relation of the focusing cup to the cathode filament, and the application of high voltage to the x-ray tube cause the electrons, which are emitted from the filament, to strike the anode target in a very small area.

The small filament (approximately 0.0085 inch in diameter) offers considerable resistance to the flow of the heating current. This heating (filament) current raises the filament temperature to a sufficiently high value to cause the electrons of the filament to *boil off* and surround the cathode in a cloud (the electron cloud). Increases in the filament current cause corresponding increases in the kinetic energy of the filament electrons, thus causing proportionately more electrons to be emitted from the coil of wire. This process of releasing electrons by heat is called thermionic emission and is further explained on pp. 46 and 47 and Fig. 4-7.

Anodes

As has been stated, the anodes of diagnostic x-ray tubes may be either stationary or rotating. In contrast, the anodes of valve tubes are always stationary. X-ray therapy tube anodes are usually stationary; however, some are rotating. The stationary anode usually consists of a copper bar or cylinder with a small tungsten *button* embedded in the end that faces the cathode. The copper rapidly conducts the heat from the tungsten target to the tube shielding.

There are several methods of dissipating the generated heat from the anode to the tube shielding. One method of anode cooling uses oil to transfer the heat to the shielding which, in turn, radiates the heat to the air. Other methods of anode cooling use fins or radiators to dissipate the heat. The fins are at right angles to the long axis of the anode. Most high-capacity radiographic tubes have a motor-driven fan attached to the shielding to aid in cooling the shielding material.

The anode is the positive plate (in the x-ray tube) for the secondary (high-voltage) circuit. When the exposure switch is closed, the cathode electrons strike the anode to complete the circuit. These electrons strike the anode in an area (actual focal spot) determined by the molybdenum focusing cup, the shape of the cathode filament, and the angle of the anode. Early radiographic tubes had the anode angle at 45 degrees. Modern stationary anode tubes have the angle at approximately 20 degrees, to decrease the *effective* focal spot size. (See Fig. 4-5.) Early focal spots included also elliptical and rectangular shapes.

The present *linear focal spot* in stationary anode tubes evolved from numerous attempts to reduce the effective focal spot size. The terms *actual focal spot*

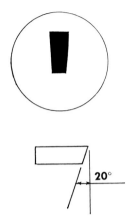

Fig. 4-5. Stationary anode. The top diagram is an end-on view of the anode (shaded) in the copper core. The lower diagram demonstrates the 20-degree angle of the bevel.

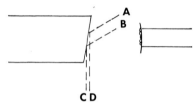

Fig. 4-6. Effective focal spot. The actual focal spot is the length (in this figure) of the line **A-B.** The projected length of the line **A-B** is imaginary line **C-D**, which is the length of the effective focus. **A-B** is 3.5 mm and **C-D** is 1 mm.

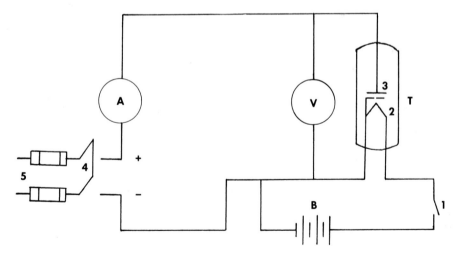

Fig. 4-7. Thermionic emission; secondary current conduction.

1. Single pole switch in battery circuit
2. Cathode filament in vacuum tube
3. Anode of vacuum tube
4. Double pole switch of alternating current
5. Fuses of alternating current line

B Battery
A Ammeter
V Voltmeter
T Vacuum tube

and *effective focal spot* are often confused and frequently misunderstood. *The actual focal spot is the actual area of bombardment by the cathode electrons. The effective focal spot is the projected area of the actual focal spot; this projected area is at right angles to the cathode electron stream.* The actual focal spot is, of course, considerably larger than the effective focal spot. The effective focal spot is the term used to describe the focal spot of a given x-ray tube. (See Fig. 4-6.)

The rotating anode is a disk approximately 3 inches in diameter (see Fig. 1-6). An external rotor induces this anode to spin upon its axis at approximately 3,000 rpm. Because of the spin, there is a constantly changing target area upon which the cathode electrons impinge. This condition permits the use of greater kilovoltages and milliampere-seconds within the safe limits of tube operation— determined on the specific tube-rating chart (see pp. 70 and 71). The circumference of the disk is the actual area of bombardment. The electrons bombard a small portion of this circumference at any specific instant. Introduction of the rotating anode tube permitted great advances in the development of high-speed radiography, which utilizes high tube current and short exposure time.

A double focal spot is used in many modern x-ray tubes (both rotating and stationary anodes). This tube usually has two cathode filaments, independent of each other. Some x-ray tube manufacturers use a single filament with two sets of connections to the filament circuit. Each connects to the continuous filament, which has a smaller portion (small filament) usually in the center of the larger. When there are two independent filaments in the cathode, they are usually side by side. Some *double-focus* tubes have a separate switch to select focal spot size. Usually the milliamperage (technique) selector incorporates this selection.

Thermionic emission

The conduction of current across the terminals of valve and x-ray tubes is made possible by thermionic emission. *Thermionic emission is the release of electrons by application of heat.*

Experiment has revealed that current flows between the cathode and anode (in a hot-filament vacuum tube) *only* when the cathode filament releases electrons. Fig. 4-7 and its text explain the necessity of electron release for current flow.

The number of electrons released (thermionic emission) depends upon the filament heat. When saturation current exists (see pp. 48 and 49), the relation between tube current and filament temperature is expressed in Richardson's equation as modified by Dushman:

$$I = AT^2e - \frac{b}{T}$$

Using tungsten as the filament material, the elements of this equation are as follows:

A and b are constants of the tungsten filament; $A = 60.2$ amps/cm^{2}degrees^2; $T =$ the absolute temperature in degrees Kelvin of the filament (for x-ray and valve tube filaments operating between 10 and 500 ma, the absolute temperatures are from 2200° K to 2700° K); $e = 2.71828$ (the approximate value of the base of natural logarithms); $- \frac{b}{T}$ (the exponent on e) is a unitless quantity since $\frac{b}{T} = \frac{e\phi}{kT}$, where $e\phi$ is work (e is the electron charge, ϕ is the work function of the metal), k is the Baltzmann constant (work per degree K), and T is in degrees; I = current density in amperes per square centimeter of the thermionically emitting surface.

The electrons flowing from cathode to anode each second constitute the tube current; the magnitude of the tube current is a function of the total number of the electrons flowing between the cathode and the anode. Tube current can be calculated as follows:

Where the charge on one electron is 4.8002×10^{-19} esu,* and one ampere-second $= 3 \times 10^9$ esu, and an electronic charge $= 4.8002 \times 10^{-10}$ esu, or 1.6019×10^{-19} coulombs:

$$1 \text{ mas} = \frac{3 \times 10^9 \text{ esu}}{10^3} \times \frac{1}{4.8002 \times 10^{-10}}$$

$$= (3 \times 10^6) \left(\frac{1}{4.8002}\right) (10^{10})$$

$$= \frac{3 \times 10^{16}}{4.8002}$$

$$= 6.24 \times 10^{15} \text{ electrons}$$

To produce x-rays, it is necessary that the liberated electrons strike the target with high velocity. This occurs when the anode is positively charged in the high-voltage circuit. Following closure of the exposure switch, the secondary voltage is quite high at the cathode in relation to the anode. Therefore, the voltage drop between the cathode and anode accelerates the liberated cathode electrons across to the positively charged anode with a force that is approximately proportional to the impressed secondary voltage. The midpoint of the high-voltage transformer is grounded to make practical insulation possible. Since the rectifier circuit is supplied from both legs of a transformer grounded at its midpoint, the result at any one moment is a high positive potential in one leg and a high negative potential in the other. This condition, with rectification of the current, provides a high potential drop between the cathode and the anode.

In a self-rectified unit, the generation of heat in the anode is usually insufficient to permit release of electrons; therefore, current cannot flow from anode to cathode in the inverse half cycle. However, if the anode becomes excessively heated from continuous or prolonged usage, it will emit electrons. Insertion of a valve tube in series between the x-ray tube anode and the high-voltage transformer prevents the rectification of current by the x-ray tube. The valve tube anode cannot reach a degree of heat that would permit release of electrons, due to a lack of appreciable potential drop.

X-rays
Characteristics of x-rays

X-rays[†] are a form of radiant energy having both a wave nature and a quantum nature. Since these rays possess a wave nature and travel with the speed of

---

*esu = electrostatic unit.

[†]The roentgen (r) is the unit of measurement of quantity of roentgen radiation (x-rays): when the secondary electrons are fully utilized and the wall effect of the chamber is avoided, a roentgen produces in 1 ml of atmospheric air at 0° C. and 760 mm of mercury pressure such a degree of conductivity that one electrostatic unit is measured at saturation point. (Actually, it amounts to the degree of ionization produced in 1 ml of air by exposing the chamber to x-rays.)

light, they are properly classified as electromagnetic waves. *An electromagnetic wave is produced by the oscillation of an electric charge.* All electromagnetic waves travel with the speed of light, which is approximately 3×10^{10} cm per second in a vacuum (186,000 miles per second is a frequently used value and is less than 1% in error).

X-rays are electrically neutral, are capable of penetrating all matter to varying degrees, and are reflected and diffracted by certain crystals. The angle of incidence equals the angle of reflection, and the dispersion by diffraction is a function of the atomic arrangement and the wavelength of the particular x-ray.

X-rays can cause numerous biologic, physical, and chemical effects. Among the biologic effects are bactericidal and lethal ones, chromosome aberration, tissue ionization, depilation, tissue desquamation, erythema production, and sterilization. Among the physical effects are the photographic effect on x-ray and other films, the ionization of nonliving substance, and the ability to penetrate matter. Among the chemical effects are the liberation of iodine from solutions of iodoform in chloroform and the discoloration of certain alkaline salts.

Since x-rays are a definite form of energy, it is necessary to expend energy to produce x-rays. Application of the heating current to the cathode filament raises the resistance of the filament to the flow of current. This resistance causes the filament to acquire a certain degree of heat in relation to the quantity of current amperage use. An increase in current causes an increase in the heat of the filament. The heat energizes the electrons of the filament atoms; some of these electrons then move away (are liberated) from the filament as a result of increased kinetic energy. Increases in the cathode filament temperature cause correspondingly greater numbers of electrons to be liberated from the filament. Application of the tube voltage (kilovoltage) drives the liberated electrons to the anode target to produce x-rays. In this manner, electric energy is expended in the production of x-rays.

In addition to the electromagnetic wave nature of x-rays, these rays have also a quantum nature and arise as discrete packets (photons) of energy (Planck's quantum theory). *A photon is a particle (quantum) of x-radiation or gamma radiation. A quantum is a definite amount of energy (hv: Planck's constant × frequency).*

Space charge and saturation current

At a given operating temperature of the filament, the total number of electrons liberated from the filament is constant regardless of the voltage. The liberated electrons surround the filament in a cloud. Each electron carries a negative electric charge; therefore, each electron repels every other electron in the cloud. Each atom that has lost an electron is then positively charged; therefore, there is an electrostatic charge between the electron cloud and the filament. The continuing heat of the filament tends to liberate additional electrons. The effect of the filament heat is sufficient to overcome the electrostatic attraction between the liberated electrons and the filament ions. *The total effect of these combined forces is the space charge.* It follows that the tube voltage necessary to drive the liberated electrons to the anode must be great enough to overcome the space charge.

When the tube voltage is low, the anode attracts only those electrons that are nearest the anode; therefore, the tube current (milliamperage) is low. When the filament temperature is constant, an increase in kilovoltage attracts greater numbers of electrons to the anode; as a result there is a corresponding decrease in the number of liberated electrons repelled to the filament.

If the kilovoltage is increased, eventually a kilovoltage value is reached at which all of the electrons are driven to the anode as fast as they are liberated and none are repelled to the cathode filament. *This kilovoltage value is the saturation voltage, and its corresponding current value is the saturation current.*

Experimental evidence reveals that *corresponding to each filament current is a maximum value of the tube current that is independent of the applied voltage.* Operation of x-ray equipment at saturation voltage and current permits independent variation of kilovoltage and milliamperage. However, when tube current values exceed 50 ma, it becomes necessary to apply sufficient tube voltage to overcome the effects of the space charge.

High values of filament current cause correspondingly greater values of the space charge. To prevent destruction or damage to the x-ray tube during application of high filament current values, a *space charge compensator* is incorporated into the circuit. The effect of this compensator if tube voltage increases is an automatic decrease in the filament current; thus the compensator maintains the correct tube current value.

Since the number of liberated electrons depends upon the heat of the filament, this number is then indirectly dependent upon the magnitude of the filament current. Thus, there can be no more electrons driven across the tube each second than there are electrons available each second from the filament. Construction of hot-filament x-ray tubes permits control of tube current either by utilization of the space charge or by total emission of the electrons from the hot filament. When saturation current is achieved, the milliamperage will depend entirely upon the total electron emission. In such an instance, increasing or decreasing the filament current regulates the milliamperage. Therefore, very slight changes in the filament current will produce quite large changes in the milliamperage. Experimental evidence reveals that in a given tube an increase in the filament current from 4 amperes to 4½ amperes will cause the milliamperage to increase from 40 to 100.

The importance of maintaining a constant filament amperage becomes evident. Consequently, voltage stabilizers of various designs are incorporated into the primary circuit. *A voltage stabilizer tends to maintain voltage fluctuations at a minimum; therefore, the amperage fluctuations are maintained at a corresponding minimum.*

X-ray production

The tungsten target contains millions of tungsten atoms. To produce x-rays, it is necessary to decelerate suddenly or stop the high-speed electrons from the cathode. When a high-speed cathode electron strikes a tungsten atom, the electron will penetrate the atom in proportion to the energy of the electron. In modern diagnostic x-ray tubes, the speed of many of the bombarding electrons, when energized by very high kilovoltages, reaches approximately 0.9 the speed of light. The impressed voltage accelerates the electrons between the cathode and anode. Thus, since the electron moves in a strong electric field, the speed of the electron becomes increasingly greater as it approaches the target. The kinetic energy can be calculated approximately if the kilovoltage is known, because energy in electron volts *(ev)* is equal to the kilovoltage: $E = ev$, where E is the energy, e is the electron charge, and v is the kilovoltage.

The formula for kinetic energy (KE) is expressed as follows:

$$\text{KE} = \frac{mv^2}{2g}, \text{ where g, the gravitational constant, is 980 gram cm/sec.}$$

According to the law of conservation of energy, when a fast-moving cathode electron is decelerated or stopped by an atom, it must give its energy to that atom. An electron expends energy to penetrate an orbital shell. This causes deceleration of the penetrating electron.

In penetrating the three outer (P, O, or N) orbits of the tungsten atom, the electron gives up energy to the atom, which emits this energy in the wavelength range of infrared (heat). It is in this manner that most of the applied energy (approximately 99%) is expended. With sufficient voltage, many of the electrons are driven to the anode with enough energy to penetrate the M, L, and even K orbits. *This very high energy given to the atom by the electrons and emitted from the atom as excess energy is in the wavelength range of the continuous x-ray spectrum.* The emitted energy is approximately 1% of the applied energy.* *The continuous x-ray spectrum is called the general or white radiation; it is also called the continuous spectrum, Bremsstrahlung or "braking" radiations, and is formed as a result of the deceleration of high-speed electrons penetrating an atom.*

When liberated from the filament, the accelerated electron may strike and dislodge an orbital electron of the target atom. When this occurs, another electron must fill the vacated space. Remember, when the cathode electron is stopped or decelerated, its energy is given to the atom. In Chapter 2 it was stated that the orbits of any atom are frequently referred to as energy levels. This statement refers to the requirement of a certain quantity of energy to remove an electron from its orbit. More energy is required to remove an electron from the K orbit than from the L orbit, from the L orbit than from the M orbit, and so on. The orbital energies are considered as *negative* energy, whereas the cathode electron energy is considered as *positive* energy. It follows that the orbits farther from the nucleus have greater *positive* energy.

Removal of an electron from its orbit usually includes removal of the electron energy also. When a bombarding electron strikes and dislodges a K electron from a tungsten atom, another electron must fill the vacated space. This atom emits energy in the form of a *characteristic x-ray* during the transition. The energy quantity is the difference between the negative energy of the K electron and the lesser negative energy of the transitional electron. *Characteristic x-rays are of definite wavelengths, are characteristic of a pure substance, and are emitted by*

---

*The efficiency of the anode may be determined from the relation of the x-ray photon energy to the cathode electron energy. This is expressed in an empirical (experimental) formula: Efficiency = (1.4) (10^{-9}) *(ZV)*; where Z is the atomic number of the target element, V is the tube voltage, and 1.4 and 10^{-9} are constants. At 100 pkv (peak kilovoltage) the efficiency of tungsten is 1.036%.

this substance when properly excited. Since a K orbit electron of tungsten represents approximately 70 kev (1 kev = 1,000 electron volts) of energy, it would require a cathode electron with approximately 70 kev of energy to dislodge a K electron. An L orbit electron of tungsten represents approximately 11 kev of energy. If an L orbit electron fills the vacated K space, the atom radiates 59 kev (the difference between 70 kev and 11 kev) of energy as characteristic x-rays; it also radiates the remaining energy as infrared rays. *The structure of the atom determines the energy of the characteristic radiation (this does not apply to the continuous spectrum, Bremsstrahlung).*

The M orbit electron of tungsten represents approximately 2.5 kev of energy. If an M orbit electron fills the vacated K space, the energy emitted during this transition is 70 minus 2.5, or 67.5 kev, which is a much greater amount of energy than that given off during an L to K transition. All this emitted energy is in the form of electromagnetic waves. When an M orbit electron fills a vacated L space, the difference in energy levels is 11 minus 2.5, or 8.5 kev of energy given up in the form of an electromagnetic wave.

Removal of a K electron causes the atom to emit a characteristic ray. *Characteristic rays of tungsten radiate from tungsten only when the tube voltage equals or exceeds approximately 70 kvp (kilovolts peak).* Elements having atomic (Z) numbers greater than 74 require greater voltages to dislodge K electrons, and the wavelengths emitted following such a transition in energy are characteristic of these more dense elements.

Corresponding rays are those rays arising from the same transition in energy level. Corresponding rays may arise from transitions between the same named orbits of any two atoms. When corresponding rays arise from transitions into the K orbits, these rays are also characteristic.

The impressed voltage controls the force of the bombarding electrons and so controls their energy. Therefore, the voltage controls the energy of the emitted electromagnetic wave, or x-ray.* Since the voltage controls the energy of the x-ray photon, the voltage peak determines the orbit from which the most energetic x-ray photon radiates and thereby determines the shortest wavelength emitted. It follows, then, that wavelength depends upon the voltage. Experimental evidence reveals that the shorter wavelengths are harder (more energetic), so hardness depends upon wavelength. If a wave is harder, the wave is capable of increased penetration; therefore, penetrability depends upon wavelength. *These three properties of x-rays—wavelength, hardness, and penetrability—are called the qualities of x-rays and are all controlled by the kilovoltage.*

Quantum nature of x-rays

Since the current of the secondary circuit is alternating, the impressed voltage must rise from zero to the predetermined peak, then return to zero, then rise to the peak, and so on. The constantly varying amounts of voltage propel the cathode electrons to the target; therefore, the resulting energy of the x-ray

---

*The energy of an x-ray photon may be determined from the formula:

$$\text{Photon energy} = \frac{12.4 \times 10^3}{\lambda \text{ Å}} \text{ electron volts}$$

photons will vary in proportion. As a result, the x-ray beam is a heterogeneous bundle of many wavelengths (the continuous spectrum).

It was previously mentioned that x-rays have both a wave nature and a quantum nature, also that x-rays originate as a heterogeneous bundle of many wavelengths. These wavelengths originate in the target from bombardment of cathode electrons possessing particular quantities of kinetic energy; therefore, the wavelengths possess a certain energy. Electrons at low energy produce longer wavelengths that are less energetic. Greater electron energy produces shorter wavelengths possessing greater amounts of energy. Thus, each individual wavelength of x-ray represents a specific quantity (quantum) of energy. Regardless of the source of a given wavelength, it invariably possesses the same quantum of energy.

The atom emits one burst of energy for each single addition of energy. *An atom cannot give off energy unless energy has been added to the atom.* If the cathode electron penetrates to the K orbit and dislodges a K electron, the atom emits a quantum of x-ray energy proportional to the K orbit energy. Since the emitted x-ray quantum originates from the K orbit, it follows that this quantum possesses a shorter wavelength than a quantum from the L orbit would possess.

Experiment proves that the shortest wavelength is solely dependent upon the maximum voltage impressed upon the x-ray tube. For the sake of convenience, x-ray wavelengths are expressed in angstrom units (Å). An angstrom unit is expressed as 1×10^{-8} cm and is 1/100,000,000 of a centimeter in length. Following is a formula to determine the wavelength of any x-ray:

$$\text{Shortest wavelength in Å} = \frac{12396.44^*}{\text{Maximum voltage}}$$

The Duane-Hunt relation. The energy of an x-ray, or light photon of frequency ν is found by experiment to be $E = h\nu$, where h is Planck's constant, equal to 6.62×10^{-27} erg-sec. In terms of wavelength:

$$E = \frac{c}{\lambda} \text{ (ergs)}$$

If metric units are used, the energy is expressed in ergs. However, a more convenient experimental energy unit is the electron volt. Since the electron charge e is equal to 4.80×10^{-10} esu (electrostatic units) and one volt = 1/300 esu of potential, 1 ev = $4.80 \times 10^{-10} \times 1/300 = 1.60 \times 10^{-12}$ ergs. Converting (1) to electron volts:

$$E = \frac{hc/\lambda}{1.6 \times 10^{-12}} \text{ (ev)}$$

But $h = 6.62 \times 10^{-27}$ and $c = 3 \times 10^{10}$. Substituting these values:

$$E = \frac{(1) (6.62 \times 10^{-27}) (3 \times 10^{10})}{(\lambda) \qquad 1.6 \times 10^{-12}} = \frac{1.24 \times 10^{-4}}{\lambda \text{ (cm)}}$$

Finally, if λ is to be in angstrom units:

$$E = \frac{1.24 \times 10^{-4}}{\lambda(10^{-8})} = \frac{1.24 \times 10^4}{\lambda} \text{ or } E = \frac{12396.44}{\lambda}$$

If the energy involved is that emitted during an electronic transition ($\triangle W$):

$$\triangle W = \frac{12396.44}{\lambda}$$

---

*Although 12.4×10^3 is a less accurate value for this constant, practical consideration permits use of this more easily remembered number. (The resulting error is less than 1%.)

Or, if the energy is known and the wavelength is desired, $\triangle W$ and λ can be interchanged (λ is in Å units; $\triangle W$ is in electron volts):

$$\lambda = \frac{12396.44}{\triangle W}$$

By the use of the formula for determining wavelength, it is possible to calculate the wavelength range most commonly used in diagnostic radiography. With a maximum voltage of 30 kvp, the minimum wavelength (λ) in angstrom units is as follows:

$$\lambda = \frac{12.4 \times 10_3}{30,000} \text{ , or } \lambda = 0.413 \text{ Å}$$

With a maximum voltage of 150 kvp, the minimum wavelength in angstrom units is as follows:

$$\lambda = \frac{12.4 \times 10^3}{150,000} \text{ , or } \lambda = 0.08 \text{ Å}$$

The above information establishes the approximate wavelength range in diagnostic radiography to be from a minimum of 0.08 Å to a maximum of 0.413 Å.

A mathematical relationship exists among the factors of wavelength (λ), velocity (v), and frequency (ν). The following formula expresses this relationship: $v = \lambda\nu$. Substituting values of wavelength from above in this formula demonstrates that shorter wavelengths possess proportionally higher frequencies: $3 \times 10^{10} = (0.413)(1 \times 10^{-8})(\nu)$; $\nu = 7.26 \times 10^{18}$ vibrations per second, approximately; $3 \times 10^{10} = (0.08)(1 \times 10^{-8})(\nu)$; $\nu = 36 \times 10^{18}$ vibrations per second, approximately.

Measurement of x-ray penetrability

Penetrability is one of the important qualities of x-rays, equally with hardness and wavelength; all three qualities are interdependent and all are dependent upon kilovoltage.

The factors for a highly satisfactory technique on one machine will not necessarily be the same as those for another machine, even though the two machines are of the same make and capacity. The differences in x-ray energy output are due to the unpredictable variations in transformers and x-ray tube targets.

Because it is almost impossible to ascertain or develop a technique by purely mathematical processes, it becomes necessary to determine the penetrability of specific x-ray photons by some standard method. The device usually employed in this determination is the *penetrometer.* A penetrometer (see Fig. 4-8, *A*) may be of any suitable metal but should be in the form of a *step wedge* with increasing thicknesses in each step. Aluminum is the usual metal of choice. In a step wedge, each successive step is ⅛ inch greater in thickness. The steps may have lead numbers on them to indicate the greatest step that a varied kilovoltage will penetrate. The milliampere-seconds used in this type of calibration must be constant in each series of exposures; it is equally important to maintain a constant distance (ffd) in each series. Fig. 4-8, *B*, represents such a series of exposures. The information gained from such a series is useful in developing techniques on new equipment or in making technique adjustments on equipment in use.

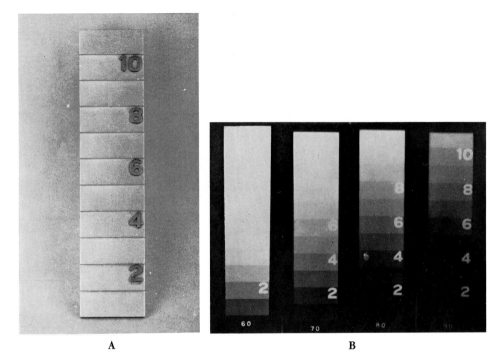

A   **B**

Fig. 4-8. A, A penetrometer. **B,** Penetrometer exposure series. The penetrometer exposure factors are 60 kvp, 70 kvp, 80 kvp, and 90 kvp; all exposures were made at a 40-inch ffd and at 50 mas.

It is usually possible to visualize density or penetration differences of 1 kilovolt in penetrometer radiographs made with 50 kvp or less. Those radiographs made at voltages between 60 kvp and 70 kvp usually require 2 kilovolts for an appreciable visualization of change in penetration; above 70 kvp, this requirement increases to 3 kilovolts.

The x-ray beam

As was mentioned earlier, the energy emerging from the x-ray tube consists of a heterogeneous bundle of many wavelengths. Since the x-ray photons arise as waves, these waves diverge from the face of the anode in all directions. Actually, x-rays radiate in all degrees of a sphere from the point of bombardment on the anode face. The protective devices that surround the x-ray tube prevent escape of most of the useless rays. Many of these rays are also so soft that they are incapable of traveling any great distance from the target.

The angle of the anode also provides for the emission of the primary (useful) x-rays through the side of the x-ray tube. X-rays emitted from small focal areas produce the sharpest radiographs since there is very little overlap of the emitted rays.

In radiography, the chief concern is with the *primary beam*. The primary beam consists of all the rays escaping from the tube shielding through the port and arising from the original bombardment of the target by the cathode electrons. Prior to penetration of the object of radiography, it is necessary to remove many of the softer rays from the heterogeneous beam to reduce unnecessary exposure.

The primary rays diverge in all forward directions with the *central ray*. The central ray is that portion of the primary rays that leaves the port at right angles to the long axis of the x-ray tube and is *the portion of the primary beam directed to the center of the film or structure to be radiographed.* It is necessary to control the divergent portions of the primary rays. Cones and diaphragms, when properly attached over the port, effectively control most of the diverging x-rays.

Secondary rays

When a beam of x-rays passes through any substance, the substance tends to absorb or remove part of the energy. Many experiments on the reduction in intensity of an x-ray beam by passage through an absorbing layer have been performed. The effect of air as an absorbing material is most important. Although air consists, for the most part, of relatively loose molecules of lighter elements, the primary rays must interact with these atoms and molecules in one or more of the three ways discussed on pp. 56 and 57. Exact data for air absorption may be obtained from the National Bureau of Standards. To obtain the exact intensity of an x-ray beam at a given distance from its target, the value obtained by calculation from the inverse-square law must be multipled by the correction factor for this distance in air. (See pp. 78 to 80.)

When the primary rays pass through the tissues of the body or other organic material, several phenomena occur. Among these phenomena is that of secondary ray production. *Secondary rays are the rays generated in the patient and surrounding objects by the passage of the primary x-rays.*

Experiment reveals that these secondary rays are usually of at least two kinds: scattered or secondary scatter rays (some possess wavelengths identical with the primary rays and others possess longer wavelengths) and characteristic fluorescent rays (these are characteristic—possess the same wavelength—of the radiator material). *Secondary scatter rays* diverge in all directions from the point of generation in the object (radiator). The greater intensity of these rays is in the forward direction. In therapy, because of the effect of these rays on human tissues, the secondary scatter rays are of extreme importance when the primary wavelength is short. *Characteristic fluorescent rays* are identical with characteristic rays, but the method of generation of each is different. *Characteristic rays result from cathode electron bombardment of the x-ray tube target; characteristic fluorescent rays result from the impact of an exciting primary x-ray photon on the radiator.* The voltage required to produce characteristic rays is proportional to the square of the atomic number of the target material.

Remnant rays

The remnant rays produce the latent image in the film (see p. 73). *Remnant radiation is that ionizing radiation which produces the radiographic image.* The total primary radiation that enters the part being radiographed diminishes in the process of interaction between these x-ray photons and matter. The remnant rays that emerge from these tissues consist of those unabsorbed primary rays and the secondary rays generated in the tissues. The quantity of the secondary rays in the remnant radiation depends upon the secondary ray wavelengths and the methods employed to control secondary ray production.

X-rays and matter

X-rays are electrically neutral and possess exceedingly short wavelengths, especially when compared with the size of the atomic nuclei and the relative spaces between the nuclei and the surrounding orbits. Because of this rather large space, many of the shorter x-ray wavelengths are capable of passing between a nucleus and the surrounding orbits without striking either the nucleus or an orbital electron. As a result, x-rays are capable of penetrating all matter. However, the material through which these photons pass absorbs much of the x-ray photon energy. This energy loss is in the form of secondary ray production.

Photons of energy may interact with and penetrate matter in any one of three different manners. These are explained in the following paragraphs (see Fig. 4-9).

1. *Photoelectric emission and true absorption.* When sufficiently high-energy photons of the primary beam collide with and remove an electron from the K orbit of an atom of the material penetrated, the atom emits a characteristic ray and another electron fills the vacated space. The removed electron receives all the energy of the photon; then the electron immediately travels away from the atom, perhaps striking and ionizing other atoms. This type of interaction is photoelectric emission with true absorption; the electron is a *photoelectron** and travels with the transferred kinetic energy of the photon. The photon has given up all of its energy.

2. *Unmodified scattering (Thompson scattering).* A high-energy photon from the primary beam may strike an atom and deflect in another path without entering the atom. The photon retains all its original energy, so it is *unmodified* (modification refers to a reduction in energy with an increase in wavelength). A photon may also pass between the nucleus and the K orbit and touch neither, but since the nucleus attracts the photon, it deflects slightly in exit direction.

3. *Compton effect.* The Compton effect is an interaction between the photon and a free (unbound) electron or between the photon and an orbital electron. A high-energy photon of the primary beam may strike an orbital electron at an angle; the photon imparts a small part of its energy to the electron to eject this electron from its orbit; the photon deflects from its original path and continues through the atom. The ejected electron is a *recoil electron* and may strike other electrons before leaving the atom and thereby cause additional ionization of this atom or other atoms in its path. *Ion pair*† formation may result

---

*The emission of negative charges by the action of light on a surface is the *photoelectric effect,* and the emitted charges are *photoelectrons.* For any given material there is a minimum light frequency (maximum wavelength) below which electrons will not be emitted; this maximum wavelength is called the *photoelectric threshold.* For a given surface, the number of photoelectrons emitted each second (the photoelectric current) is directly proportional to the intensity of the light; also, the kinetic energy of the emitted photoelectrons depends only on the light frequency and is independent of light intensity.

†When an atom loses an electron that attaches to another atom, each becomes an ion and the two are called an ion pair. Some authorities consider ion pair formation as an additional method of interaction of photon energy and matter.

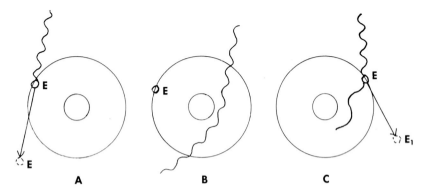

Fig. 4-9. Interactions of energy photons and matter. **A,** True absorption with photoelectron emission. **B,** Unmodified or true (Thompson) scattering. **C,** Compton effect: the Compton photon, less some of its energy, travels onward in a different direction; the recoil electron (E_1) continues in a different direction from the Compton photon; the recoil electron possesses less energy than the Compton photon.

from such action. The photon retains the major portion of its original energy and may cause additional ionization. *This modified photon is a Compton photon.*

According to the degree of penetration by x-rays, animal tissues are classified as follows: *radiopaque*—bones and other tissues containing calcium salts; *intermediate*—muscle, the epidermis, blood, cartilage and other connective tissues, and stones containing either cholesterol or uric acid; or *radiolucent*—adipose tissues, gas, and air.

The degree to which x-rays penetrate tissues depends upon the atomic and molecular structures of the tissues and the energy of the primary photons; the physical condition of the patient also affects the penetration. This characteristic of x-rays to penetrate matter to varying degrees makes x-rays useful as a diagnostic tool in medicine and in industry. The fact that x-rays do not penetrate all animal tissues equally permits the use of x-rays in the demonstration of the varying densities of these tissues.

X-rays and filters

It has been explained that passage of x-ray photons through matter results in a decrease in the emerging photon energy because of absorption.

In radiography, it is necessary to reduce unwanted wavelengths in the primary beam by inserting an aluminum filter in the tube-shielding port (see p. 96). *Present requirements are that at least 2 mm of aluminum be used in addition to the inherent filter.* Additional thicknesses of aluminum require a slight upward adjustment in the kilovoltage, as discussed on p. 96. Aluminum filters are used because the characteristic fluorescent rays of this element are so soft that the energy of these rays is expended in a few centimeters of air. As a result, there is no visible effect on the film.

Other pure-substance materials have been employed experimentally as filters, and in certain instances such materials present potential advantages. The use of iron as a filter in diagnostic radiography was explored by Bösche and Frik in

1962, and results of experimentation with it are reported in an article by Schanze. The experimental evidence reported in this article indicates that between 60 and 120 kvp iron absorbs equal quantities of soft (primary) rays as the same thickness of pure aluminum and increases the total energy striking the film by from 6 to 20%. The increase is obtained through the production of hard secondary rays that cannot be absorbed by the patient.

Filters are used in therapy to control x-ray beam quality. The use of filters in therapy requires absolute exactness. It is necessary to measure the quality and quantity of the primary beam to determine the dose delivered to the patient. In this measurement, it is also necessary to determine the exact

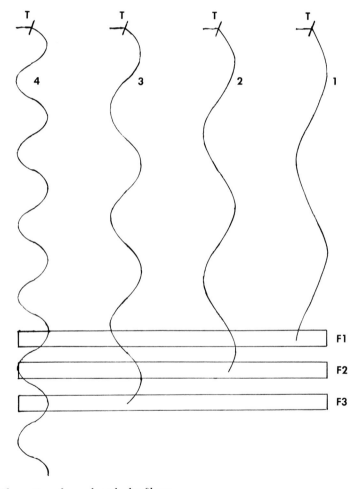

Fig. 4-10. Absorption of wavelengths by filters.

T.	Target of x-ray tube	**1.**	Wavelength whose energy is absorbed by filter no. 1
F1.	Filter No. 1	**2.**	Wavelength whose energy is absorbed by filter no. 2
F2.	Filter No. 2	**3.**	Wavelength whose energy is absorbed by filter no. 3
F3.	Filter No. 3	**4.**	Wavelength whose energy is great enough to penetrate all three filters

thickness of a given metal that will reduce the intensity of the beam to exactly one half; such a thickness is the *half-value layer (hvl)*.

Fig. 4-10 is a schematic representation of the manner in which filters absorb certain of the weaker x-ray photons and permit other photons to penetrate the filter. If sufficient filters were added in the primary beam, the resulting x-ray beam would contain waves of all the same length. Such an x-ray beam is *monochromatic* or *homogeneous*: all of the waves are of the same length and contain identical energy quanta.

The materials used in therapy filters are tin, copper, aluminum, and sometimes lead. A Thoraeus filter is frequently employed in therapy. According to dosage specifications, the *Thoraeus filter consists of varying thicknesses of tin, copper, and aluminum.* Tin is usually the filter nearest the tube; *aluminum must be the external filter* (filter nearest the patient). Supervoltage therapy may require the use of lead as a filter, in which case lead precedes tin as the filter nearest the tube.

Filtration controls the photons of energy emitted from radioactive materials in essentially the same manner as it controls x-ray photons, since both are high-energy electromagnetic waves. All electromagnetic waves respond to filtration according to absorbing coefficients of the absorbing layer.*

X-ray intensity

Radiographic processes depend upon the quantity of radiographic intensity that strikes the x-ray film; however, x-ray therapy processes depend upon the total quantity of intensity absorbed by the tissues. Intensity of radiation is that energy carried by the radiation in a unit of time through a small surface perpendicular to the direction of the radiation, divided by the area of the surface. The quantity of radiation is the product of *intensity times time*. The nature (intensity) of an x-ray beam depends upon both the current and voltage between the cathode and anode.

The number of cathode electrons generating x-rays during anode bombardment has a direct relation to the intensity of this beam of x-rays. If this number increases there will be corresponding increases in the number of x-rays generated. Increases in number of available electrons are achieved either by increasing time or by raising current.

It follows that intensity is associated with milliamperage. Then quantity of radiation (exposure) is the product of milliamperage times time. Milliampere-seconds is an expression of radiographic (intensity) exposure. Milliamperage times time in seconds equals milliampere-seconds. Stated algebraically this becomes ma $\times$ s = mas.

If ma and mas are known:

$$s = \frac{mas}{ma}$$

---

*The use of the words *filter* and *filtration* in relation to the absorption of the photon energy must not be confused with the same terms as used in chemistry. Chemical filtration refers to the actual holding back of some of the material in suspension. Physical filtration refers to absorption of some of the energy by the filter (absorbing layer).

If both s and mas are known:

$$ma = \frac{mas}{s}$$

Experimental evidence reveals that there are two types of radiation: continuous and characteristic (see pp. 50 and 51). Continuous radiation consists of the several wavelengths and does not require excessively high voltage. Characteristic radiations occur *only* when the voltage is sufficiently high. The continuous (general) radiation intensity (1) is directly proportional to the millamperage; (2) varies approximately with the square of the voltage; and (3) varies with the Z number of the target material.

Each type of radiation, continuous and characteristic, affects tissues similarly. No biologic change can occur from energy acting upon living tissues *unless energy is absorbed by these tissues*. The degree of ionization is a measure of the quantity of interaction of energy and matter. Many methods of x-ray intensity measurement have been developed. Probably the most satisfactory of these is the one that depends upon the measurement of the degree of ionization of air at a given distance from the x-ray tube target; measurements of this type must be made in air to avoid back-scatter (the radiation scattered back from the underlying materials).

Common radiation measurement and detection instruments

The **condenser r-meter** (r is the unit of measure of quantity of roentgen radiation) is commonly used to measure the radiation intensity of x-ray therapy machines (see Fig. 4-11). A brief explanation follows. The r-meter consists of a

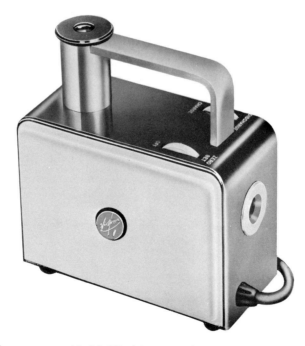

Fig. 4-11. Condenser r-meter, Model 570. (Courtesy The Victoreen Instrument Co.)

box containing an electroscope that is insulated from the box, a device for charging the electroscope and its attached electrode, and a battery-operated lamp to illuminate the scale, which reads directly in roentgens. A movable scale marker is attached to the electroscope and a small microscope permitting visualization of the illuminated scale. The ionization chamber tube fits into a receptacle in one end of the box. When the tube is placed in contact with the electroscope electrode, a connection is made between this electrode and a second electrode in the ionization chamber in the opposite end of this tube. When operated, the electrometer is charged so the scale marker points to zero. Insertion and contact of the tube, whose chamber has been ionized by the passage of x-rays, causes a loss in potential of the electrometer according to the degree of ionization in the chamber. The scale marker then moves from zero to indicate a certain number of roentgens. After operation, the air in the ionization chamber returns to its normal state and the electroscope is again charged. Measurements are made by exposing the chamber to a certain quantity of radiation at a specific distance from the x-ray tube target for a *specific* (usually 1 minute) *period of time.*

The **dosimeter pencil** (pocket dosimeter) is another device used to measure

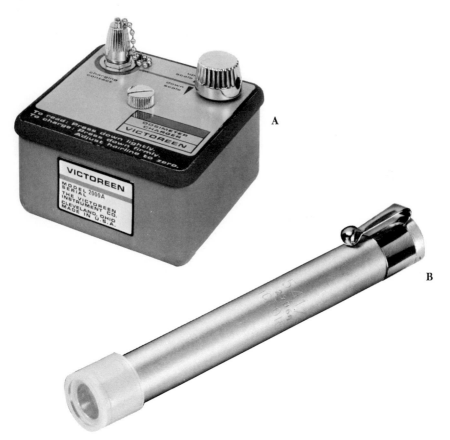

Fig. 4-12. A, Victoreen dosimeter charger. **B,** Victoreen direct reading pocket dosimeter. (Courtesy The Victoreen Instrument Co.)

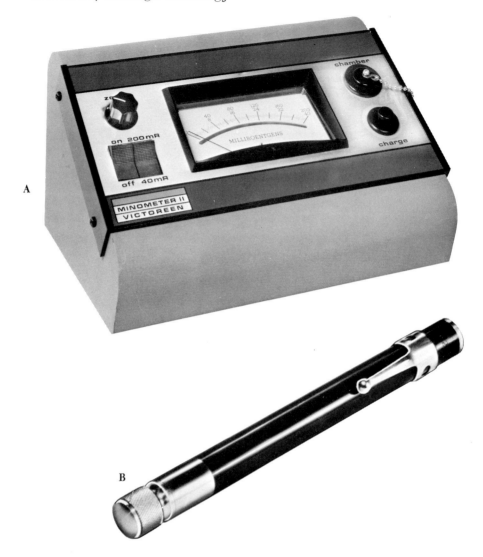

Fig. 4-13. A, Victoreen Minometer II. **B,** Victoreen indirect reading pocket dosimeter. (Courtesy The Victoreen Instrument Co.)

ionization by radiation (Fig. 4-12). This device, carried in the pocket of the personnel when they are around sources of radiation, operates somewhat differently from the r-meter. The particular advantage of this device is that the wearer can read it at any time, simply by placing one end to his eye and the opposite end to a light. The device nearly always has a *drift*, so that any measurement accruing over a one-day period is somewhat in error.

A dosimeter pencil is essentially a small Lauritzen electroscope to be worn on the person for recording the quantity of ionizing radiation encountered. This electroscope consists of a fine fiber loop attached to an insulated electrode that is encased in a tube containing lenses and a graduated reticle for viewing and calibrating the motion of the fiber. A refinement of this instrument in the dosimeter pencil is the provision of a reticle scale for determining the rate of radiation received. The rate is determined by the movement of the fiber for a set period of time.

Another device used similarly to the dosimeter pencil is the **minometer** (Fig. 4-13). This instrument can be read only when it is applied (connected) to the charger.

R-meters and dosimeter pencils are operated *after* they are given a static charge. The quantity of charge given to the instrument varies, and there is usually some means of *bleeding off* any excess charge prior to use of the instrument. Dosimeter pencils are charged by use of a battery-powered electronic circuit. The r-meter charger produces a static charge by friction, and any excess placed on the instrument is bled off through high resistance.

The foregoing instruments are employed principally in conjunction with relatively constant x-ray intensities. Ionization—type radiation detectors used to detect high or varying radiations are the ionization chamber, proportional counter, and the Geiger-Müller counter.

The **ionization chamber** consists of a gas-filled envelope and two electrodes of different electrical potentials. The envelope may be one of the electrodes, and the gas may be any number of materials, including air. An ionizing radiation particle or photon entering the gas-filled envelope produces ions, which, because of the applied potential, drift toward the electrodes. The ions drift to the oppositely charged electrode. The applied potential causes an electric current to flow until the potential balance is restored. The current from the chamber is very small, requiring electronic amplification of the signal before it can be recorded on a meter. Ionization chambers do not record individual radiation particles or photons but integrate (add up) the signals produced as an electric current.

The **proportional counter** consists of a gas-filled envelope with two electrodes, one of which is a cylinder concentric with very fine wire that acts as the other electrode. A potential difference drives radiation-formed ions through the gas with sufficient energy to produce new ions.

The **Geiger-Müller counter** (commonly called the Geiger counter or GM counter) is similar in design to the proportional counter. The chief differences are in the mode of operation and the gas in the detector tube. The potential across the electrodes of a Geiger counter detector tube produces enough gas multiplication* from a single radiation particle to discharge the tube below its operating threshold. The detector tube is then recharged by the high-voltage supply and is again ready to record another particle. Since the Geiger tube discharges below its operating threshold each time it functions, the tube does not discriminate between types of radiation. Furthermore, the Geiger tube operate over a range of several hundred volts without gross changes in its counting rate. The *Geiger plateau* is the voltage range over which only small changes in the counting rate occur.

Other instruments employed for varying radiation intensity measurements include the Cutie Pie and scalers (see Figs. 4-14 and 4-15).

---

*The formation of new ions by driving the original ions through the gas is called *gas multiplication*.

Film badges

Although they are not measuring instruments, film badges are worn by persons engaged in work with radiation to record the quantity of radiation received.* Film badges may be for x-rays and gamma rays, for neutrons, or for beta particles. Wedged, laminated filters (material depending upon the type of radiation to be measured) are employed in film badges so that radiation quantity between certain levels may be determined.

Periodic blood counts

Periodic blood counts on all personnel employed in radiation areas are made so that changes in the hemogram that may be the result of excessive radiation may be determined. However, periodic blood counts are *not* a measure of quantity of radiation received.

Natural radiations

Some of the more complex elements possess the ability to emit either particles of matter or electromagnetic waves or both from their nuclei. These elements

---

*Any device worn to detect or measure radiation will measure only that radiation received by the device and simply serves to indicate the radiation received by the wearer.

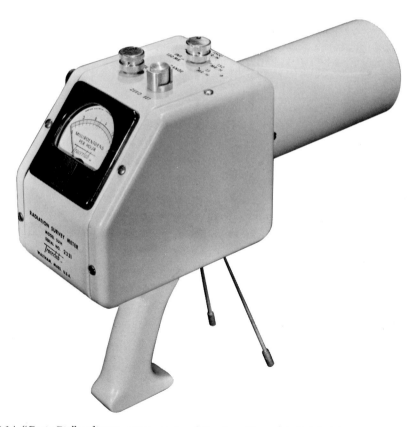

Fig. 4-14. "Cutie Pie" radiation survey meter. (Courtesy Tracerlab-Keleket.)

are *radioactive** and include three major families: actinium, thorium, and uranium. Each of these families finally *decays* into one of the three isotopes of lead.

The fact that the nucleus becomes much larger with the increase in atomic number is indicative of the increased complexities of these nuclear structures. Experimental evidence reveals that such complex structures may not always be stable; therefore, it is logical that the arrangements of these nuclei may change under certain circumstances. Due to nuclear instability, elements having an atomic number of 83 and over are naturally radioactive. All elements can be made radioactive by artificial means.

Three types of radioactive emission have been found to exist. These are alpha and beta particles and gamma rays. Alpha particles consist of two protons and two neutrons. Actually, an alpha particle is nothing more than the nucleus of an atom of the common helium isotope. It is strongly positive and quite heavy when compared to a single atomic mass unit (AMU). Alpha particles are ejected at speeds of from 9,000 to 20,000 miles per second, are slowed down in matter very rapidly because of their size, and are stopped by a thin sheet of paper. These particles are capable of intense ionization and travel in erratic paths. If the alpha particle does not collide with other matter, it will collect two free electrons and become an atom of helium.

Present information indicates that the beta particle is also ejected from the nucleus of certain atoms. However, there are no free electrons in the nucleus, so the beta particle must be ejected from a neutron in the nucleus. The neutron is somewhat larger than the proton, so the neutron probably consists of a proton and an electron (according to certain theories). *Beta particles are high-speed electrons* that possess strong negative charges, or they may have positive charges and are then called *positrons*. These particles have much greater speeds than the alpha particles. Some beta particles may possess as much as 5 mev (million electron volts) of energy. Beta particles cause less ionization than alpha

---

*Radioactivity is the emission of radiant energy; this is a property of certain elements and includes ejection of alpha and beta particles and gamma rays.

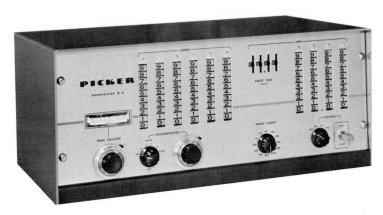

Fig. 4-15. Picker Magnascaler II A. (Courtesy Picker Nuclear.)

particles, travel in straight paths for much greater distances than alpha particles, and, depending upon the energy of the particles, are capable of penetrating tissues up to about 1 cm in thickness.

Electric and magnetic fields deflect both alpha and beta particles. Gamma rays are true electromagnetic waves that possess no electric charge and travel with the speed of light. Gamma rays are capable of extreme penetration and cause less ionization than beta particles. The wavelengths of gamma rays are in general shorter than the wavelengths of most x-rays. The chief difference between gamma rays and x-rays is in their origin: gamma rays are natural, x-rays are not. Gamma rays are approximately 1/100 as effective in causing ionization as the beta particle and 1/10,000 as effective as the alpha particle.

Gamma rays, like all photons, are absorbed exponentially. This exponential absorption is a direct result of the nature of gamma ray energy loss. In contrast with alpha and beta particles, gamma rays do not lose their energy continuously in small amounts; they lose their energy by absorption during interactions with matter.

Like x-rays, gamma rays are used extensively in therapy. Beta particles are quite limited as therapeutic agents, and alpha particles are of even less use in therapy. (However, production of alpha particles by neutron bombardment for treatment of localized tumors in such inaccessible parts of the body as the brain is being more widely accepted.)

Table 4-1. Decay processes of the uranium family

Substance	Atomic number	Atomic weight	Half-life	Energy form
Uranium 1	92	238	4.5 billion years	α, γ
Uranium X_1	90	234	24.5 days	β, γ
Uranium X_2	91	234	1.14 minutes	β, γ
Uranium 2	92	234	2 million years	α, γ
Ionium	90	230	7.6×10^4 years	α, γ
Radium	88	226	1,600 years	α, γ
Radon	86	222	3.8 days	α, γ
Radium A	84	218	3 minutes	α, β
Radium B	82	214	26.8 minutes	β, γ
Radium C*	83	214	19.7 minutes	α, β, γ
Radium C′	84	214	2×10^{-4} seconds	α
Radium D	82	210	22.2 years	β, γ
Radium E	83	210	4.85 days	α, β
Radium F (polonium)	84	210	139.5 days	α, γ
Radium G (lead)	82	206	Stable	0

*Radium C may decay into either C′, as in the table, or as below:

Radium C″ (thallium)	81	210	1.32 minutes	β, γ

When radium C emits a beta particle and a gamma ray, the new element is radium C′ with atomic number 84 and atomic weight 214. Radium C′ then emits an alpha particle and the new element is radium D with atomic number 82 and atomic weight 210. When radium C emits an alpha particle, the new element is radium C″ with atomic number 81 and atomic weight 210. Radium C″ then emits a beta particle and a gamma ray and the new element is radium D with atomic number 82 and atomic weight 210.

Depending upon its energy, the alpha particle can penetrate approximately 1 cm of air; the beta particle, approximately 12 to 15 meters of air; the gamma ray, approximately 500 meters of air.

Natural decay

Knowledge of radioactivity is of increasing importance to x-ray technicians. Radioactivity includes the processes of natural radioactive decay, which is explained briefly as follows.

Natural decay is the process by which radioactive elements lose nuclear particles and energy and become stable elements. This process requires periods of time ranging from a few minutes (even less in some artificial elements) to a few billion years.

If an element ejects an alpha particle, there will be a decrease of two in atomic number and a decrease of four in atomic weight. When an element ejects a beta particle, there is an increase of one in atomic number but no change in atomic weight. Since the beta particle is ejected from the neutron, the nucleus is left with an additional positive charge. Gamma rays are usually emitted at the time of alpha or beta particle emissions; however, it is not known if the gamma ray is emitted simultaneously with the particle or if one phenomenon follows the other. Radiations occur *only* during energy transfer, and the gamma ray emissions occur probably as a result of the reorganization of the nuclear material.

*The time required for a given quantity of radioactive element to lose exactly one half its activity is the half-life of that substance.**

The isotope of lead that occurs from actinium decay has the atomic weight 207; the isotope of lead that occurs from thorium decay has the atomic weight 208.

---

*Various authorities disagree about some of the radioactive emissions, e.g., radium B, C″, E, and F.

REFERENCES

Clark, George L.: Applied x-rays, ed. 4, New York, 1955, McGraw-Hill Book Co.

Glasser, Otto: Medical physics, Chicago, 1950, Year Book Publishers.

Glaser, Otto, Quimby, Edith H., Taylor, Lauriston S., and Weatherwax, J. L.: Physical foundations of radiology, ed. 2, New York, 1957, Paul B. Hoeber, Inc.

Hodgman, C. D., editor: Handbook of chemistry and physics, ed. 28, Cleveland, 1944, Chemical Rubber Publishing Co.

Meschan, Isadore: Normal radiographic anatomy, Philadelphia, 1951, W. B. Saunders Co.

Reimann, Arnold L.: Thermionic emission, New York, 1934, John Wiley & Sons, Inc.

Robertson, John Kellock: Radiology physics, ed. 3, Princeton, N. J., 1955, D. Van Nostrand Co., Inc.

Schanze, Ulrich O.: Iron filters in diagnostic radiology, Radiologic Technology 37(3):137, 1965.

Chapter 5

Preventive maintenance

Equipment failure

It is not within the province of the radiologic technologist to make major repairs to the radiographic equipment. It is necessary that the technologist be able to explain to the x-ray service personnel the probable cause of failure or its source so that repair can be completed expeditiously. Under normal circumstances, time is a major factor in most departments, and any time saved will be beneficial. Useful information relayed to service personnel *before* they leave their office could save much time lost in obtaining the proper repair parts. For the x-ray technologist, knowledge of preventive maintenance must include the ability to *isolate* the problem, through a logical sequence of checks and evaluations, and, whenever possible, to notice the beginning of trouble so that it can be corrected before serious damage occurs.

The checking sequence

1. Since the technologist is the usual operator of the equipment, he becomes the logical person to call the service man. Prior to the call, evaluation of the problem in the following manner will usually expedite the necessary repair. Make a series of astute observations regarding the problem. Repeat these observations to the service man, with the reason for such observations.
2. At the time of exposure:
   (a) Observe the various meter readings.
   (b) Listen carefully for the normal sounds of the equipment in comparison with the unusual sounds.
   (c) Be aware of that "intangible" sense or feeling of normal operation compared with the same type of sense regarding abnormal operation.
3. Verify the exposure problem with all circuit conditions:
   (a) Radiography with Potter-Bucky diaphragm in and out.
   (b) Fluoroscopy in and out.
4. Appearance of the radiograph:
   By logical deduction, account for the radiographic deviation according to prime factors, distance, structures penetrated, and film and film holder combination.
5. Sequence of timing sounds:
   (a) Was the operation of the equipment normal in regard to the sequence of sounds?

(b) Did the meters read normally?
    If there were abnormal readings, why and how were they abnormal? How much deviation from normal was observed?

(c) Have the controls been checked? (Move each control and reset to same value. The reason for this is that the stop that mechanically centers the contacts may have been temporarily out of alignment or adjustment, or it may have been broken.)

6. The circuit breaker:
    Circuit breakers may be operated:
    (a) By high milliamperage.
    (b) By high kilovoltage or high kilovoltage in conjunction with time and milliamperage.
    (c) By means of any short circuit to the ground.
    If the circuit breaker "kicks out" during an exposure, there may be a temporary overload resulting from settings too high for safe operation. Repeating the exposure with reduced settings may pinpoint this type of difficulty. The condition of the circuit breaker should be checked if the panel board fails to light up.

7. The x-ray tube:
    Most installations make use of an x-ray tube with a transparent port for observation of the cathode filament. If the filament fails to heat, perform steps a and b:
    (a) With the filament circuit closed and while observing the cathode filament through the port, rotate the tube or move the cathode cables. The purpose of such movements is to localize, if possible, a broken wire inside the high-voltage cable or a poor connection in the "plug-in" cable jack.
    (b) If the cable is attached with a hand-tightened thread or screw device, attempt to tighten the device.

8. If the machine is full-wave rectified and one of the rectifying valves is burned out, the milliammeter will register somewhat more than one half the selected milliamperage during the exposure.*

9. If one of the high-tension cables is punctured:
    (a) There will usually be a strong odor of burning rubber.
    (b) There will seldom be a "flash" seen or a "hissing" sound heard.

10. Fuses:
    The fuse panel is usually located in an easily accessible area. With the main power supply disconnected, examine each fuse carefully to ascertain which fuse is burned out.

11. A check of all accessible "plug-in" electric connections including the main power cable, if so connected, sometimes will reveal that the trouble is caused by a connection inadvertently loosened by cleaning or by unusual cable movements.

12. Precaution: *Do not* make repeated exposures if the trouble is not readily apparent; further damage may result.

---

*See p. 36 for additional discussion of valve-tube failure.

Tube-rating charts

A tube-rating chart is supplied with each installation. In the event of an x-ray tube replacement, be certain to obtain the correct tube-rating chart for the new x-ray tube.

Focal spot size is the principal factor governing the quantity of energy applied to the diagnostic x-ray tube. The (maximum) rate of heat conduction through the target and dissipation from the anode limits the quantity of energy applied as a result of electron bombardment of this small area. It is readily seen that energies producing heat quantities greater than that tolerated by the tungsten target material can melt the tungsten at the focal spot. The rate of conductivity of heat through the target and from the anode of one tube may not necessarily be the same as that for another tube having the same focal spot size.

Proper use of the tube-rating chart tends to prevent overloading the tube; overloading usually necessitates an expensive replacement. The radiographic tube-rating chart is designed to indicate maximum "safe" exposure values for any one exposure. Repeated exposures having these same maximum values can still overload the tube. New combinations of exposure factors should be checked on this chart prior to exposure. From the tube-rating chart it may be found that the required milliampere-second value using relatively high milliamperage is unsafe at the desired kilovoltage. Usually, this same milliampere-second value will

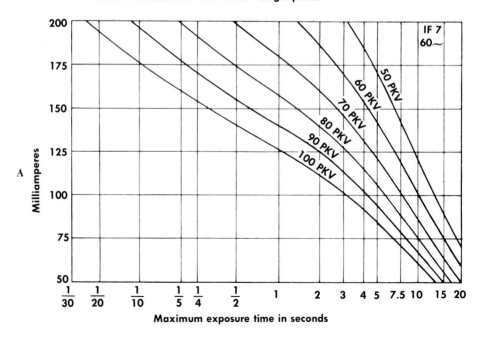

Tube type Dynamax — stator frequency — 60 cycles
Focal size small (1.0 mm)
Kind of rectification full wave — single phase

Fig. 5-1. Tube-rating charts. **A,** 1.0 mm focal spot. **B,** 2.0 mm focal spot. (Courtesy The Machlett Laboratories, Inc.)

be safely obtained if the milliamperage is reduced to one half value and the time is doubled in value, assuming that the load on the large filament is not switched to the small filament. This would make it necessary to check the rating on the small filament-rating chart. (See Fig. 5-1.)

A tube-thermal characteristics chart is developed at the factory from values of maximum anode heat storage capacity and heat dissipation of the anode. The heat units developed in the anode may be calculated from the product of the kilovoltage and the milliampere-seconds.

The rating charts in Fig. 5-1 are for the Dynamax 25 x-ray tube. Two examples of technique factor selections are given.

1. An exposure of 200 ma, for $\frac{1}{20}$ second, and at 90 pkv can be used safely on the small focal spot. It is seen on the chart that the maximum allowable energy for $\frac{1}{20}$ second is for 200 ma and 97 pkv.
2. An exposure of 100 ma. for 4 seconds, and at 100 pkv cannot be used on the small focal spot. It is seen on the chart that the maximum allowable energy for 4 seconds is for 100 ma and 92 pkv. The technologist may elect either of two options:
   a. Use the large focal spot.*
   b. Use the small focal spot but use 50 ma for 8 seconds.

---

*However, this increases the penumbra effect.

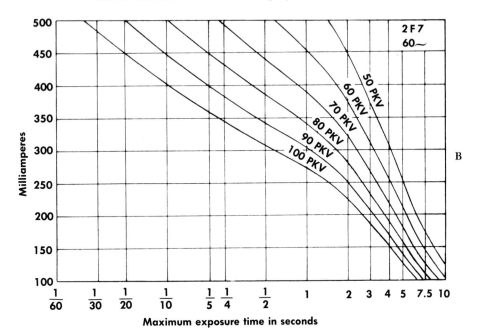

Tube type Dynamax — stator frequency — 60 cycles

Focal size large (2.0 mm)

Kind of rectification full wave — single phase

Fig. 5-1, cont'd. For legend see opposite page.

To prevent unnecessary evaporation of the cathode filament, *always open the filament circuit when it is not in use, that is, between patients and between exposures of a single patient,* except during certain special radiographic procedures.

Routine care

An x-ray machine represents a large financial investment to the owner. It is the technician's responsibility to maintain this equipment in a state of peak efficiency.

Protect the tabletop from scratches and sticky dirt by use of a cotton sheet, except during sinus and skull radiography. The patient is made more comfortable with the use of a smooth sheet. Use a good grade of waxless furniture polish to maintain the tabletop finish. When blood, grease, or other material has inadvertently been spilled on the table, wipe if off with warm water and surgical or green soap. Dry the area thoroughly and then wipe clean with a second disinfectant such as 70% alcohol. Dry again, and apply furniture polish.

The tube housing, table ends and sides, and parts of the control panel that are blackshould undergo daily cleaning with a cloth dampened with furniture polish. Monthly attention should be given the counterbalance cables of the fluoroscopic tube and screen and of the Potter-Bucky diaphragm. Any "fraying" or broken strands should be immediately called to the attention of the service personnel. The tube stand and other parts of the equipment that are bright or chrome finished should be cleaned frequently with a special chrome polish to prevent tarnish. Keep the tube stand track clear of dust and lint.

Spilled barium should be removed immediately after the patient is dismissed. If there is crinkled black surface paint on parts of the equipment, use a cloth dampened with warm water to wipe the surface and then rub with a fiber or medium stiff bristle hairbrush and then with a dry cloth.

Some radiographic equipment requires a "warm-up" period prior to use. Allowing this period to elapse ensures greater consistency in radiographs.

The wall power safety switch to stationary equipment should be opened at the end of the work period. When not in use, the power supply cord of portable equipment should be removed from the outlet and coiled on the hooks provided.

In using either portable or stationary equipment, avoid unnecessary bending of the high-tension cables.

Chapter 6

Radiographic principles

The radiographic image
Chemical considerations

Many radiographic phenomena are quite similar to, and many are the same as, comparable photographic phenomena. A considerable degree of useful and practical information concerning radiography may be attained by making proper comparison with photography. In each art the first image on the film is achieved through a physical principle, the result of which is the latent image. *The latent image is the invisible image produced by a physical effect of electromagnetic wave energy upon certain members of a family of chemicals called the halogens.** This image can be rendered visible by the subsequent chemical developing process. A property of the halogen family, that of *photosensitivity*, sets these elements apart from all others.

Chief interest in the halogens is restricted to bromine, which combines readily with silver to form silver bromide (AgBr). This particular silver halide is probably the principal silver salt used in the film emulsion, although the silver salts of iodine and chlorine are often used in conjunction with silver bromide.

Modern x-ray film base may be either cellulose acetate or one of the newer synthetic materials. When it is cellulose acetate, the base is approximately 0.0075 inch thick; the synthetic material is approximately 0.0073 inch thick. The finished film consists of the base coated on both sides with a dehydrated suspension of silver bromide in gelatin. The structure of the silver bromide crystals may be explained simply as a combination of positive silver ions and negative bromine ions. Both coats are of constant thickness, approximately 0.001 inch, and the dispersion of the photosensitive crystals is homogeneous. A blue tint is usually added to the sheet of cellulose acetate to increase the diagnostic quality of the radiograph. Most manufacturers apply a scratch-deterring coating to both surfaces.

Different proportions of silver salts are used in the production of different types of x-ray films. With most no-screen film, the photosensitive coating is slightly greater in thickness than the same coating on plain film. The no-screen film coating is more sensitive to x-ray energy than to light energy, and it contains about 40% more silver crystals than the plain film coating. The plain film coating is highly sensitive to light energy.

Formation of the latent image in the photosensitive coating of the film results from the action of the energy passed through the object radiographed when this energy (remnant radiation) strikes the silver bromide crystals. When the latent

---

*The halogen family of elements includes fluorine, chlorine, bromine, iodine, and astatine.

73

image is developed, it is called the actual image (*manifest image*). Upon striking the silver bromide crystals, the x-ray energy causes the crystals to separate into positive silver ions (Ag^+) and negative bromine ions (Br^-). This reaction may be written simply as follows:

$$Light^* + AgBr \rightarrow Ag + Br(gas) \uparrow$$

The complete *lattice structure* of silver bromide provides a situation in which the silver is free to move. This is probably the principal reason for the selection of this particular silver halide in these photosensitive emulsions. The lattice structure of silver bromide consists of alternate silver and bromide ions:

$$
\begin{array}{ccccccccc}
Ag^+ & Br^- & Ag^+ & Br^- & Ag^+ & Br^- & Ag^+ & Br^- & Ag^+ \\
Br^- & Ag^+ & Br^- & Ag^+ & Br^- & Ag^+ & Br^- & Ag^+ & Br^- \\
Ag^+ & Br^- & Ag^+ & Br^- & Ag^+ & Br^- & Ag^+ & Br^- & Ag^+ \\
Br^- & Ag^+ & Br^- & Ag^+ & Br^- & Ag^+ & Br^- & Ag^+ & Br^+ \\
 & & & Ag^+ & & & & & \\
Ag^+ & Br^- & Ag^+ & Br^- & \square & Br^- & Ag^+ & Br^- & Ag^+ \\
\end{array}
$$

This is a uniform structure except for the misplaced Ag^+ ion (in italics). This condition is known as *Frenkel's disorder;* the misplaced silver ion is known as an *interstitial ion.*

Physical considerations

The degree of density in the radiograph probably depends upon the total number of silver ions present in each specific area of the radiograph; i.e., where greater energy absorption occurred, greater tissue density existed; therefore, fewer silver ions were available for eventual development.

The theory of latent image productions is very involved; therefore, only a portion of the theory is presented.

The x-ray energy striking the silver bromide crystals releases electrons from the crystals. Some of the electrons collect as *sensitization specks*[†] on or near the surface of the crystals. The silver particles migrate to the specks and collect in the form of atomic silver. The number of electrons collecting at the sites of sensitization determines the number of silver particles attracted to these sites. Silver particles will not collect if electrons are absent; hence, there would be no potential development sites.

In general, it is correct to assume that milliampere-seconds control *radiographic density,* since the number of cathode electrons made available to bombard the target controls the number of x-ray photons in any exposure. Radiographic density *is the amount of film blackening—the degree of gradation of blackness in the radiograph.*

It is also correct to assume that kilovoltage controls *contrast,* since the voltage impressed upon the tube controls the energy of the bombarding cathode electrons, thereby controlling the resulting photon energy. Contrast may be explained as the comparative difference in transmitted light between the lighter and darker areas in the radiograph.

---

[*]X-ray energy is substituted for light energy when cardboard holders are used and is augmented by light energy when intensifying screens are used.

[†]Sensitization specks is an expression used in the explanation of the latent image formation. In theory, more of these specks form when greater energy strikes the silver halide crystal.

Contrast, which must be considered with density, *is the visible difference between adjacent densities resulting from subject and film characteristics.* Tissues of different structural characteristics and different compositions are never penetrated to the same degree in any one exposure.

The greater the number of high-energy photons contained in the primary beam, the greater will be the degree of penetration of the object being radiographed; therefore, the numbers of silver and bromine ions liberated in the film will be greater.

A radiograph is a permanent photographic record of the structures through which a beam of ionizing radiation has passed. However, it may be rendered useless by lack of visibility of detail. This condition may be caused by either overexposure or underexposure. Consequently, radiographic sharpness (definition) may be present but obscured.

Radiographic sharpness

Radiographic sharpness is also called definition (sharpness of detail). *Detail may be defined as the quantity of visibility of fine structures and over-all sharpness that is radiographically demonstrated.* Definition depends upon many factors, which include object-film distance (ofd), focal-film distance (ffd), umbra and penumbra, motion of part, focal spot size, and screen crystal size. In this section, four of these factors are considered. (Note that definition and visibility of detail are *not* the same. If visibility of detail is lacking, it may prevent the "seeing" of definition.)

The object-film distance is the distance between the object being radiographed and the film. Since the art of radiography involves the use of three-dimensional subjects, it is impossible to radiograph a part of the human anatomy that possesses no thickness. Study of Fig. 6-1, *A,* will reveal that as the object-film distance is increased, the size of the resulting image is proportionally increased. The necessity of keeping the film as close as possible to the structure under radiographic consideration cannot be overemphasized.

The focal-film distance is the distance (usually in inches) between the focal spot of the x-ray tube and the film. Many radiographic techniques presently require a 40-inch focal-film distance. Fig. 6-1, *B,* demonstrates the varying effects of increased and decreased focal-film distances, using the same length line for the object as used in Fig. 6-1, *A.* Study of Fig. 6-1, *B,* will reveal that longer focal-film distances (when practical) are highly desirable (as in teleroentgenography) since longer focal-film distances tend to produce an image size approximating the size of the object.

The radiographic image size may be enlarged or reduced within certain limits by using either of two methods. The enlargement is achieved when object-film distance is increased or when focal-film distance is decreased. The reduction is achieved when object-film distance is decreased or when focal-film distance is increased. An increase of object-film distance will blur the radiographic image, producing *unsharpness.* The same effect results from a decrease of focal-film distance. The formula for determining the quantity of magnification is written:

$$\frac{\text{ofd}}{\text{ffd} - \text{ofd}} = \% \text{ magnification}$$

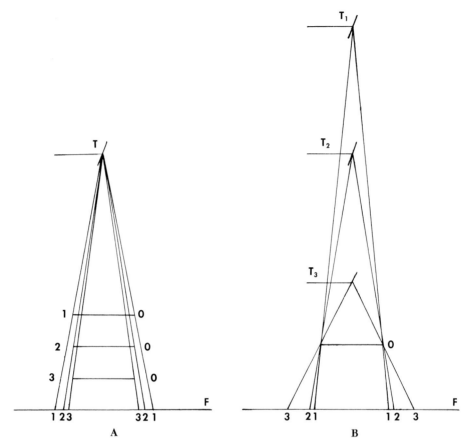

Fig. 6-1. Effects of object-film distance, focal-film distance, and focal spot size on the radiographic image. In **A**, *T* is the focal spot at a constant distance from the film *F*. *O* (the object) is of constant length in the three positions, but as ofd is decreased from position *1* to *3*, the size of the image of *O* is decreased. In **B**, *O* is the object at a constant distance from the film *F*. As *T* (the focal spot) is brought closer to the film from position *1* to *3*, the size of the image of *O* is increased.

Magnification is desirable in certain instances, e.g., to emphasize certain bone sections, hairline fractures, or other suspected diseased areas. A good procedure is to strive for the same percentage of magnification in each successive radiograph of a sequence of a fracture. To use the magnification formula, ofd and ffd must be converted to the same unit of measure. Either multiply inches by 2.5 or divide centimeters by 2.5. (One inch = 2.54 cm; however, 2.5 is a satisfactory conversion factor.)

Example: ffd is 36 inches, ofd is 15 cm. What is the percentage of magnification?

$$\frac{15}{2.5} = 6; \quad \frac{6}{36-6} = \% \text{ magnification}; \quad \frac{6}{30} = 20\% \text{ or } 0.20$$

In terms of light and shadow, umbra is a complete shadow within which no light is received from a given source. Penumbra is the space of partial illumina-

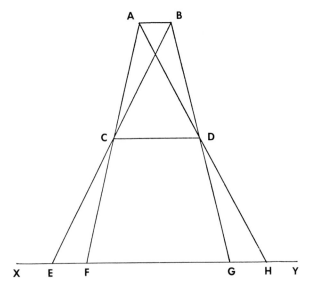

Fig. 6-2. Penumbra. The penumbra effect is demonstrated by the lines *E-F* and *G-H*. *F-G* is the true shadow, *A-B* is the light source, and *C-D* is the object. *X-Y* is the film.

tion on all sides, between the umbra, and the full light. In radiography, the x-ray energy can be compared to light energy, but it must be remembered that although light energy does not pass through an opaque object, x-ray energy will. The light umbra may be compared with the sharp radiographic image and the light penumbra with the degree of radiographic unsharpness caused by object-film distance, focal-film distance, and focal spot size. Study of Fig. 6-2 will reveal certain of these principles.

In Fig. 6-2, the line *A-B* (or a point source in the center of this line) represents the light source; line *C-D* represents the object; *F-G* represents the umbra or true shadow on the film *X-Y;* and *E-F* and *G-H* represent the areas of penumbra or radiographic unsharpness. (Because the objects of radiography possess three dimensions, completely sharp reproduction of them is not possible. *This lack of perfect sharpness in radiography is called unsharpness.*) It is evident that smaller light sources will produce proportionally less penumbra. Also, smaller focal spot sizes will produce less areas of unsharpness when both object-film distance and focal-film distance are optimum. Use of smaller effective focal spots (see Figs. 4-4 and 4-5) results in sharper radiographs.

Impingement of the cathode electrons on very small focal spots causes less blurring and improves proportionally the definition in the resulting image in the x-ray film. In most stationary anode tubes, the small spot range is from 1.8 to 2.6 mm and the large spot from 2.8 to 4.6 mm. In a rotating anode tube, the small spot is usually 0.8 to 1.0 mm and the large spot usually 2.0 mm. A fairly recent innovation is the fractional focus tube, which possesses a small focal spot of 0.3 mm. This tube is designed to permit the use of rather long object-film distances, not only to obtain maximum radiographic enlargement but also to retain definition.

A certain degree of unsharpness* is inevitably present in radiographs. In special cases some sharpness is sacrificed in favor of magnification. In some of the standard techniques, a low degree of unsharpness is expected. When using the unsharpness formula, all numerical values may be used as found and need not be converted to a common unit.

Distance and radiographic intensity

X-ray intensity diminishes at a rapid and predictable rate as the distance from the source (focal spot) increases. This reduction in intensity is in accordance with the *inverse square law*,† which states that the *intensity is inversely proportional to the square of the distance.*

If any degree of accuracy in the description of a beam of x-rays is to be achieved, both the *quality* and *intensity* of the beam must be considered. The qualities of x-rays are discussed on p. 51. The intensity of x-rays is discussed on pp. 59 and 60. Intensity measurements are necessarily made at a specific distance from the source. As has been pointed out, x-rays diverge in all directions from the point of origin, but their escape, except through the port provided, is prevented by the tube shielding. At this time proper consideration should be given to the primary beam and its intensity at a given point. Proper measurements of the beam intensity must include consideration of the fact that x-rays travel in straight lines and that passage through any substance (including air) causes a reduction in intensity as a result of scattering and/or absorption. In other words, true measurements of intensity must be made in air at specific distances from the origin and in the central portion of the direct primary beam.

Fig. 6-3, *A*, represents a geometrically perfect four-sided pyramid 4 feet in height and 4 feet square at the base. This figure illustrates all of the intensity energy entering at point *P* and passing through planes *ABCD* and *A'B'C'D'*. If 100 units of intensity fall upon plane *ABCD*, which is an area of 4 square feet, each square foot will receive one fourth of 100, or 25 units, of intensity per square foot. The same quantity will pass through plane *ABCD* and fall upon plane *A'B'C'D'*, which is an area of 16 square feet. Thus, each square foot here receives 6.25 units of intensity. In summary, doubling the distance reduces the intensity

---

*A formula to determine the quantity of unsharpness has application only when marginal sharpness and detail (see p. 75) are too blurred for diagnostic purposes The optimum value of unsharpness is 1.0; however, any value for unsharpness of 2.0 or less is satisfactory.

$$U = \frac{dF + DM}{D - d} + S;$$ where U is the quantity of unsharpness, d is the ofd, F is the focal spot size

in millimeters, D is the ffd, M is motion of part in millimeters, and S is the factor for screen blurring. The blurring factor for most modern screens is 0.15.

†The *radiographic effect formula*, an empirical formula, has been derived from the inverse square law and is written as follows:

$$re = \frac{(ma)(s)(kvp^2)}{d^3}$$

Use of this formula will obtain approximate results when applied to plain film in cardboard holders. The values for *re* may be of any numerical quantity and have no specific relation to radiographic intensity.

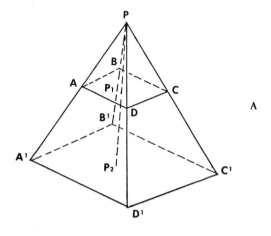

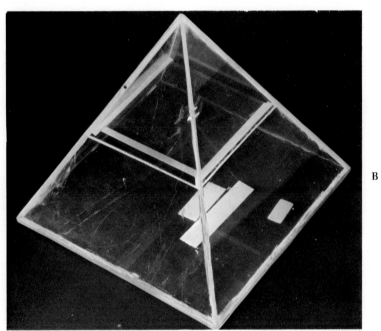

Fig. 6-3. Four-sided pyramids. In **A,** the distance from P to P_1 is 2 feet. It is 2 feet from P_1 to P_2. *ABCD* is a square, side *AB* being 2 feet long. *A'B'C'D'* is a square, with side *A'B'* being 4 feet long. **B** is a clear plastic construction. Its dimensions are as follows: base sides, 1 foot; vertical height, 1 foot. The small base (at the 6-inch vertical point) is removable.

to one fourth of the original per unit area for unit time. The methods for measuring intensity are discussed on pp. 59 to 63.

The inverse square law is written algebraically as:

$$I :: \frac{1}{d^2},$$

where I is the intensity of the radiation, and d is the focal-film distance (ffd).

Since intensity and milliampere-seconds are used as being equal, the formula is then written as:

$$\frac{\text{Old mas}}{\text{New mas}} = \frac{\text{Old ffd}^2}{\text{New ffd}^2}$$

The formula may be applied as in the following example:

In a given examination the mas employed is 10, and the ffd used is 6 feet. What will be the new mas value at an ffd of 8 feet? (Of course, the intent is to achieve a film whose density is approximately that of the original.)
Substituting in the second formula, we obtain:

$$\frac{10}{x} = \frac{(6)^2}{(8)^2}$$

$$= \frac{(3)^2}{(4)^2}$$

$9x = 160$
$x = 17.77$; that is, the new mas at an 8-foot ffd is 17.77

Parallel rays

As x-rays radiate outward from the point of origin in the x-ray tube target, the weaker x-rays radiate at wider angles form the central ray than the stronger x-rays. As a result fewer of the weaker primary rays strike the object and film at increased target-film distances. The stronger primary rays strike the object and film at increased target-film distances and travel in paths more nearly parallel to each other. (See Fig. 6-8.) These are called parallel rays.

Parallel rays are employed in *teleroentgenography* to present image shadows of the various viscera in nearly correct relative size. Since the various viscera of the thoracic cavity are situated at remarkably different distances from the film in routine chest radiography, the parallel rays avoid, to a great extent, the enlargement obtained when the more angular rays are employed in producing the radiographic image.

Grids and Potter-Bucky diaphragms

A grid is a stationary arrangement of thin lead strips interspaced with a radiolucent material. The purpose of the grid is to remove (absorb) a considerable quantity of the secondary (scattered) rays, which cause unnecessary density in the radiograph. (See pp. 55 and 56, secondary rays and remnant rays.) Since the lead strips of the grid absorb the rays that strike them, inevitable shadows (*grid lines*—absence of radiation effect upon the film) will appear in the radiograph.

Experiment proved that proper arrangement of the lead strips (parallel with the long axis of the grid and table) in a grid that moved in the direction of the short axis of the x-ray table prevented these grid lines in radiographs. This work of Dr. Potter and Dr. Bucky resulted in the Potter-Bucky diaphragm which is commonly called the Bucky. Grids are used where the use of the Bucky is either impractical or impossible. The grid is light and portable and may be used in conjunction with mobile radiographic equipment. Lysholm and wafer are common names of grids. (See Fig. 6-4.)

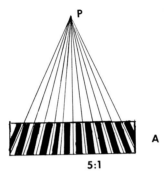

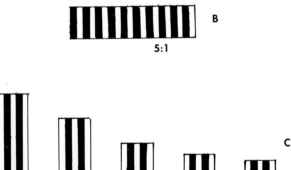

Fig. 6-4. Grid ratios. Arbitrarily the relation between the width of the lead strip (black) and the intervening radiolucent material has been drawn as being equal. This is done for purposes of easy comprehension. Actually, the lead strips are exceptionally thin.

The Bucky is beneath the x-ray tabletop and moves a flat grid in the direction of the short axis of the table. A cassette tray is below the grid, and the entire device is placed upon a pair of tracks so that the entire Potter-Bucky diaphragm can be moved the length of the x-ray table. The purpose of the Bucky is to facilitate radiographic exposure of thick or dense anatomic parts and to decrease the scattered or secondary rays that strike the film. As a result, a Bucky improves detail visibility and contrast. Because the grid moves, grid lines are not produced in the radiograph. The lead strips in a grid are exceedingly thin. A distinct relationship, expressed as the *grid ratio*, exists between the height of the lead strips and the width of the intervening spaces.

A grid ratio has been defined as follows: *"The grid ratio is the relation of the height of the lead strips to the distance between them."** Thus a grid in which

———
*From Characteristics and applications of x-ray grids, Cincinnati, 1958, The Liebel-Flarsheim Co.

the thickness or vertical height is 8.0 mm and in which the space between each two lead strips is 1.0 mm would have a ratio of 8:1. The other ratios are 16:1, 12:1, 6:1, 5:1, and 4:1.

In Fig. 6-4, *C*, the comparative heights of the five grids are diagramed and greatly enlarged (1 mm = 0.1 inch). To reach the film, the x-rays must travel between the lead strips in the grid. The required distance that x-rays must travel in a 16:1 grid is twice that in an 8:1 grid. A 16:1 grid absorbs twice as many scatter rays as an 8:1 grid. Everything else being constant, radiographs made with a 16:1 grid will be considerably less dense than those made with an 8:1 grid. Increased scatter-ray absorption improves radiographic contrast. From the above, three conditions are evident: *film contrast varies directly with grid ratio; scatter-ray absorption varies directly with grid ratio; film density varies inversely with grid ratio.*

The distance between the tube target and the grid surface becomes more critical with the use of higher ratio grids because fewer primary rays are capable of passing between the lead strips of the grid.* For example: a 36-inch focal film distance is quite satisfactory with an 8:1 grid in the Bucky, whereas a 40-inch focal-film distance is equally satisfactory with a 12:1 or 16:1 grid in the Bucky. This principle is explained in terms of the *grid radius. The flat grid radius is the vertical distance from the center of the tube side of the grid to the target of the tube.*

Fig. 6-4, *A*, is a diagram of a *focused (aligned) grid* in which the x-ray beams pass between the lead strips. Fig. 6-4, *B*, is a diagram of a *parallel grid.* A focused grid absorbs more scattered rays than a parallel grid; also, the focused grid is more critical than the parallel grid. Parallel grids inevitably absorb more of the useful rays than focused grids.

Although there is a definite optimum distance (radius) for a specified grid, usually sufficient latitude exists with each grid to permit minimum distances of 26 to 28 inches and maximum distances of 44 to 48 inches before the problem of *off-distance cutoff* becomes serious. If an aligned grid is employed at a distance other than that specified by the radius, certain areas of the film may not be exposed because the x-rays have been absorbed or "cut off" by the lead strips.

Off-center and off-level cutoff may occur when aligned grids are used and the tube or table is angled or not centered.

The grid radius determines the optimum distance between the x-ray tube and the grid. The use of these grids at this distance permits a maximum penetration by the useful rays because of the arrangement of the thin lead strips.

Although the *crossed grids* are not shown in Fig. 6-5, some discussion of them is pertinent. Crossed grids are usually constructed as two linear (parallel) grids; one grid is placed directly above the other with its lead strips at right angles to those of the lower grid. Crossed grids have both advantages and disadvantages when compared with linear grids.

> In general, the crossed grid will remove more secondary radiation than a linear grid of ratio equal to the combined ratios of its two equal parts; e.g., a crossed grid each of whose parts has 5:1 ratio will remove more secondary radiation than a linear grid of 10:1 ratio. This advantage is most striking at voltages under 100 kvp.

---

*Reference is made to a situation where interchangeable grids are available.

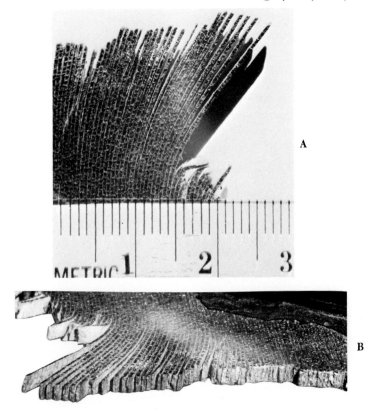

Fig. 6-5. A, Photograph of the lead strips and intervening radiolucent substance of an 8:1 focused grid. **B,** View of the lead strips.

The advantage of the linear grid over the crossed grid is that it may be used in tilted tube techniques without undue "cutoff" in the radiograph.*

A Bucky is operated by any of three methods: mechanical cocking followed by mechanical release; mechanical cocking followed by electronic release; and complete electronic control of reciprocation.†

The following is an explanation of the grid travel in a manually cocked Bucky. Cocking the Bucky moves the grid in position at one edge of the table. Closing the exposure switch electronically releases the grid, which then begins to travel to the opposite side of the table. A spring regulates the rate of travel. The Bucky timer determines the total travel time. The actual radiographic exposure occurs only during the grid travel.

The recipromatic Bucky differs from the manually cocked Bucky in that the grid travels in both directions across the table during the exposure. The manually cocked Bucky requires two selections: one of exposure time on the control panel and a corresponding one on the Bucky. The recipromatic Bucky requires select-

---

*From Characteristics and applications of x-ray grids, Cincinnati, 1958, The Liebel-Flarsheim Co.

†Oscillating grids are incorporated as a part of certain specialized equipment.

Table 6-1. Grid (Bucky) and nongrid conversion table

Nongrid to grid				
5:1	6:1	8:1	12:1	16:1
add 10-12 kvg	10-15 kvp	12-18 kvp	15-21 kvp	18-24 kvp
	or mas multiplied by			
2	3	4	5	6
Grid to nongrid				
5:1	6:1	8:1	12:1	16:1
subtract 10-12 kvp	10-15 kvp	12-18 kvp	15-21 kvp	18-24 kvp
	or mas divided by			
2	3	4	5	6

ing only the exposure time; the length of the exposure determines the number of times the grid travels.

Since there is a considerable amount of useful as well as scatter-ray absorption when a grid is used, more penetrating x-rays must be made available; this is accomplished by increasing the peak kilovoltage. (Increasing the milliampere-seconds frequently accomplishes a comparable result; however, it is more practical to add to the peak kilovoltage because increasing the milliampere-seconds markedly increases the exposure intensity.)* The conversion factors for nongrid to grid (Bucky) technique and for grid (Bucky) to nongrid, along with conversions for lower to higher and higher to lower grid ratios, are listed in Table 6-1.

In converting technique from higher grid ratio to lower, it is advisable to reduce the milliampere-seconds, which also reduces the quantity of radiographic exposure to the patient.†

Higher kilovoltage requires still higher ratio grids, and probably a change from moving grids to stationary grids with increased numbers of lines per inch. The modification of existing technique factors to compensate for changes in grid ratio should allow for changes in the number of lead strips per inch.

Radiographic cones

Cones are used to limit the field of exposure, to decrease the amount of secondary scatter, and generally to improve detail visibility in the radiograph. Although cones differ in size, length, and shape, all are used for the same three purposes.

Cones are made of a light metal with a radiopaque liner material. They may have a round, flared end that permits a round field of exposure, or they may be

---

*When the standard, high-contrast technique is routine, the thickness of the part penetrated determines the kv to employ. In such instances it is better to compensate for changes in grid ratio with corresponding changes in mas.

†An empirical formula based on the grid index is as follows:

$$\text{Known mas} \, \frac{(\text{index of grid desired})}{(\text{index of grid used})} = \text{New mas}$$

The grid index is the numerical value by which the nongrid mas is multiplied to obtain the desired mas for a specific grid.

Table 6-2. Cone-technique conversion

Size of cone, inches	Increase kvp by	or	Increase mas by
3 × 10	6 to 8		60%
5 × 10	2 to 4		20%
8 × 10	None		None
Fully extended	6 to 8		60%
Nonextended	4 to 6		40%

designed to provide a rectangular field of exposure. There are also modifications that vary the field of exposure by manipulation of single or double diaphragms built into the device. There is a choice of field shape in these single- and double-diaphragm devices; the shapes may be round, square, or rectangular and of variable size within the shape of the diaphragm.

Cones should be used, except in extremely rare instances. The trend in radiologic practice is for all radiographs to possess *corner cutoff* (equal in all corners) so that there is visual demonstration of a limited field of exposure.*

In instances that require numerous exposures over a specific area, *coning down* is highly desirable. Coning down refers to the use of an extension, dental, or mastoid cone to emphasize certain structures by eliminating secondary scatter. Coning down on a specific structure is recommended for certain areas of the body, e.g., for a lateral or posterior (A-P) view of the lumbosacral joint (even when a single view for emphasis is requested following a routine exposure).

Use of very small cones necessitates an increase in the exposure quantity. This may be accomplished by an increase in peak kilovoltage or in milliampereseconds; however, it is preferrable to increase the peak kilovoltage. Table 6-2 lists the required increases for the various-sized cones.

Various types of collimating devices are replacing the standard "set of cones." The use of cones requires accuracy in alignment and direction of the central ray to prevent the condition called *cone cutoff*. The use of collimators requires even greater accuracy for the same reason. When a circular cone or collimator is employed, the *cone coverage formula* may be used to predetermine the diameter of the field of exposure at different distances:

$$\frac{(L)(d)}{l + z} = D$$

where L is the focal-film distance, l is the length of the cone, z is the distance between the cone slot and the focal spot, d is the large diameter of the cone, and D is the diameter of the field of exposure.

Example: $L = 40$ inches, $l = 10$ inches, $z = 3$ inches, $d = 8$ inches.

$$\frac{(40)(8)}{10 + 3} = D$$

$$\frac{320}{13} = D$$

$$D = 24.61 \text{ inches}$$

---

*This practice is of course determined by the radiologist in charge of the department.

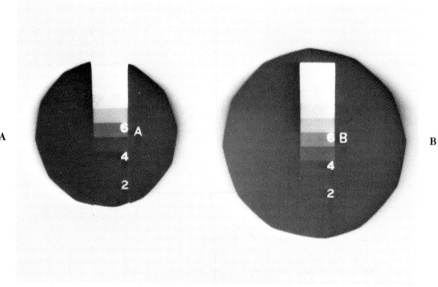

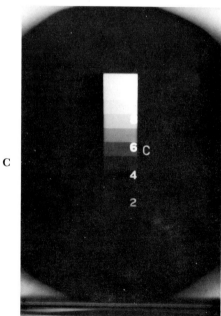

Fig. 6-6. Effects of cone size on film density. In **A, B,** and **C,** kvp was 45; mas was 5; and ffd was 40 inches. Par-speed screens, cassettes, and plain film were used. (Note: Density readings were made between the **A, B,** or **C** and the number 6 on the step-wedge.)

Film	Field size	Density	Background density
A	7³⁄₁₆ inches	3.15	1.95
B	10¼ inches	3.18	1.95
C	16⅛ inches	3.20	1.95

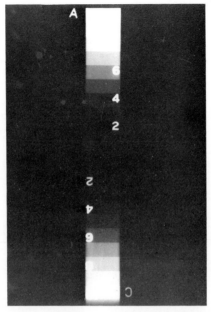

Fig. 6-7. Cathode heel effect on radiographic density. Kvp here was 65; mas, 10; and ffd, 40 inches. Par-speed screens and plain film were used. Density value at anode end on step 6 = 3.08. Density value at cathode end on step 6 = 3.14.

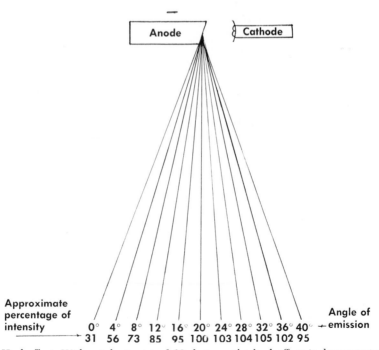

Fig. 6-8. Heel effect. With a tube target of 20 degrees, the heel effect is demonstrated in this diagram by comparing the angles of emission (upper numbers) with the percentages of intensity (lower figures). The greatest percentage of intensity occurs with the 32-degree angle of emission and is 105%.

When no cone is employed, remove the *l* from the formula. When a square or rectangular collimator is employed, *d* becomes one of the aperture sides and *D* becomes the corresponding side in the field of exposure.

Heel effect

In modern equipment, the heel effect is of no great significance; however, it may be employed to maintain, in the same radiograph, comparable density of both thick and thin anatomic parts. *The heel effect obtains a slightly more penetrated image on the cathode side of the radiograph than on the anode side;* this increased density is just visible. This is the result of the emission of the more intense rays from the part of the anode nearest the cathode. (See Fig. 6-8). When the long axis of the x-ray tube is parallel with the long axis of the table, the heel effect is seldom visible. It is greater when shorter focal-film distances are used.

In a posterior (A-P) view of the thoracic spine, it is possible to employ the heel effect to advantage. The patient should be so positioned that the anode end of the x-ray tube is nearest the patient's head. This permits the stronger rays to penetrate the thicker parts of the spine.

Stereoradiography

Stereoradiography is the process of making stereoscopic radiographs. A three-dimensional effect of these radiographs is obtained by the proper mounting and viewing of two very slightly dissimilar exposures of the same structure. A special device called a *stereoviewer* is employed for this purpose.

The two radiographs required for this projection are made at angles of the same degree but on opposite sides of a vertical line through the center of the structure radiographed. Consequently, the tube is shifted from approximately 1¼ inches from one side of center to the same distance on the opposite side of center, a total shift of 2½ inches. In each shift, the tube is angled to the same point in the structure being radiographed.[*] For a shift of 2½ inches, the optimum distance between the radiographs and the reflecting mirrors of the viewer is 25 inches. Also, a 2½-inch tube shift is best employed with a 25-inch focal-film distance. Approximately 2½ inches represents the distance between the pupils of the eyes (interpupillary distance).

Most tabletop and Bucky radiography is performed at a 40-inch focal-film distance, and most chest radiography at a 72-inch focal-film distance. When the focal-film distance is greater than 25 inches, an adjustment in the distance of the tube shift will improve three-dimensional visualization of the structures. Dr. Joseph Selman presents a proportion that explains the interrelationship of tube shift, focal-film distance, interpupillary distance, and viewing distance:

Tube shift : ffd : : Interpupillary distance : Viewing distance[†]

Practical application of this proportion will develop an appreciation of the relationship. When the viewing distance is 25 inches, the tube shift is one tenth the focal-film distance. An increase of the focal-film distance to 40 inches requires

---

[*]Completely satisfactory results are obtained when the central ray is angled at 90 degrees to the film surface, especially if the tube shift does not exceed 2½ inches.

[†]From Selman, Joseph: The fundamentals of x-ray and radium physics, Springfield, Ill., 1954, Charles C Thomas, Publisher.

a tube shift of 4 inches, although a tube shift of 2½ to 3 inches will obtain useful results.

Stereoradiographs may be viewed in any one of several devices. Probably the most commonly used device is the Wheatstone Reflectoscope or a modification. This device has two adjustable mirrors and two connected viewing boxes (illuminators) mounted on a sliding carrier so that each illuminator is always the same distance from its corresponding mirror.

Stereoradiography is employed chiefly for medical interpretation of structures within the body. Stereographic visualization makes apparent the separation of overlapping structures and/or the depth and shape of a single structure.

In stereoradiography, varying conditions govern the direction of the tube shift. Among these conditions are structures under consideration, heel effect (if a grid is used), and mechanical devices available on the equipment. The tube shift is usually at right angles to the dominant anatomic lines. If the tube shift is at right angles to the Bucky or grid lines, there will be no change in density in comparable anatomic parts. However, if the tube shift is parallel with the grid lines, density variations may exist in the resulting radiographs unless the heel effect is properly employed. Proper coning and the use of correctly sized cones are highly important in stereoradiography. There will be noticeable differences in density in the radiographs if the effective focal spot size is different in the two exposures.

Tomography

Other methods of producing radiographs to demonstrate internal structures have been developed. Although the principle is essentially the same in most of these methods, numerous names are applied to the patented apparatus: planigraph, laminagraph, stratigraph, tomograph, etc. The basic principle employed is that of maintaining an exact focus at one depth of structure while the tissues above and below this structure are blurred. The relationship between the ffd and the ofd remains constant, although both distances change during the exposure (and during tube travel in the planigraph). Fig. 6-9, *B*, is a diagram of the basic geometry in this type of radiography. In this procedure, the patient must remain motionless while both the tube and cassette are moved in opposite directions throughout a specific time interval. The exposure time in this procedure will vary, in accordance with the equipment and requirements, from a few tenths of a second to several seconds.

Intensifying screens

Intensifying screens are one of the greatest aids to the production of high quality radiographs. Use of these screens can reduce exposure time, reduce exposure quantity, and minimize motion of part.

Intensifying screens are composed of a dehydrated suspension of x-ray excitable phosphors* coated on one side of a sheet of radiolucent material. These phosphors are finely divided and of uniform size (0.015 mm or less) in the suspension, which is of constant thickness. The screens are mounted within the cassette to increase the effect of the applied x-ray energy. This increased effect is achieved

---

*A phosphor is a phosphorescent substance or body, that is, it shines in the dark.

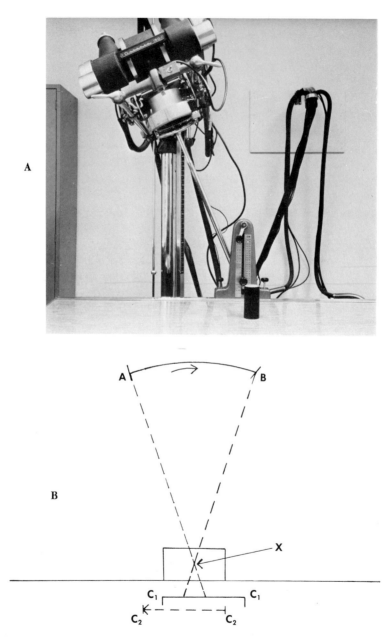

Fig. 6-9. A, Planigraph attached to x-ray machine. Planigraph rod is seen angled and between tube arm and Bucky tray. Planigraph rod is attached at fulcrum to the depth selection. Depth cylinder is positioned in center of x-ray table in front of fulcrum. **B,** Body section radiographic principle. A fulcrum is attached on the level of structure *X.* As the x-ray tube is moved from *A* to *B* during the exposure, the cassette is moved in the opposite direction from a position as in C_1 to a position as in C_2; the cassette is moved in the same horizontal plane. The structure at *X* is in constant focus; all other structures are blurred.

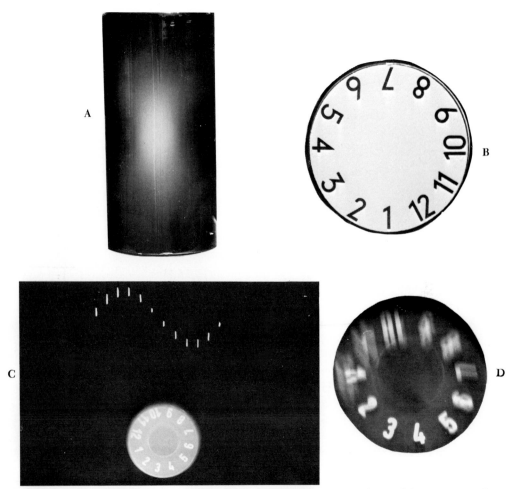

Fig. 6-10. A, Depth cylinder used for **D** here. **B,** Top of depth cylinder used for **D. C,** Depth cylinder radiographs. **D,** Depth cylinder radiograph with fulcrum at 4 cm above tabletop.

because x-ray energy causes the phosphors of the screen to glow with a blue-white light.

The radiographic effect upon the film in a cassette is achieved by a combination of the x-ray energy plus the fluorescent light energy of the phosphors. In general, the screens may increase from ten to sixty times the applied energy of the x-rays as they pass through the screens. The quantity of intensification depends upon the type and size of the phosphors in the screen emulsion. The x-ray energy accounts for approximately 2% of the total exposure in intensifying screen cassettes through actinic action.*

Quantity of intensification means the same as speed of intensification and is called *screen speed.* Phosphor size affects speed and sharpness of detail in the

---

*The results of one series of experiments indicated that 98.3% of the total exposure was the result of screen intensification.

Table 6-3. Intensifying screen types

Screen speed	Purpose
Detail Slow or High definition	Requires greater exposure but produces excellent detail, contrast, and sharpness
Average Medium or Par	Requires moderate exposure and produces good sharpness and detail
Fast or High	Requires very short exposure and produces slightly less sharpness and detail

radiograph. The three standard speeds of intensifying screens are listed in Table 6-3.

Some manufacturers use the same size phosphors in both the average and detail-speed screens. The addition of a yellow dye to the coating in the detail-speed screens suppresses the speed of intensification. One manufacturer uses the calcium tungstate phosphor in all his screens. Another uses the barium lead sulfate phosphors for the high-speed screens and the medium-sized phosphors of calcium tungstate for both the average and detail-speed screens; the later, however, includes the yellow dye. A fourth speed of intensifying screen produced by at least one manufacturer is called extra fast (Lightning Special), and is designed to use with low voltage equipment (under 60 kvp) to reduce exposure to the patient. The speed of this screen is like that of the high-speed screens above 60 kvp; below 60 kvp the extra fast screen requires approximately one third the exposure (mas) of the high-speed screen.

In general, the high-speed intensifying screen may be used as a standard. With an arbitrary value of 1.0 as its speed (of intensification), the intensification speed and unsharpness values of the other screens are as follows:

Screen	Relative speed	Average unsharpness
Average speed	2	0.3
High resolution	4	0.25
Detail speed	8	0.15

The application of the preceding information is very simple. If 10 mas are used with high-speed screens, then 80 mas must be used with detail-speed screens to obtain the same radiographic density. It is seen that sharpness improves with the use of slower screens; however, the improvement is very slight.

In addition to the speed of intensification, it is also important to reproduce sharp image detail in a radiograph. Sharpness in a radiograph (and in photographs) is said to be present when no point in the reproduced subject has a *circle of confusion* of diameter greater than 1/1,000 its distance from the eye. Stated differently, radiographs appear perfectly sharp if the circles of confusion corresponding to all single points in the object shadow converge at the eye with angles not exceeding three minutes of an arc. The circle of confusion is the disk, of measurable diameter, by which a point in the object is represented in the image formed by a lens. (X-ray beams follow light beam laws to the extent that these photographic principles apply.)

Sharp radiographic detail is achieved through the resolving power of the screen expressed in lines per millimeter. The resolving power of a film or plate is the ability of this film or plate to reproduce the fine detail of the optical image. Resolution is the act or property of rendering visible the separate parts of an object. The resolving powers of the commonly used intensifying screens are as follows: detail, 9 to 10; par, 7 to 8; high speed, 6 to 7; and extra fast, 5 to 6.

Intensifying screens perform several distinct functions in radiography. Since the screens increase the effect of the applied energy to the film, it is possible to use less electric energy, which results in lower roentgen output (smaller roentgen doses) to the patient—a safety factor. The same increased effect upon the film permits the use of relatively low voltage equipment to obtain good radiographs. Use of intensifying screens decreases exposure time considerably and, as a consequence, minimizes motion of part.

When film is placed in cassettes, extreme care must be taken to achieve good *screen-film contact*. This term means that the two screen surfaces that sandwich the film must be in total contact with the film and must exert equal pressure over the entire surfaces of the film. The condition of poor screen-film contact is seldom consistent throughout the cassette; the film is in good contact with the screens in some areas and in poor contact in others. A film exposed in such a cassette will have sharp shadows with good detail in one area and blurred, indistinct image shadows in another. (See Fig. 6-11.)

Several methods of screen-film contact determination have been developed.

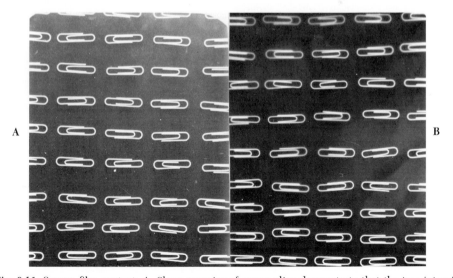

A   B

Fig. 6-11. Screen-film contact. **A,** Sharp margins of paper clips demonstrate that the two intensifying screens are in good contact with the film throughout the entire surfaces. **B,** Unsharp paperclip shadows in the upper and left upper parts of the radiograph demonstrate that at least one screen is in very poor contact, if it is in contact at all, with the film in this area of the cassette.

Among them is one that is quite simple. New paper clips are placed in any pattern desired over the surface of the cassette to be tested, being certain that all paper clips are *lying flat* and singly on the tube-side surface. The cassette contains an unexposed film. A routine exposure for average (par) speed intensifying screens, as used in Fig. 6-11, is as follows: 55 kvp, 5 mas, and 40-inch ffd. The film is processed in the usual manner. If the screens are in good contact with the film *on both sides,* the shadows of the paper clips will be quite sharp; if not, noticeably blurred shadows of some paper clips will be seen in certain areas of the film.

Since the intensifying screens are quite expensive and easily damaged, they must be handled with care. If dirt is attracted to the screen surface, the dirt should be removed with a camel's hair brush. If this is not successful, a lint-free cloth should be dampened with pure grain alchohol and gently wiped over the affected area. Screens should be kept free of splashed water, developer, or fixer, since any of these agents may cause spots, which are removable only from certain newer type screens. Light spots in the radiograph occur from decreased activity of spotted areas in the screens.

There are certain phosphors that will continue to glow after the source of energy has ceased; phosphors containing impurities will do this. This *afterglow* is called *screen lag* and would be present only if intensifying screens contained such phosphors. Screen lag is not encountered if the screens are obtained from reputable suppliers and manufacturers.

Fluoroscopic screens

Intensifying screens are used to aid in the production of a permanent image in the film. *Fluoroscopic screens are used by the radiologist to observe actions of the various viscera with or without the presence of contrast media.*

A fluoroscopic screen is generally made of a layer of a phosphor (zinc sulfide) coated on a piece of durable plastic. This screen, to seal out dirt, is sandwiched between a protective cover on the tube side and a sheet of leaded glass, which is the viewing side. The protective cover on the tube side permits x-ray penetration; the lead in the glass *partially* protects the operator from direct radiation.

Zinc sulfide is used in a modified state so that the generated light rays are between 5,200 Å and 5,400 Å; maximum sensitivity of the eye to light rays is from 5,000 Å to 6,000 Å. The color of the light from a fluoroscopic screen is usualy modified to a greenish yellow.

A device called an *image amplifier* was developed to increase the relatively dim light from fluoroscopic screens. This device, attached to the fluoroscopic screen, intensifies and reflects the image brilliance by means of mirrors. Such a piece of equipment is of invaluable aid to the radiologist in making his evaluations of the patient's condition.

Frequently, the doctor employs a *spot-film device* in conjunction with fluoroscopic examinations. Such a device includes a carrier for an 8″ × 10″ or 10″ × 12″ cassette and either mechanical releases or electronic relays for moving the cassette under the screen during fluoroscopic examinations. Other relays automatically switch the tube voltage and tube current to produce radiographic images in the film of the particular area of examination.

When the x-ray machine includes such a device, it usually has a second x-ray tube mounted beneath the tabletop as a part of the fluoroscopic device. This tube has its own relays and factor selections separate from the main radiographic tube.

Phototimers

A phototimer is a device beneath the Potter-Bucky diaphragm and cassette tray used to duplicate radiographic density in successive exposures. A phototiming device has its separate controls on the control panel; however, the milliamperage and kilovoltage selectors are the same ones used in routine radiography.

The following statements explain the principle of the phototimer. A special cassette with no radiopaque material in the back permits x-ray energy to penetrate the cassette. A fluorescent screen mounted directly below the cassette tray receives the remnant rays from the cassette. The energy of these rays causes

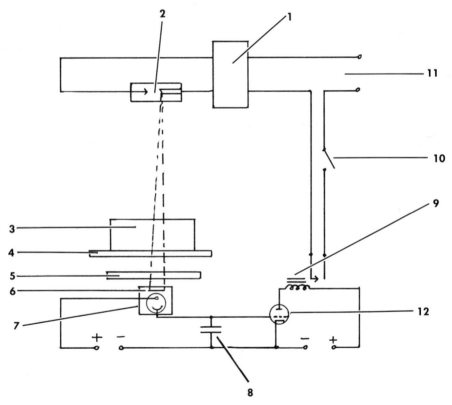

Fig. 6-12. Schematic diagram of a phototimer circuit.

1. X-ray power supply
2. X-ray tube
3. Object x-rayed
4. Tabletop
5. Cassette (with no lead backing)
6. Fluorescent screen
7. Phototube
8. Capacitor (condenser)
9. Relay
10. Exposure switch
11. Power line
12. Thyratron

fluorescence in the screen. The fluorescent light energy falls on a photoelectric cell. The electricity generated in the cell flows to a condenser until it has sufficient current to permit discharge. Upon discharge of the condenser, a Thyratron tube ionizes, causing a relay to open and terminate the x-ray exposure. It is in this manner that a phototimer controls radiographic density. (See Fig. 6-12.)

Filters

Filters are inserted into the filter slot in the tube shielding to remove the softer rays, which cause increased and undersirable densities in the radiograph. These softer rays cause needless radiation to the patient and are therefore objectionable. *Filters are used in radiography to improve radiographic quality and to protect the patient.*

Aluminum filters of 1 to 3 mm total thickness are used in addition to the inherent filter. Too much reliance on the inherent filter is hazardous. Prior to all exposures, an inspection is essential to determine the presence of 2 mm of aluminum in the filter slot. (See p. 57.) The use of 3 mm of aluminum requires a slight increase in kilovoltage; 2 to 4 kvp are added to the technique for every 1 mm of aluminum in excess of 2 mm.

Filters absorb the softer x-ray photons (see p. 57). If the filter material is aluminum, any secondary rays will be so weak that they expend their energy in a very few centimeters of air. (See Fig. 4-9.)

Protection in radiography

It is extremely important to use filters in radiography to control radiographic quality and to furnish adequate protection to the patient. *The ability to avoid retakes is the best protective device the technician can employ to benefit the patient.*

The increasing use of radioactive materials and x-rays affects *all persons*. The present recommended maximum weekly dose for radiologic technologists is 0.1 r (100 mr) in a 48-hour week. The MPD (maximum permissible dose) in any 13-week period must be no greater than 25 rems (roentgen-equivalent-man) to the hands, forearms, feet, head, neck, and ankles, and in any 13-week period no greater than 3 rems to the skin of the whole body, the gonads, blood-forming organs, and lens of the eye.*

All animal tissues are sensitive to radiation; i.e., absorption of radiation doses above certain minimum roentgen values will change or alter the tissue. The following tissues (the sequence in which they are listed is not significant) are most readily affected by the ionizing energy of x-rays and gamma rays: dermis, lymphatics, hemopoietic and leukopoietic (blood-forming) tissues, bone (especially the epiphyses in growing children), and the specialized germinal epithelium (gonads). These tissues are also equally sensitive to alpha and beta particles and other high-energy particles.

Aluminum has a marked effect upon filtration of the softer x-rays. Insertion of an additional 1 mm of aluminum into the path of the primary beam increases the permissible milliampere-seconds from two and one-half to three times. This does not indicate a required increase in milliampere-seconds. It does ef-

---

*From NCRP Report no. 33.

Table 6-4. Milliroentgens per milliampere-second*

Added filter (mm al)	*Radiation intensity using a high-voltage rotating anode tube* Kvp						
	50	60	70	85	100	130	
None	7.6	10.2	13.3	18.4	22.5	29.6	
0.5	4.8	6.8	9.2	13.2	15.8	20.4	mr/mas
1.0	3.2	4.6	6.3	9.6	12.0	15.9	at 40″ fsd
2.0	1.5	2.2	3.2	5.3	8.0	11.3	
3.0				3.1	5.8	9.2	

	Radiation intensity using a stationary anode tube					
None	8.2	11.6	14.9	19.8	25.0	
0.5	5.0	7.4	9.8	14.0	17.0	
1.0	3.3	4.8	6.7	10.0	12.8	mr/mas, 40″ fsd
2.0	1.5	2.3	3.4	5.6	8.4	
3.0				3.2	5.8	

Multiplying factors to determine radiation intensity at distances other than 40 inches

FSD, inches	35	34	33	32	31	30	29	28	27	26	25
Multiplying factor	1.30	1.38	1.47	1.56	1.72	1.79	1.9	2.04	2.19	2.37	2.56

FSD, inches	24	23	22	21	20	19	18	17	16	15
Multiplying factor	2.78	3.02	3.31	3.63	4.0	4.44	4.94	5.87	6.25	7.1

*From Trout, E. D., Kelly, J. P., and Cathey, G. A.: Am. J. Roentgenol. **67**:946, 1952.

fect a reduction in radiographic intensity to the patient, thus permitting an increase in milliampere-seconds without an increase in the roentgen dose to the patient.

It is impractical to measure radiation intensity during radiographic procedures. Such practice would also unduly alarm the patient. However, it is practical to have a working knowledge of radiation dose in terms of milliroentgens per milliampere-second. Trout, Kelley, and Cathey have developed a table containing some of this information (see Table 6-4). Since the patient receives the direct x-ray beams, it is necessary that the technician be aware of the milliroentgens per milliampere-second delivered to the patient. Should the radiographic request require large amounts of milliroentgens or roentgens, the technician should consult his radiologist or other supervising physician.

Both the quality and quantity of radiation increase in proportion to a corresponding increase in kilovoltage. Doubling the kilovoltage increases the roentgen output approximately four times.*

Therapy is to be administered only by, or under the direct supervision of, a radiologist. It is recommended that a period of 4 weeks (minimum) should

---

*A standard electrical formula states that $E = IR$, electromotive force equals current intensity multiplied by conductor resistance. The power formula states that $P = EI$, power equals electromotive force multipled by current intensity. Substituting IR for E, the power formula becomes $P = IRI$ or $P = I^2R$.

elapse after specific areas of the body have received certain maximum roentgen values in radiography or therapy before there is additional exposure to the same areas. This period of time is considered sufficient in most instances to allow the injured tissues to recuperate and form new cells.

X-rays are cumulative in effect. They can destroy all living tissue. Scattered radiation is less harmful than primary radiation but still very harmful. A cone that is small enough to expose only the required area effectively controls scattered radiation. The use of such cones is extremely important to adequately protect the patient's gonads. The male infant's gonads are especially susceptible to x-rays because of their location. *When possible, cover the gonads in both sexes with pliable leaded rubber* during radiographic exposures, especially in those cases in which the primary rays can strike the gonads.

Good radiographic practices

1. Always use a cone when possible, and always use the smallest cone (or cone opening) possible.
2. Limit the cone size or diaphragm opening when using a round cone so that a small and identical amount of cutoff is visible in each corner of the radiograph. Limit the diaphragm opening when using a rectangular cone so the the field of exposure is slightly less than the film size.
3. Avoid *retakes:*
   a. By being absolutely certain of proper positioning.
   b. By being absolutely certain of proper exposure factors.
   c. By being absolutely certain of correct patient, film, and part identification.
   d. By observing proper immobilization procedures. Use sandbags or other such devices to achieve patient comfort and proper immobilization and positioning.
4. Be sure to use the protective lead screen (or cubicle) to protect yourself. If this is impossible, stand a minimum of 6 feet from the widest primary beam. (All portable equipment should have a timer cord at least 6 feet long or other arrangement to achieve a distance of 6 feet between x-ray table or bed and the operator.)
5. Never stand in the direct x-ray beam or hold the part to be radiographed.
6. Be certain, when using personnel from other departments to help in holding the patients, that they are not called upon too frequently. These persons must also wear leaded aprons and gloves.
7. Always wear a leaded apron when assisting in fluoroscopy; always wear leaded gloves if your hands are in the direct beam.
8. Be sure to supply the doctors with red goggles at least 20 minutes prior to fluoroscopy so that they are enabled to *accommodate* (dilate the pupils of) their eyes. Supply the doctors with leaded aprons and gloves for the fluoroscopic examination.

X-rays generated at voltages up to 100 kvp require 1.5 mm of lead as protection in the walls of the control booth (or in a portable protective screen); for x-rays generated at voltages between 100 kvp and 150 kvp, the lead thickness requirement is 2.5 mm. Certain therapy installations require various combinations of poured concrete, concrete blocks, and lead.

Ionized particles are capable of producing both deleterious and desirable results. Since x-rays ionize the air as they pass through it, it is necessary that therapy, radiographic, and fluoroscopic rooms be well ventilated.

The technologist should lock the doors into the fluoroscopic room to prevent entrance of unnecessary light. Entrance of light will prolong the fluoroscopic examination and increase the radiation exposure to the patient and the department personnel.

The minimum precautions to observe with ionizing radiations are stated in the NCRP Report No. 33, *Medical X-ray and Gamma-ray Protection for Energies up to 10 mev.*

The following statements are of particular interest regarding fluoroscopy. The minimum distance between the fluoroscopic tube target and the tabletop must be at least 12 inches. The total filtration placed permanently in the useful beam must be equal to that in a radiographic tube primary beam, 2.5 mm of aluminum or its equivalent. The source-skin distance of image intensifier equipment *should not* be less than 15 inches. The exposure rate of fluoroscopes operated at 80 kvp *shall not* exceed 3.2 r/mA-min and *should not* exceed 2.1 r/mA-min with the exposure measurement made in air at the position where the beam enters the patient. The exposure rate employed in fluoroscopy *shall not* normally exceed 10 r/min measured as above. The maximum permissible milliamperage to be used during fluoroscopy is 5; the recommended range of fluoroscopic milliamperage is from 3 to 5.

In addition to being aware of the effects of x-rays, one must also remember that radiographic procedures require extremely high voltages. Therapy voltages are, of course, much greater. Be careful to prevent accumulation of dirt, dust, and moisture around high-voltage equipment, as these can cause short circuits.

Practical technique changes

Working knowledge of radiographic principles enables the technician to perform efficiently, i.e., to produce radiographs of consistently high diagnostic quality at top speed and under all conditions. No two radiologists will desire necessarily the same degree of contrast and latitude, so each technician must finally produce radiographs to satisfy the particular requirements. Keeping these qualifying statements in mind, the following items may be employed to enable quick and practical technique changes.

1. Practical use is made of the inverse square law in changing technique factors: a normal chest radiographed at 6 feet requires 10 mas with a given kvp. The same kvp at a 3-foot distance requires 2.5 mas (one fourth the mas at one half the distance).
2. In the normal diagnostic range of kilovoltage, each increase or decrease in thickness of 1 cm of anatomic part requires the addition or subtraction of 2 kvp for plain film and 3 kvp for no-screen film. (See p. 54.)
3. Each inch of distance change, for a maximum of 10 inches, requires the addition or subtraction of 1 kvp.
4. If the mas is halved, 10 kvp must be added; if the mas is doubled, 10 kvp must be subtracted. (In either instance, the quantity of kvp added or subtracted depends upon the kilovoltage range.)

5. To penetrate a grid whose ratio is 8:1, increase exposure four times; for 12:1, increase five times; for 16:1 or 17:1, increase six times.

6. To cone down, i.e., to reduce the field of exposure to an area less than 8 inches by 10 inches, and to maintain radiographic density, increase exposure from 20% to 60%.

7. To maintain constant radiographic density when using screens of different intensification: from medium to detail, increase exposure three and one-half times; from medium to high speed, decrease exposure approximately one half; from medium to extra fast, decrease exposure to approximately one third if kvp is less than 60; otherwise there is no change.

REFERENCES

Characteristics and applications of x-ray grids, Cincinnati, 1958, The Liebel-Flarsheim Co.

Fuchs, Arthur W.: Principles of radiographic exposure and processing, Springfield, Ill., 1958, Charles C Thomas, Publisher.

Longmore, T. A.: Medical photography, ed. 5, London and New York, 1955, The Focal Press.

Mees, C. E. Kenneth: The theory of the photographic process, ed. 2, New York, 1954, The Macmillan Co.

Selman, Joseph: The fundamentals of x-ray and radium physics, Springfield, Ill., 1954, Charles C Thomas, Publisher.

The fundamentals of radiography, ed. 8, Rochester, N. Y., Eastman Kodak Co.

Trout, E. D., Kelly, J. P., and Cathey, G. A.: The use of filters to control radiation exposure to the patient in diagnostic roentgenology, Am. J. Roentgenol. **67**:946, 1952.

Chapter 7

Film processing

The preceding chapters have presented the principles of x-ray production, the pertinent properties of x-rays, and the principles of latent image formation. It is now necessary to explore the chemical processes occurring in the formation of the manifest image and the areas of artifact formation related to this process.

The exposed film emulsion contains the latent image. It is necessary to make this latent image manifest by reducing the exposed silver salts to (black) metallic silver in the shape of the image. Following reduction (development) in the developing solution, it is necessary both to fix the manifest image and to clear the emulsion of the silver bromide.

Processing room chemistry

A modern manual processing room usually contains the following solutions: developer, water bath, acid stop bath, fixer, water bath, and photoflow solution. (Note: If the fixer tank is positioned in the wall between the processing and drying rooms, the last water bath and the photoflow will then be in the drying room.)

Composition of the developer

Chemicals	Function
1. Elon-hydroquinone	Brings out the latent image in the film emulsion by action of the Elon (an activator) and hydroquinone (a developer). Elon is a trade name for metol. The developer removes bromine ions from the energy-struck silver bromide and leaves black metallic silver in the emulsion. Metol is strong and stable and brings out the *softer* tones. Hydroquinone is weak and unstable and brings out the *brilliant* blacks.
2. Sodium carbonate	Produces a developer pH of approximately 11.0. It also accelerates the reducing action and softens the emulsion.
3. Potassium bromide	Acts as a restrainer.
4. Sodium sulfite	Acts as a preservative; slows down oxidation.

Developing agents are used to produce a visible image corresponding to the latent image. Development is accomplished through either of two methods: *physical*, wherein the developing solution supplies the silver to form the developed image, or *chemical*, wherein the silver is in the film emulsion and the developing solution reduces the silver to metallic silver, which is black. Our interest is in chemical development, in which each silver halide grain is either developable as a unit or is not developable. The process of development is one of an oxidation-reduction reaction. The formula for the oxidation of silver bromide grains is:

$$\text{Silver bromide} + \text{Hydroquinone} \longrightarrow \text{Free bromine} + \text{Quinone} + \text{Hydrogen}$$
$$\text{and silver} \qquad \text{ions}$$
$$\text{ions}$$
$$2AgBr + C_6H_4(OH)_2 \longrightarrow 2Ag^+ + 2Br^- + C_6H_4O_2 + 2H^+$$

The total density of a radiograph depends for the most part upon the number of silver halide grains struck by the exposure energy. Each grain in the emulsion is protected by a chemical layer that breaks down in one or more sites depending upon the total energy striking the grain. The number of these sites determines the speed with which the developing agent reduces the grain. As a result, some grains may not develop simply because of insufficient time. However, all silver halide grains will develop (reduce) when left in contact with the developing agent for a long enough period of time. Density resulting from reduction of unexposed grains is a form of fog, which is discussed later in this chapter.

Water bath

The water bath is just as important as the developer and fixer. After the film has been removed from the developer, the water bath washes out the alkaline developer in the film emulsion.

Acid stop bath

Improved radiographic quality results when the films are immersed for 30 seconds in an acid stop bath consisting of a 28% solution of acetic acid.

Composition of the fixer

Chemicals	*Function*
1. Sodium thiosulfate	Dissolves the excess silver bromide salts in inverse proportion to the amount of exposure in a given area. In the area where a part of the object radiographed did not cover the film, no silver salts will be dissolved. This part of the film will be totally black.
2. Potassium alum	Hardens the film emulsion by a shrinking and *tanning* action on the gelatin.
3. Acetic acid	Acts as an acidifier of this fixing solution and as a neutralizer of the alkalinity of the wet film when an acid stop bath is not used. It tends to remove animal fats from the gelatin.
4. Sodium sulfite	Acts as a preservative.

Water bath

After the fixer, the water bath removes the excess fixer and helps prevent streaking of the films.

Under normal conditions, it requires approximately 1 hour to process a radiograph in proper manner if a hot-air dryer is available in the darkroom. At least two manufacturers have developed automatic processing machines. A belt feeds the exposed film into the machine, which completely processes and dries the radiograph in approximately 6 to 10 minutes.

Troubleshooting
General information

The *optimum* developing temperature for x-ray films is 68° F. Most films require a minimum of 2½ minutes for development. Plain and high-speed film may be developed in 5 minutes at 68° F. (or 4 minutes at 70° F.). No-screen film requires from 2 to 3 minutes longer. All films should be fixed for a minimum of 10 minutes, although *fixing time is considered to be twice the "clearing time."**

When removed from the developer, a single 14″ × 17″ film will have absorbed approximately 3 ounces of solution in its emulsion; hence, it is necessary to replenish the solution frequently.

In certain areas, especially in high altitude, algae may grow in the water bath. This condition may be improved by suspending a small sheet of pure copper in the water bath. Both sides of the copper sheet must be scoured each day for greatest effectiveness.

Fog

Film fog, which may be caused by a physical force or a chemical reaction, is a condition of cloudiness or partial opacity of a developed film that should be clear. By definition, *fog is undesirable cloudiness of a radiographic image.* Exposing the film to stray light or other radiant energy or using incorrect development procedures causes fog on a film.

The condition of fog on a film may be localized in one area or it may be general. Film fog tends to obscure some of the minute details of the demonstrated structures and thereby interferes with the ultimate diagnostic quality of the radiograph.

Oxidation may weaken or partially exhaust the developer, and the use of such a developer may result in chemical fog because prolonged developing time is required. Overdevelopment and normal development at excessively high temperatures† may cause chemical fog. Also, it is likely that development at lower than proper temperatures will cause chemical fog.

Prolonged inspection of films during development is a frequent cause of fog, due to a combination of light and accelerated oxidation of the developer.

Fog frequently occurs on films that are outdated when exposed.

Fog is controlled by the following: radiation, chemicals, and light; fog is influenced by these factors: temperature, film storage, and film age.

Physical forces capable of causing film fog include heat, daylight, artificial light, x-rays, and gamma rays.

---

*Clearing time is the minimum time required in a given fixing solution for removal of all the unexposed silver halides.

†Special mixing formulas and/or solution concentrates in which the restrainer is partially or wholly absent are available from the film manufacturers. Such solutions are used for rapid development and fixation in conjunction with surgical procedures. These techniques are designed for rapid processing at high temperatures for 1 minute in each solution.

Heat. Prolonged storage of x-ray film in rooms where temperature is much above 80° F. may cause fog.

Light. White light that leaks around doors or through cracks in the walls will cause fog. The wrong type of safelight filter will permit passage of rays that cause fog. Wattage beyond specifications in the safelight globes will cause fog. Overlong exposure of films to the "safe" rays of the safelight will cause fog.

X-rays and gamma rays. When x-ray film is stored in the darkroom or other areas that are not adequately protected from x-rays in adjacent therapy or diagnostic rooms, it is possible that x-radiation or gamma radiation and even beta particles from isotopes may cause fog. X-rays may penetrate improperly protected pass boxes and fog the films either before or after exposure.

Static

Static marks on radiographs are the result of electric discharge on the film surface. Static electricity may collect on the person or clothing of the technologist who processes the film. This is especially true in high altitude. Static marks may occur as *tree* or *branching* static: the static marks resemble the branching of tree limbs. Other forms of static include *smudge* marks and small black pinpoint areas on the finished radiograph (see Fig. 7-1). Films need to be stored in an upright position to prevent static marks that would result from pressure.

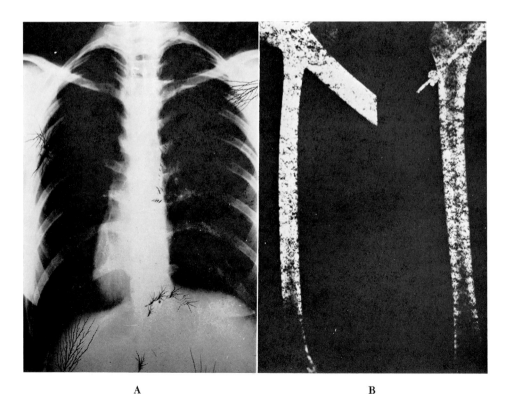

A   **B**

Fig. 7-1. **A,** Tree or branching static. **B,** Smudge static.

Exhaustion

Exhaustion of the developer and fixer occurs progressively in spite of proper replenishment of solutions. Exhaustion of these solutions refers to a gradual decline in strength as a result of several conditions.

The process of reducing atomic silver to metallic silver liberates bromine ions from the silver bromide crystals. These bromine ions combine with sodium in the developer to form sodium bromide. The presence of sodium bromide tends to impede or decrease the rate of activity of the remaining developing solution. Another deleterious result of the reducing action is the release of hydrogen ions in the developer, which also occurs as a result of time. The release of hydrogen ions tends to lower the pH of the developer and therefore a longer time is required for development. Age contributes considerably less to the exhaustion of the fixer than to the exhaustion of the developer.

To maintain maximum efficiency in the processing room, the technician should incorporate the following into his routine. He should stir the solutions each morning before use to prevent uneven development and fixation. He should always cover the developer tank since light and air tend to decrease the effectiveness of this solution rapidly. He should adhere strictly to the *time-temperature* method of processing. This method uses a constant-temperature control device (such as a thermostat) in the incoming water supply to maintain a definite optimum time of processing.

Since exhausted solutions may be the cause of colored stains on the radiograph, the technologist should make frequent checks for exhaustion. He should check periodically the pH of both the developer and the fixer. A milky appearance of the developing solution denotes gross exhaustion. The fixer pH ranges between 4.5 and 4.8. To check the fixer for exhaustion, add one drop of the fixer to 1 or 2 ml of a 10% solution of potassium iodide. If the solution turns milky or cloudy, the fixer is exhausted and should be discarded.

Stains

Routine inspection for accumulation of fixer in the corners and top of the hangers should be made. The accumulation should be scrubbed off with a stiff brush and a nonabrasive scrubbing compound. Such an accumulation may cause colored streaks and stains on an otherwise good radiograph. Stains can also be caused by incomplete fixation and incomplete washing after fixation and by improperly cleaned tanks.

Artifacts

As the films are placed in the developer, they should be agitated for at least 1 minute to loosen any air bubbles that may be on the film surface. If these bubbles were left on the film, there would be undeveloped areas at the site of each air bubble.

Rough handling of the films prior to exposure, especially bending, will cause black crescent marks on the finished film surface. These crescents will be surrounded by definite white or lighter areas. Similar handling after exposure produces distinct black crescents in the emulsion of the processed and finished radiograph; however, the latter crescents are often only slightly more dense than the

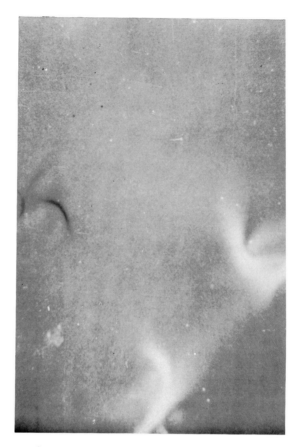

Fig. 7-2. Pressure crescents.

surrounding parts. (See Fig. 7-2.) The manufacture of certain films tends to prevent the formation of these crescents.

Improperly stirred solutions cause layers of increased or decreased film density as a result of increased or decreased activity of the developing or fixing solutions.

A rather serious but infrequent artifact of improperly processed film emulsions is that of reticulation. *Reticulation is defined as a network of corrugations produced accidentally or intentionally by a treatment producing rapid expansion and shrinkage of the swollen gelatin in processing.* Reticulation occurs as a result of a too great difference in temperature between any two of the several darkroom solutions.

The emulsion on a film suspended in the developing solution becomes quite loose as a result of the quantity of solution absorbed. The parts of the emulsion containing large quantities of metallic silver are heavier than surrounding areas of emulsion containing less metallic silver; the heavier emulsion may slide downward in the less heavy emulsion and cause typical streaking. (See Fig. 7-3.) This artifact may occur in areas of density greater than the surrounding area and so contribute to a loss in visibility of detail, and even to a loss in definition.

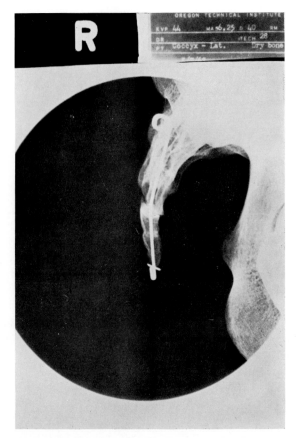

Fig. 7-3. Streaked silver deposit. The black line extending vertically downward from the tip of the coccyx is a heavy deposit of metallic silver.

Graininess is a mottling of the radiographic image and is controlled by screen and film emulsion composition. Graininess is influenced by processing.

REFERENCES

Files, Glenn W.: Medical radiographic technic, Springfield, Ill., 1956, Charles C Thomas, Publisher.

Longmore, T. A.: Medical photography: radiographic and clinical, ed. 5, London and New York, 1955, The Focal Press.

Selman, Joseph: The fundamentals of x-ray and radium physics, Springfield, Ill., 1954, Charles C Thomas, Publisher.

Chapter 8

Principles of radiographic quality

The production of radiographs of high diagnostic quality depends upon many elements. Radiographic quality is the characteristic summation of the various elements that combine to produce a radiograph and is determined by the degree of tissue diffierentiation. Tissue differentiation in the radiograph occurs because x-ray energy quantity is absorbed in proportion to the tissue density. *Maximum tissue differentiation is present only when the radiograph demonstrates maximum sharpness (definition) and maximum visibility of detail.*

Since the radiologist, or other physician, reads the radiographs, it is within his province to determine the degree of quality or tissue differentiation required in any radiograph; therefore, it becomes necessary to understand each of the methods by which radiographic quality may be modified to satisfy a particular requirement. The following material is a condensed version of those elements pertaining to radiographic quality. In many instances a detailed discussion of a single element may be found in Chapter 6.

The end result of a given series of a radiologic technologist's professional endeavors is one or more radiographs of the maximum tissue differentiation consistent with circumstances. Diagnostic quality depends directly upon the quantity of tissue differentiation. When the exposure and processing are complete, and when the finished radiograph is viewed, the technologist should look at it analytically and critically. The items contributing to this radiograph include the primary factors of radiography (kilovoltage, milliamperage, and time), the patient, the film and the film holder employed, and the method and equipment including accessories employed in exposing and processing. Of all these items, the technologist can best vary the primary factors to his advantage.

Analytic evaluation of a given radiograph can be applied if the radiograph elements are reviewed separately. These eight elements are definition, blurring, magnification, distortion, visibility of detail, latitude, density, and contrast.

Definition

Definition (sharpness of detail) *refers to the distinctness with which images of anatomic structures are recorded.* Definition is controlled by the following: motion, focal spot size, both focal-film and object-film distances, and screen composition. Definition is influenced by the following: fog, film emulsion composition, processing, density, and contrast.

This and the following three paragraphs present a special analysis of the effects upon definition of blurring, magnification, and distortion. Although magnification and distortion are frequently associated with each other in influencing

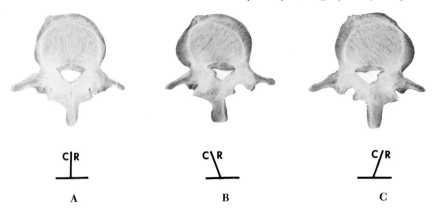

Fig. 8-1. Distortion. In **A**, **B**, and **C** the kvp was 45; the mas, 1.25; and the ffd, 40 inches. All used a cardboard filmholder with plain film. In exposure **A** the central ray is directed to a 90-degree angle with the filmholder surface. In exposure **B** the central ray is directed 20 degrees to the right and to the center of the vertebra. In exposure **C** the central ray is directed 20 degrees to the left and to the center of the vertebra.

definition, experimental evidence leads to a conclusion that each of the above three conditions requires separate consideration.

It therefore becomes necessary to establish definitions and/or limitations for each condition. *To blur is to make indistinct or vague in outline or character, as a blurred picture or image.* To distinguish blurring from both magnification and distortion it is necessary to establish that blurring affects the marginal sharpness visibly in the image of the object radiographed. Factors affecting marginal sharpness are: focal spot size, motion of part, the chemical nature and physical size of the crystals used in both the intensifying screen and film emulsions, screen-film contact, and parallax* of the two film coatings.

Magnification usually is accompanied by a degree of blurring, but is caused by the following: variations in focal-film distance and in object-film distance. *Magnification is the symmetrical enlargement of the image on the radiograph.* (See pp. 75 to 78.)

Distortion is the perversion of shape in a radiographic image. Foreshortening and/or elongation are the manifestations of distortion resulting from the change in radii of the two sides of an object. Distortion may result when the central ray is angled or when the object is not centered to the vertical central ray. (See Fig. 8-1.)

Focal spot size

The x-ray tube focal spot (target) is the most important mechanical factor affecting definition. The smaller the focal spot size, the sharper the image. (See p. 77.) In order to maintain sharpness when focal spot size is increased because of a different machine or x-ray tube, it becomes necessary to compensate for this difference by an increase in the focal-film distance.

---

*Parallax is the apparent displacement of an object as seen from two different points. When a film is wet, the emulsions are swollen, and unsharpness due to parallax may be significant. Modern film bases are so thin as to cause negligible unsharpness from parallax.

Motion

During exposure, motion of the part blurs the image and results in a loss of definition. There are four methods by which motion may be minimized: (1) by the use of immobilization devices such as sandbags, compression bands, etc.; (2) by the use of the shortest possible exposure time, which usually necessitates the use of intensifying screens (the slight decrease in sharpness caused by intensifying screens is not objectionable in the attempt to minimize motion); (3) by requiring the patient to suspend respiration during the exposure, except during extremity radiography; and (4) by the elimination of possible motion of the tube support arm and stand.

Magnification (see pp. 75 to 78)

Magnification inevitably causes losses in varying degrees of definition. However, magnification may be reduced to a minimum by two factors: object-film distance and focal-film distance. These are usually considered the major factors affecting magnification. As focal-film distance is increased, magnification is decreased. Conversely, as object-film distance is decreased, sharpness is improved. In some instances, magnification is desirable when visibility of a part is more important than maximum sharpness.

Distortion

Distortion, like magnification, causes losses in varying degrees of definition (detail sharpness). (See Fig. 8-1.) Distortion is controlled by proper alignment of focal-object-film. In radiography of certain parts, such as a lateral mandible, it is necessary, and permissible, to distort slightly the object image in a desired radiograph. In this particular instance, the target angulation distorts (elongates) the image of the mandible.

Intensifying screens (see pp. 89 to 94)

The use of intensifying screens contributes to loss in definition; however, this loss is minimal. The loss of definition depends upon the size and chemical nature of the crystals used in the emulsion. Since all screens are manufactured to specific standards, there is little noticeable difference in sharpness between any two speeds of the same brand (manufacture) of screen. Most screens are manufactured with the emulsion crystal size comparable to earlier standards for medium speed. This size crystal is small enough to permit excellent detail and large enough to respond quickly to a relatively intense exposure.

Regardless of the minimal amount of lost detail caused by the use of intensifying screens, the probability of motion is greatly reduced as a result of shorter required exposure time.

Screen-film contact (see pp. 93 and 94)

Poor screen-film contact affects definition considerably since the area of poor contact produces a blurring effect on the film. There are several conditions that cause poor contact. Among these are a warped cassette, improperly installed intensifying screens, and improper tension of the cassette clamps. Some of these conditions can be corrected; in other instances, new casettes or screens must be purchased. (See p. 94 for methods of checking the screen-film contact.)

Cardboard holders (see pp. 17 and 18)

Cardboard holders are used in the radiography of relatively thin parts; the maximum thickness of the part usually recommended is 13 cm. (For parts thicker than 13 cm, it is more practical to use cassettes with intensifying screens.) No-screen film is most commonly used in cardboard holders. The coating on this type of film is much more sensitive to x-radiation than the coating on screen film.

No-screen film in cardboard holders gives excellent detail of both soft tissue and bone when a somewhat longer exposure time than cassette exposure is used.

Visibility of detail
Latitude

A radiograph of extreme densities and opacities (blacks and whites) has high (short-scale) contrast. The contrast in such a radiograph may be so great as to obscure small but significant shadows. Reduction in contrast is a move toward several shades of gray instead of extreme blacks and whites; such a change is toward *latitude* (long-scale contrast). Latitude in a radiograph is the extreme range of demonstrated tissue densities over which diagnostic potential is present; it represents the maximum and minimum deviations from optimum tissue differentiation in a single radiograph. By definition *latitude is the range in exposure factors that will produce a diagnostic radiographic image.*

Latitude is controlled by density, contrast, and film type and may be considered as related directly to visibility of detail.

Density and contrast

Density and contrast are considered two very important factors contributing to visibility of detail. Many factors contribute to the control of both density and contrast, whereas few factors singly affect density or contrast.

The density of a radiograph is the darkened or light opaque area of the film caused by radiation or light striking the film. The silver salts in such radiated or light-struck areas, by action of the developing agent, are reduced to black metallic silver.

By definition *density is the amount of film blackening.* Density is controlled* by milliampere-seconds, or variations in either milliamperage or time in seconds.

Two sets of conditions influence† (affect) density. The factors of primary influence are the following: processing, kvp, film type, focal-film distance, heel effect, and pathology of structure. The factors of secondary influence include the following: fog, screen composition, grids, filters, and the type of beam restrictor employed, such as cones, collimator, or diaphragm.

Milliampere-seconds

In general, milliampere-seconds are considered to affect only the density; however, in radiography of some of the more dense structures, a change in milliampere-seconds will affect both density and contrast. Kilovoltage determines the penetrability, and milliamperage determines the intensity of the x-ray beams.

---

*By *controlled* is meant the ideal primary method of producing a major change.

†*Influenced* refers to methods other than the primary one that may intentionally or unintentionally produce change.

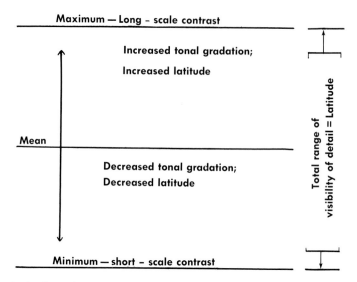

Fig. 8-2. Latitude chart. As x-ray energy increases and exposure quantity decreases, the radiograph demonstrates many shades of gray. Conversely, as x-ray energy decreases and exposure quantity increases, the radiograph demonstrates sharply distinct blacks and whites.

Kilovoltage

Kilovoltage (penetrability) controls both density and contrast. If the peak kilovoltage is increased, the density is increased and the contrast is decreased. Conversely, if the peak kilovoltage is decreased, the density is decreased and the contrast is increased.

Recognizing that kilovoltage has a definite effect in control of *both* contrast and density, the *standard* practice has been to maintain a constant milliampere-second value (relative to the structure) and vary the peak kilovoltage according to the thickness of the part. With the current emphasis on decrease of radiation to the patient and greater latitude in the radiograph, a different concept in radiographic practice is gaining wide acceptance, that is, using a constant, *optimum peak kilovoltage** (usually 120) with the milliampere-seconds as the variable. It is generally preferable to vary the time and maintain a constant milliamperage.

Focal-film distance

Varying the focal-film distance may be useful in affecting only density. The shorter the focal-film distance, the greater the amount of radiographic intensity reaching the film; therefore, the greater the film density. (However, when the focal-film distance is decreased, definition is sacrificed.) (See pp. 75 to 78.)

The following factors, which influence both contrast and density, are discussed in order of importance.

---

*Recent experimental evidence indicates that there may be a maximum kilovoltage optimum for a given anatomic part or structure. Further research may establish kilovoltage levels as optimum to employ for specific structures, with milliampere-second selections between established minimums and maximums. On this theory it can be assumed that high kv technique does not necessarily imply 90, 100, 120, or even 150 kv.

Potter-Bucky diaphragms and stationary grids

It has previously been stated (p. 80) that the use of a Bucky or grid will increase contrast because of the reduced amount of secondary (scattered) radiation reaching the film. If a grid or Bucky is not used, the film will have greater density because of the scattered radiation. It is, then, correct to assume that if a grid or Bucky increases contrast, density is decreased.

Cones and diaphragms

The use of cones and other devices to limit the area of exposure increases contrast and decreases density. If a small cone such as an extension cone is used, the primary radiation can enter the patient in an area proportional to the size of the cone and the distance between the patient and the cone. Therefore, the use of a small cone limits the amount of secondary radiation generated in the patient. When the amount of secondary radiation is so limited, there is less remnant radiation. As a result, density is decreased and contrast is increased. In order to maintain density while using small cones, peak kilovoltage or milliampere-seconds must be increased.

Film holders, intensifying screens, and films

With the use of cardboard holders in routine procedures a radiograph of less contrast and density but with improved visibility of both soft tissue and bone is obtained. The various types of film holders were discussed on pp. 17 and 18. Refer also to p. 111.

On p. 110 it was mentioned that the use of intensifying screens affects definition to a certain degree. However, when intensifying screens are employed, there is a measurable increase in contrast as a result of an increase in density. The increased density is a result of the screen fluorescence from x-ray energy and the sensitiveness of the film emulsion to the blue-violet and ultraviolet light from the calcium tungstate (or other phosphor) crystals.

If high peak kilovoltage (in the 80 to 120 range) is employed, it is advisable to use cassettes with barium lead sulfate intensifying screens, which are rated as fast screens. These phosphors have proved superior in this kilovoltage range over calcium tungstate phosphors. The crystal size of the fast (high-speed) barium lead sulfate phosphors is comparable to that of the medium-speed calcium tungstate phosphors.

There are three types of x-ray film: regular (screen) film, no-screen film, and the comparatively new fast-speed film. The regular and fast-speed films, which are very sensitive to light energy, are used with intensifying screens. The contrast and density obtained in plain (regular) and high-speed films are superior to that obtained in no-screen film. No-screen film is quite sensitive to x-ray energy and usually demonstrates more latitude, with excellent soft tissue and bone detail.

Filters (see pp. 57 to 59 and 96)

Filters should be used with all diagnostic x-ray equipment. The minimum recommended filtration is 2 mm of aluminum in addition to the inherent filter. Usually, the addition of 1 mm of aluminum beyond this requirement necessitates an increase of 2 kvp since additional filtration decreases the film density.

In high kilovoltage techniques, the use of additional filtration improves film contrast.

Contrast media

Because most of the internal viscera possess essentially the same radiographic densities as the surrounding structures, it becomes necessary to add some contrast medium to the viscera for purposes of radiographic demonstration. In some instances, a contrast medium that is opaque to x-rays is used; in other instances, contrast media that are radiolucent are employed. Some of the viscera studied by use of contrast media include the gallbladder, kidneys, ureters, urinary bladder, esophagus, stomach, small and large bowels, arteries, veins, ventricles of the brain, spinal canal, heart, etc. The use of contrast media increases contrast because of the differences in relative absorption of x-ray energy between the tissues and the medium employed. The radiopaque media absorb the x-rays, whereas the radiolucent media are more easily penetrated than the surrounding tissues.

The contrast media are prepared in several forms, each according to requirements of visualization of a specific viscus or structure. The various forms include solutions, suspensions, emulsions, pastes, powders, tablets, and gases. The viscera or structures visualized, the examination name, and the media employed are listed in Table 16-1.

General body considerations

Consistent production of high quality radiographs requires development of an easily followed technique that is satisfactory in most instances. It is useful to develop a technique chart that shows the maximum permissible deviations from the norm. *The best total results can be obtained only when the time-temperature method of film processing is employed.*

All possible anatomic and physiologic variations in patients cannot be explicated here. Listed below are some of the variations requiring consideration. The exposure percentage changes are approximate and are to be varied within set limitations according to the requirements of the patient.

Physical condition	*Exposure change*
Extremely obese	Increase exposure
Muscular	Increase exposure (kilovoltage)
Very thin	Reduce exposure
Child	Reduce exposure
Elderly person	Reduce exposure
In wet cast	Increase exposure 3 to 4 times
In dry cast	Increase exposure 2 times
Pathologic condition	
Sclerosis	Increase exposure (kilovoltage)
Osteomyelitis	Increase exposure slightly
Osteoporosis	Reduce exposure
Paget's disease	Increase exposure
Bone atrophy	Decrease exposure

Elements of diagnostic quality

The eight elements affecting diagnostic quality are the following: blurring, magnification, distortion, definition, visibility of detail, contrast, density, and latitude. The effects of a single technique change on any or all of these elements are more readily understood when presented in tabular form. (See Table 8-2 for the elements affecting radiographic quality.)

Table 8-1. Film critique table

Factors: kvp—62, mas—100, focal spot—1.0 mm, al filter—2.5 mm, ffd—40″, ofd—4″, screens—med., plain film, 8:1 grid, dev. time—5′, dev. temp.—68°F., acid stop bath—yes, cone—collimator. No change, 0; increase, +; decrease, −.	Blurring	Magnification	Distortion	Definition	Visibility of detail	Contrast	Density	Latitude
Examination of lateral skull—change to be made (single change each time):								
1. Raise to 12:1 grid	0	0	0	0	−	−	−	−
2. Raise kvp to 75	0	0	0	0	−	−	+	−
3. Use 48″ ffd	−	−	0	+	−	−	−	−
4. Use fast film	0	0	0	0	−	−	+	−
5. Use 3.5 mm al filter	0	0	0	0	−	−	−	−
6. Use 150 mas*	0	0	0	−	−	−	+	−
7. Use cardboard holder	0	0	0	+†	−	−	−	−
8. Use fast screens	0	0	0	−‡	−	−	+	−
9. Use 2.0 mm focal spot	+	0	0	−	−	0	0	0
10. Develop 2′ @ 68° F.	0	0	0	0	−	−	−	−
11. Patient uncooperative	+	0	+	−	−	0	0	0

*This change assumes an increase in focal spot size.
†The increase indicated in definition is not readily visible.
‡Modern screens will not produce a measurable loss in definition.

Table 8-2. Diagnostic quality factors*

Radiographic quality			
Photographic properties	Density	Controlled by	Ma, time (mas)
		Primarily influenced by	Processing, kvp, film, target-film distance, heel effect, pathology
		Secondarily influenced by	Fog, screens, grid, filter, beam restrictor (cone, collimator, diaphragm)
	Contrast	Controlled by	Kvp
		Primarily influenced by	Fog
		Secondarily influenced by	Processing, patient, film, grid, screens, mas, filter, compression
	Definition	Influenced by	Density, contrast, fog, film, processing
		Controlled by	Motion, target-film distance, focal spot size, screens, film-screen contact
Geometric properties	Magnification	Controlled by	Object-film distance, focal-film distance
	True distortion	Controlled by	Target-object-film alignment

*Courtesy Dr. James P. Steele, Chairman, Committee on standardization of radiographic terminology.

For example, in Table 8-1, Change No. 1, changing the grid from one with an 8:1 ratio to one with a 12:1 ratio has no effect on image blurring; therefore, the correct mark in the blurring column is a zero. Continuing, the greater grid ratio has no effect upon magnification, since a grid was used originally; therefore, this column is marked with a zero. The greater grid ratio has no effect upon distortion or definition; therefore, these columns are also marked with a zero. The grid with the greater ratio absorbs an increased quantity of scattered rays, along with a minimal amount of primary rays; these combined are the remnant rays. Since more remnant rays are absorbed, fewer remnant rays strike the film emulsion to produce the latent image, which will make the manifest image less visible. An increased grid ratio, then, causes a decrease in visibility of detail, so this column is marked with a minus sign. Also, because grid with greater ratio absorbs more remnant rays, permitting fewer remnant rays to strike the film emulsion and produce the latent image, there will be an overall reduction in the dark black and gray areas in the image shadow to contrast with the lighter white areas in the image shadow; consequently, this column is marked with a minus sign. Since greater grid ratio permits fewer remnant rays to form the latent image, an overall reduction in energy striking the film results in decreased image and film density; this column, then, is also marked with a minus sign. Finally, greater grid ratio permits fewer remnant rays to strike the film and cause the latent image, so there is a reduction in visible image shadow and a decrease in latitude, indicated by the minus sign in the latitude column.

To consider another change, it is necessary that all conditions revert to the original example; it is of the utmost importance to consider *one change at a time.*

As a second example, consider a change (not shown in Table 8-1) in which the part (object) is raised above the tabletop in a second exposure, i.e., there is an increased ofd, and blurring and magnification are each increased remarkably. Blurring and magnification are each marked with a plus sign; distortion with a zero; and definition and visibility of detail with a minus sign. Contrast and density would be marked with a minus sign, since an increased ofd permits fewer remnant rays to strike the film (as demonstrated in a recent experiment). Finally, latitude would be marked with a minus sign since there is a decreased quantity of visible image shadow.

Another example that is readily demonstrable is as follows. When an object is rayed at a 40-inch table-top ffd, and then re-rayed at a 40-inch ffd using the Bucky diaphragm and a grid (and compensating with increased mas), the increased ofd in the second exposure results in an increase in image shadow size (magnification) of approximately one quarter inch.

REFERENCES

Files, Glen W.: Medical radiographic technic, Springfield, Ill., 1956, Charles C Thomas, Publisher.
Fuchs, Arthur W.: Principles of radiographic exposure and processing, Springfield, Ill., 1958, Charles C Thomas, Publisher.
Longmore, T. A.: Medical photography, ed. 5, London and New York, 1955, The Focal Press.
Mees, C. E. Kenneth: The theory of the photographic process, ed. 2, New York, 1954, The Macmillan Co.
Selman, Joseph: The fundamentals of x-ray and radium physics, Springfield, Ill., 1954, Charles C Thomas, Publisher.

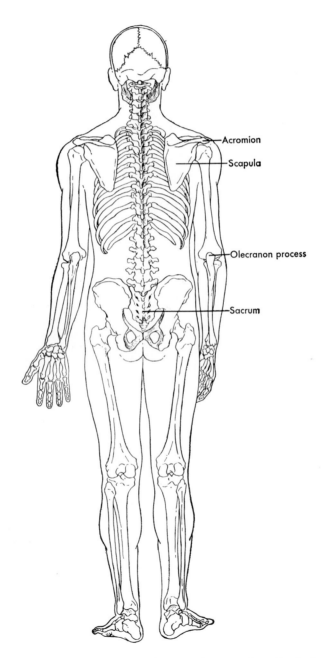

Fig. 9-2. Skeleton—posterior view. (From Anthony, Catherine Parker: Textbook of anatomy and physiology, St. Louis, 1967, The C. V. Mosby Co.)

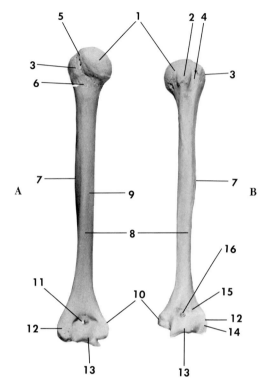

Fig. 9-3. Left humerus. **A,** Posterior surface. **B,** Anterior surface.

1. Head
2. Lesser tubercle
3. Greater tubercle
4. Intertubercle groove
5. Anatomical neck
6. Surgical neck
7. Deltoid tuberosity
8. Shaft
9. Radial groove
10. Medial epicondyle
11. Olecranon fossa
12. Lateral epicondyle
13. Trochlea
14. Capitulum
15. Radial fossa
16. Coronoid fossa

Radius and ulna

The bones of the forearm are called the radius and ulna. The radius is the bone on the lateral side. It is quite small at its proximal end and quite large at its distal end. The ulna lies on the medial side and is quite large at its proximal end and small at the distal end. The radius begins at the proximal end with the head, followed by the neck and the radial tuberosity, which is inferior and medial to the head. The midportion is called the body or shaft. The distal end, which forms the greater portion of the wrist joint, has a styloid process on the lateral surface and a small notch, the ulnar notch, on the medial surface. The ulna begins proximally with the olecranon process, which contains, anteriorly, the semilunar notch. Inferior to the olecranon process is the coronoid process, which is anterior and superior on the anterior surface of the ulna. The radial notch is located on the lateral surface of the coronoid process. The midportion of the ulna is termed the body or shaft and terminates in the small distal end. The distal

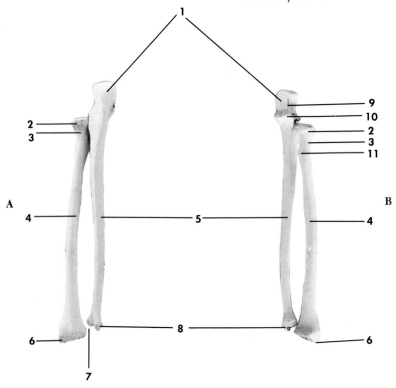

Fig. 9-4. Left radius and ulna. **A,** Posterior surface. **B,** Anterior surface.

1. Olecranon process
2. Head of radius
3. Neck of radius
4. Shaft of radius
5. Shaft of ulna
6. Styloid process of radius
7. Articulates with radius
8. Styloid process of ulna
9. Semilunar notch of ulna
10. Coronoid process of ulna
11. Tuberosity of radius

end includes the head of the ulna laterally and the styloid process medially. (See Fig. 9-4.) In addition to the articulations with the humerus, which were previously mentioned, the olecranon process of the ulna articulates with the olecranon fossa of the humerus; the coronoid process articulates with the coronoid fossa of the humerus; and the head of the radius articulates with the radial fossa of the humerus and with the radial notch of the coronoid process of the ulna. The distal ends of the radius and ulna articulate with each other in the ulnar notch of the radius, which is located on the medial surface of the radius. The distal end of the radius, in addition, articulates with the scaphoid and lunate of the carpus. The distal end of the ulna, in addition, articulates with a triangular-shaped cartilage.

Carpals, metacarpals, and phalanges

The carpus consists of eight bones in two rows: proximal row (from the lateral to the medial side)—scaphoid (navicular), lunate, triquetrum (triangular), and

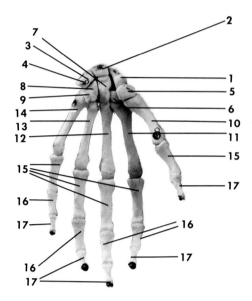

Fig. 9-5. Left-hand, palmar surface. (Note: Tufts of the terminal phalanges are obscured by the metal washers used in articulation.)

1. Scaphoid
2. Lunate
3. Triquetrum
4. Pisiform
5. Trapezium
6. Trapezoid
7. Capitate
8. Hamate
9. Hamulus process of hamate
10. First metacarpal
11. Second metacarpal
12. Third metacarpal
13. Fourth metacarpal
14. Fifth metacarpal
15. Proximal phalanges
16. Middle phalanges
17. Distal (terminal) phalanges

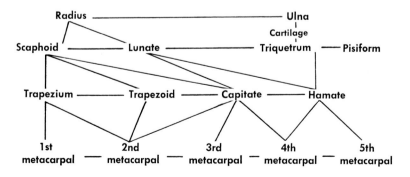

Fig. 9-6. Carpal articulations.

Table 9-1. Articulations of the carpus

Bone	Number of articulations	Articulations
Scaphoid	5	Radius, trapezium, trapezoid, capitate, and lunate
Lunate	5	Radius, capitate, hamate, triquetrum, and scaphoid
Triquetrum	3 and disc	Lunate, pisiform, hamate, and triangular-shaped cartilage
Pisiform	1	Triquetrum
Trapezium	4	Scaphoid, trapezoid, 1st and 2nd metacarpals
Trapezoid	4	Scaphoid, trapezium, capitate, and 2nd metacarpal
Capitate	7	Scaphoid, lunate, 2nd, 3rd, and 4th metacarpals, trapezoid, and hamate
Hamate	5	Lunate, 4th and 5th metacarpals, triquetrum, and capitate

pisiform; distal row (from the lateral to the medial side)—trapezium (greater multangular), trapezoid (lesser multangular), capitate, and hamate, which has a hook-shaped process on its volar surface called the hamulus. (See Fig. 9-5.) Articulations of the carpal bones are listed in Table 9-1 and are diagramed in Fig. 9-6. There are five metacarpals, which are numbered one through five from the lateral to the medial side. At their distal ends are the phalanges. There are three phalanges in each of the last four digits and two in the first digit, or thumb, making a total of fourteen phalanges in each hand. The carpals form the wrist, the metacarpals form the hand, and the phalanges form the digits, or fingers.

Lower extremity
Femur

The lower extremity begins with the femur, the long bone of the upper leg. At its proximal end are the head, anatomic neck, and greater and lesser trochanters. The intertrochanteric crest (ridge) extends obliquely between the trochanters on the posterior surface. The intertrochanteric line is on the anterior surface. It, too, lies between the trochanters. The midportion is called the body or shaft. The lateral epicondyle, lateral condyle, patellar surface, medial condyle, and medial epicondyle are located on the distal end. The intercondylar fossa is between the condyles on the posterior surface. (See Figs. 9-7 and 9-8.) The head of the femur articulates with and in the acetabulum of the pelvis, the distal end articulates with the tibia, and the patella articulates with the patellar surface.

The patella is the only sesamoid bone in the body that is essential. It is the largest of all the sesamoid bones. (See Fig. 9-9.)

Tibia and fibula

The bones of the lower leg are the tibia and fibula. The tibia is quite large. Proximally, the tibial plateau lies between the medial and lateral condyles. This plateau is divided into the medial and lateral facets by the intercondylar eminence (spine). The intercondyloid fossae are anterior and posterior to the spine.

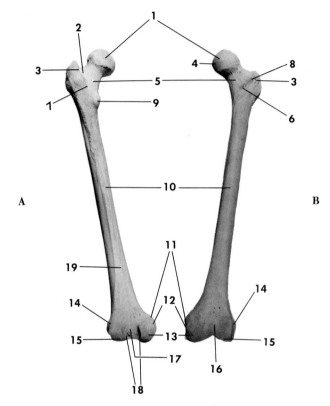

A   B

Fig. 9-7. Left femur. **A**, Posterior surface. **B**, Anterior surface.

1. Head	11. Adductor tubercle
2. Trochanteric fossa	12. Medial epicondyle
3. Greater trochanter	13. Medial condyle
4. Fovea capitis	14. Lateral epicondyle
5. Neck	15. Lateral condyle
6. Intertrochanteric line	16. Patellar surface
7. Intertrochanteric crest	17. Intercondylar fossa
8. Tubercle of femur	18. Intercondylar notch
9. Lesser trochanter	19. Popliteal surface
10. Shaft	

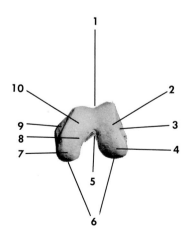

Fig. 9-8. Left femur, distal surface.

1. Patellar surface
2. Lateral groove
3. Lateral epicondyle
4. Lateral condyle
5. Intercondylar fossa
6. Intercondylar notch
7. Medial condyle
8. Semilunar area
9. Medial condyle
10. Medial groove

Fig. 9-9. Left patella. **A**, Anterior surface. **B**, Posterior surface.

1. Quadriceps femoris attachment
2. Area covered by a bursa
3. Patellar ligament attachment
4. Facet for articulation with medial condyle of femur
5. Facet for articulation with lateral condyle of femur

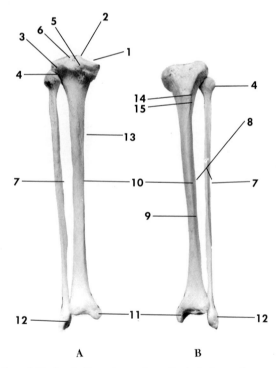

Fig. 9-10. Left tibia and fibula. **A**, Posterior surface. **B**, Anterior surface.

1. Medial condyle
2. Intercondylar eminence (structure obscured by articular device; not shown in anterior surface photograph)
3. Styloid process of fibula
4. Head of fibula
5. Posterior intercondylar fossa of tibia
6. Lateral condyle of tibia
7. Body of fibula
8. Attachment site of interosseous membrane
9. Anterior crest of tibia
10. Body of tibia
11. Medial malleolus of tibia
12. Lateral malleolus of fibula
13. Popliteal line of tibia
14. Tuberosity of tibia
15. Attachment site of patellar ligament

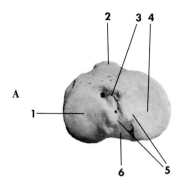
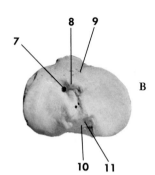

Fig. 9-11. Left tibia, proximal end. **A**, Structures. **B**, Attachment sites.

1. Lateral condyle
2. Tuberosity
3. Anterior intercondylar fossa
4. Medial condyle
5. Intercondylar eminence
6. Posterior intercondylar fossa

7. Lateral meniscus attachment
8. Anterior cruciate ligament attachment
9. Medial meniscus attachment
10. Posterior cruciate ligament attachment
11. Medial meniscus attachment

Table 9-2. Articulations of the tarsus

Bone	Number of articulations	Articulations
Calcaneus	2	Talus, cuboid
Talus	5	Lateral and medial malleoli, distal end of tibia, navicular, and calcaneus
Cuboid	4 (5)	Calcaneus, lateral cuneiform, 4th and 5th metatarsals, and sometimes navicular
Navicular	4 (5)	Medial, intermediate and lateral cuneiforms, talus, and sometimes cuboid
Medial cuneiform	4	Navicular, intermediate cuneiform, and 1st and 2nd metatarsals
Intermediate cuneiform	4	Navicular, medial and lateral cuneiforms, and 2nd metatarsal
Lateral cuneiform	6	Navicular, intermediate cuneiform, cuboid, and 2nd, 3rd, and 4th metatarsals

The articular facet for the fibula is on the posterior surface of the lateral condyle. The tibial tuberosity is on the anterior surface of the tibia inferior to the plateau. The midportion of the tibia, called the body (shaft), extends into the distal end. At the distal end on the medial surface is the medial malleolus. The head of the fibula (the fibula is lateral to the tibia) has a styloid process that projects superiorly from the posterior part of it. The midportion is called the body. The distal end of the fibula is called the lateral malleolus. (See Figs. 9-10 and 9-11.) In addition to the articulations with the femur, which were previously mentioned, the head of the fibula articulates with the lateral condyle of the tibia, but the fibula does not enter into the formation of the knee joint. The distal ends of the tibia and fibula articulate with the talus.

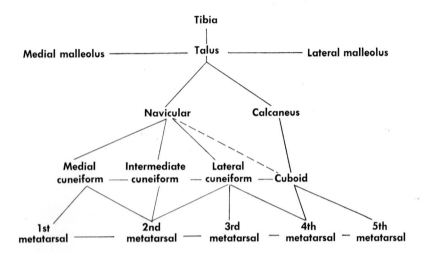

Fig. 9-12. Tarsal articulations.

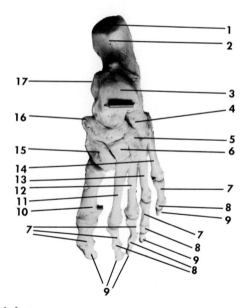

Fig. 9-13. Dorsum, left foot.

1. Calcaneal tuberosity
2. Calcaneus
3. Talus
4. Cuboid
5. Lateral cuneiform
6. Intermediate cuneiform
7. Proximal phalanx
8. Middle phalanx
9. Distal (terminal) phalanx
10. First metatarsal
11. Second metatarsal
12. Third metatarsal
13. Fourth metatarsal
14. Fifth metatarsal
15. Medial cuneiform
16. Navicular
17. Sustentaculum tali

Tarsals, metatarsals, and phalanges

The tarsus consists of seven bones: talus, calcaneus, navicular, medial (first) cuneiform, intermediate (second) cuneiform, lateral (third) cuneiform, and cuboid. The articulations are listed in Table 9-2 and are diagramed in Fig. 9-12. There are five metatarsals, which are numbered one through five from the medial to the lateral side. At their distal ends are the phalanges. There are two phalanges in the first digit, or great toe, and three phalanges each in the last four digits. (See Fig. 9-13.) The tarsals, metatarsals, and phalanges comprise the foot. The ankle articulation is that between the tibia, lateral and medial malleoli, and the talus. The phalanges, although part of the foot, comprise the toes (digits).

REFERENCES

Anthony, Catherine Parker: Textbook of anatomy and physiology, ed. 7, St. Louis, 1967, The C. V. Mosby Co.

Best, C. H., and Taylor, N. B.: The living body, New York, 1952, Henry Holt & Co., Inc.

Best, C. H., and Taylor, N. B.: The human body, New York, 1956, Henry Holt & Co., Inc.

De Coursey, Russell Myles: The human organism, New York, 1955, McGraw-Hill Book Co.

Goss, Charles M.: Gray's anatomy, ed. 28, Philadelphia 1966, Lea & Febiger.

Greisheimer, Esther M.: Physiology and anatomy, Philadelphia, 1950, J. B. Lippincott Co.

Kimber, Diana Clifford, and Gray, Caroline E.: Textbook of anatomy and physiology, New York, 1928, The Macmillan Co.

Meschan, Isadore: Normal radiographic anatomy, Philadelphia, 1951, W. B. Saunders Co.

Chapter 10

Positioning for the extremities

Routine

The routine steps are listed as follows:

1. Know the desired position.
2. Select all factors except kilovoltage.
3. Conduct the patient into the radiographic room. If cooperation of the patient is possible, have him assume the desired position.
4. After deciding what size film to use, place the film on the tabletop beneath the part to be radiographed. Use proper identification and an *R* or *L* to denote the right or left side.
5. If possible, explain to the patient what is going to be done.
6. Center the part to be radiographed to the proper film holder division.
7. Center the tube both lengthwise and crosswise to the part to be radiographed.
8. Measure the patient for thickness of the part. From the technique chart, determine the kilovoltage and select it on the control.
9. Close the primary switch and check the line voltage.
10. Give the patient instructions concerning breathing.
11. *Observe* the patient's movement *until the moment that the exposure is made.*
12. During the exposure, ascertain that the machine is delivering the desired milliamperage by watching the milliampere meter.
13. Instruct the patient to resume normal breathing.

If another view is required, select the proper factors on the control panel. Remove the exposed film (in the film holder), and replace it with the proper-sized film holder and film for the next exposure. If more than one view is to be taken on one film, simply change the location of the lead half or third blanks and reposition the part to be radiographed. With the first exposure of a series of multiple exposures on a single film, mark the part of the anatomy that is even with the center mark of the film holder; keep this mark even with the center mark in all subsequent exposures of this series.

Be sure to complete the identification procedure. The starting factors stated for all the following techniques are for a *12:1 grid* when a Bucky is used. For tabletop work, back-scatter radiation can be reduced by placing a sheet of leaded rubber beneath the film holder. Bone radiography requires the use of the small focal spot. Extremity radiography usually requires two or more views on each film. The method of division of the film holder face is demonstrated in Fig. 10-1.

In this chapter reference is made to one of these four methods of division in each set of positioning instructions.

Several devices are employed to mark or identify the radiographs. These devices include radiolucent metal plates with slots for lead numerals and letters, radiopaque plates with numbers and letters cut out in small wheels, and *flashcards* to be used with identifying lamps in the darkroom. The last device permits a variety of data to be typed on the card and then stamped into the film emulsion. To enable use of this device, a piece of leaded rubber, or other radiopaque material, is placed in one of eight positions, either on the film-holder surface or in a precut area in the intensifying screens. These positions are shown in Fig. 10-2.

It is necessary that the greatest possible protection from extraneous radiation be given both the patient and the operator. In addition to collimation of the primary beam, numerous other devices may be employed for gonadal protection. Among these are leaded rubber gloves and aprons and specially cut pieces of leaded rubber sheeting, which is available through x-ray supply houses.

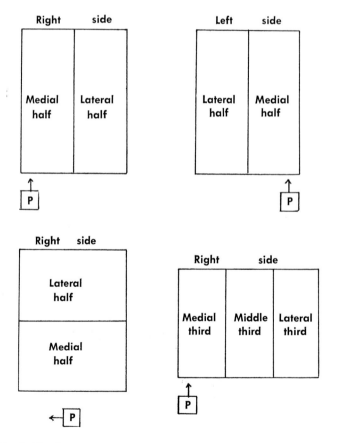

Fig. 10-1. Film holder face divisions. The square containing the letter *P* denotes the position of the patient in relation to the film on the tabletop. The arrow indicates the direction the patient faces.

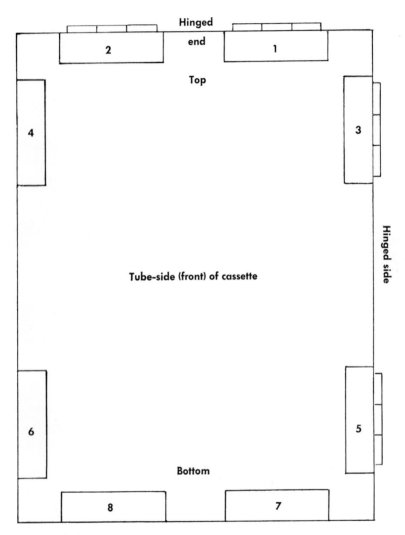

Fig. 10-2. Lead blocker positions.

Thumb

Thumb—posterior (A-P), oblique, and lateral views (Figs. 10-3 and 10-4)

Film size—8″ × 10″	*Tabletop*	
Cardboard	*Cone to cover*	
Crosswise		

Technique

Factors	Screen film cassette (par)	Screen film cardboard	No-screen film cardboard
Ma	100	100	100
Time	0.1	0.75	0.2
Mas	10	75	20
Thickness in cm	3	3	3
Kvp	43	56	52
Distance	40	40	40

Patient preparation

Remove all jewelry from the patient's hand.

Palpation point

Distal end of proximal segment.

Procedure

Posterior (A-P)—Seat the patient at the end of the table. Place the hand in internal rotation with the midposterior surface of the thumb in the center of the lateral side of the film holder.

Oblique—Place the palm flat on the film holder with the midportion of the thumb in the center of the film holder.

Lateral—Place the palm flat on the film holder with the midportion of the thumb in the center of the film holder. Flex the fingers to rotate the thumb into the true lateral position.

Central ray

Direct the central ray perpendicular through the distal end of the proximal segment of the thumb to the center of the film holder.

Immobilization

Posterior (A-P)—Place sandbags or sponges under the elbow. Instruct the patient to support his fingers with his other hand.

Oblique—Place sandbags on the elbow and fingertips.

Lateral—Place sandbags on the elbow and against the fingertips.

Right-left markers

Place the correct marker on the lateral view of the first metacarpal and phalanges.

Technical tips

Keep the long axis of the thumb parallel with the film to open the joint space.

Structures demonstrated

Posterior (A-P), oblique, and lateral views of the first metacarpal and phalanges.

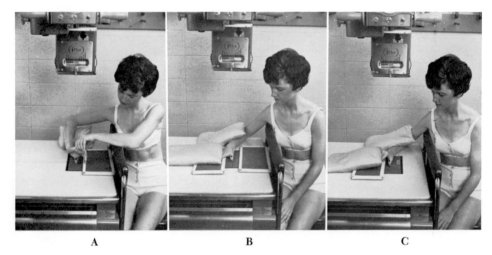

Fig. 10-3. Thumb positions. **A,** Posterior (A-P) position. **B,** Oblique position. **C,** Lateral position.

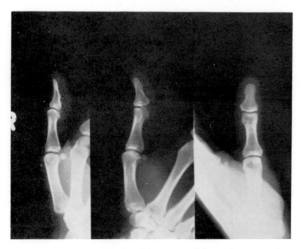

Fig. 10-4. Thumb views. Posterior (A-P), oblique, and lateral views. (Courtesy Dr. E. I. L. Cilley, Dr. T. W. Crowell, Dr. R. E. Waud, and Dr. G. H. Hoffman.)

Hand

Hand—anterior (P-A) and oblique views (Figs. 10-5 and 10-6)

    Film size—10″ × 12″   *Tabletop*
    Cardboard   *Cone to cover*
    Crosswise

Technique

Factors	Screen film cassette (par)	Screen film cardboard	No-screen film cardboard
Ma	100	100	100
Time	0.1	0.75	0.2
Mas	10	75	20
Thickness in cm	4	4	4
Kvp	46	59	56
Distance	40	40	40

Patient preparation

Remove all jewelry, if possible.

Palpation points

Distal ends and shafts of metacarpal bones.

Procedure

Anterior (P-A)—Seat the patient at the end of the table. Place the hand in the prone position, with the fingers and thumb extended and slightly separated. Center the midshaft of the third metacarpal in the center of the medial half of the film holder.

Oblique—With the palm on the film, rotate the hand externally approximately 35 degrees. Flex and separate the fingers, and extend the thumb. Center the midshaft of the third metacarpal in the center of the lateral half of the film holder.

Central ray

Direct the central ray perpendicular through the midshaft of the third metacarpal to the center of the film holder.

Immobilization

Place a sandbag on the forearm.

Right-left markers

Place the correct marker on the oblique view, lateral center border of the film holder.

Structures demonstrated

Anterior (P-A) and oblique views of the carpals, metacarpals, and phalanges.

Technical tips

Relax the fingers to position the long axis of the metacarpals parallel with the film surface.

Technical tips

On P-A view, relax fingers and hand to position long axis of wrist parallel with film surface.

Structures demonstrated

Anterior (A-P), oblique, and lateral views of the distal ends of the radius and ulna, the carpal bones, and the proximal ends of the metacarpals. The ulnar flexion view better demonstrates scaphoid fractures.

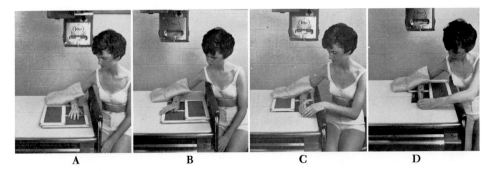

Fig. 10-7. Wrist positions. **A,** Anterior (P-A) position. **B,** Radial deviation (ulnar flexion) position. **C,** Oblique position. **D,** Lateral position.

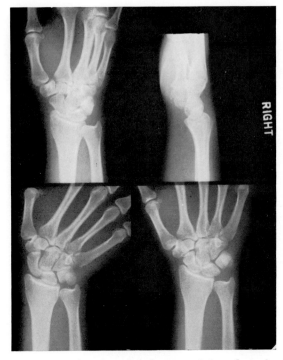

Fig. 10-8. Wrist views. Anterior (P-A), radial deviation (ulnar flexion), oblique, and lateral views. (Courtesy Dr. E. I. L. Cilley, Dr. T. W. Crowell, Dr. R. E. Waud, and Dr. G. H. Hoffman.)

Forearm

Forearm—posterior (A-P) and lateral views (Figs. 10-9 and 10-10)

> *Film size—10″ × 12″*   *Tabletop*
> *Cardboard*   *Cone to cover*
> *Lengthwise*

Technique

Factors	Screen film cassette (par)	Screen film cardboard	No-screen film cardboard
Ma	100	100	100
Time	0.1	0.75	0.2
Mas	10	75	20
Thickness in cm	5	5	5
Kvp	49	62	61
Distance	40	40	40

Patient preparation

Remove all jewelry.

Palpation points

Radial and ulnar styloid processes; lateral and medial epicondyles of humerus.

Procedure

Posterior (A-P)—Seat the patient at the end of the table. Place the forearm in the supine position on the lateral half of the film holder with the joint nearer the injured site included on the film holder. A line through the radial and ulnar styloid processes is parallel with the film surface.

Lateral—From the posterior (A-P) position, rotate the forearm internally 90 degrees, at the same time flex the elbow 90 degrees, and rest the upper arm on the table. Place the forearm on the medial half of the film holder with the included joint in the same plane as in the posterior view. A plane through the radial and ulnar styloid processes and the humeral epicondyles is perpendicular to the film surface.

Central ray

Direct the central ray perpendicular through the shaft of the forearm to the center of the film holder.

Immobilization

Posterior (A-P)—Place a 1-inch sponge or sandbag under the hand and a heavy sandbag on the palm of the hand.

Lateral—Place sandbag on each side of the hand.

Right-left markers

Place the correct marker on the lateral view, center border of the film holder.

Technical tips

The P-A position of the hand and wrist with elbow extended presents an untrue forearm position with the radius crossing over the ulna.

Structures demonstrated

Posterior (A-P) and lateral views of the radius and ulna and elbow, and/or wrist joints.

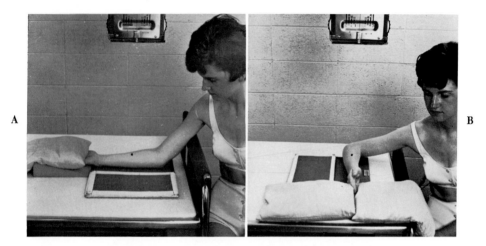

Fig. 10-9. Forearm positions. **A,** Posterior (A-P) position. **B,** Lateral position.

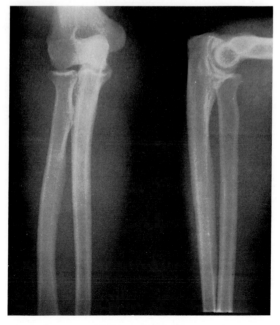

Fig. 10-10. Forearm views. Posterior (A-P) and lateral views. (Courtesy Dr. E. I. L. Cilley, Dr. T. W. Crowell, Dr. R. E. Waud, and Dr. G. H. Hoffman.)

Elbow

Elbow—posterior (A-P) and lateral views (Figs. 10-11 and 10-12)

> *Film size—10″ × 12″*   *Tabletop*
> *Cardboard*   *Cone to cover*
> *Crosswise*

Technique

Factors	Screen film cassette (par)	Screen film cardboard	No-screen film cardboard
Ma	100	100	100
Time	0.1	0.75	0.2
Mas	10	75	20
Thickness in cm	7	7	7
Kvp	52	67	65
Distance	40	40	40

Patient preparation

Remove sleeve from part.

Palpation points

Radial and ulnar styloid processes; lateral and medial epicondyles of humerus.

Procedure

Posterior (A-P)—Seat the patient at the end of the table on a low stool. Place the elbow in the supine position on the lateral half of the film holder with the shoulder and elbow in the same horizontal plane. A plane through the radial and ulnar styloid processes and the humeral epicondyles is parallel with the film surface. Center the midpoint of the elbow (a point 1 inch distal to the epicondyles) to the film holder.

Lateral—From the posterior (A-P) position, rotate the elbow internally 90 degrees; at the same time flex the elbow 90 degrees, and rest the upper arm on the table. The humerus projects off the medial aspect of the film holder. A plane through the radial and ulnar styloid processes and humeral epicondyles is perpendicular to the film surface. Center the midpoint of the elbow to the film holder.

Central ray

Direct the central ray perpendicular through the elbow to the center of the film holder.

Immobilization

Posterior (A-P)—Place a 1-inch sponge or sandbag under the hand and a heavy sandbag on the palm of the hand.

Lateral—Place sandbags on each side of the hand.

Right-left markers

Place the correct marker on the lateral view, above the humerus, center border of the film holder.

Technical tips

In the A-P view, if the elbow cannot be extended more than 110 degrees, make two exposures: one, an A-P of the proximal forearm, and the other, an A-P of the distal humerus on one film.

Structures demonstrated

Posterior (A-P) and lateral views of the elbow joint, distal humerus, proximal radius, and ulna.

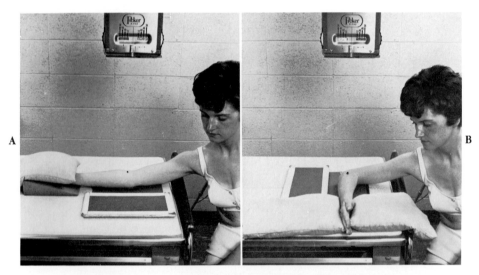

Fig. 10-11. Elbow positions. **A,** Posterior (A-P) position. **B,** Lateral position.

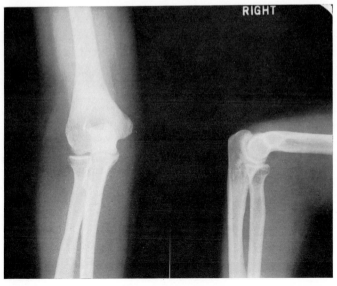

Fig. 10-12. Elbow views. Posterior (A-P) and lateral views. (Courtesy Dr. E. I. L. Cilley, Dr. T. W. Crowell, Dr. R. E. Waud, and Dr. G. H. Hoffman.)

Humerus
Humerus—posterior (A-P) view (Figs. 10-13 and 10-14)

> *Film size—10″ × 12″*   *Bucky*
> *Cassette*   *Cone to cover*
> *Lengthwise*

Technique

Factors	Screen film cassette (*par*) Bucky	Screen film cassette (*par*) tabletop
Ma	100	100
Time	0.2	0.1
Mas	20	10
Thickness in cm	10	10
Kvp	66	54
Distance	40	40

Patient preparation
Remove clothing from part.

Palpation points
Lateral and medial epicondyles of humerus; acromion process of scapula.

Procedure
Place the patient in the supine position with the long axis of the humerus over the center line of the table. Rotate the arm into the supine position so that a line through the humeral epicondyles is parallel with the film surface. Include the joint nearer to the injured site, and place the edge of the cassette 2 inches beyond this joint.

Central ray
Direct the central ray perpendicular through the shaft of the humerus to the center of the film holder.

Immobilization
Place sandbags under and over the hand. Employ suspended respiration.

Right-left markers
Place the correct marker on the lateral side, center border of the film holder.

Technical tips
The distal humerus may best be demonstrated by seating the patient at the end of the table with his elbow extended on the tabletop and the upper arm in external rotation.

Structures demonstrated
Posterior (A-P) view of the upper two thirds or of the lower two thirds of the humerus.

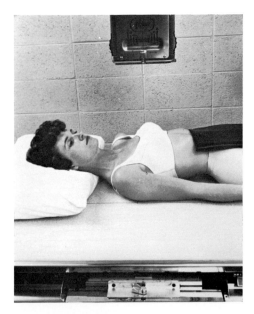

Fig. 10-13. Humerus—posterior (A-P) position.

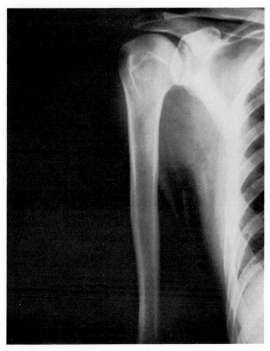

Fig. 10-14. Humerus—posterior (A-P) view. (Courtesy Dr. E. I. L. Cilley, Dr. T. W. Crowell, Dr. R. E. Waud, and Dr. G. H. Hoffman.)

Humerus—lateral view (Figs. 10-15 and 10-16)

> *Film size—10″ × 12″*   *Bucky*
> *Cassette*   *Cone to cover*
> *Lengthwise*

Technique

Factors	Screen film cassette (par) Bucky	Screen film cassette (par) tabletop
Ma	100	100
Time	0.2	0.1
Mas	20	10
Thickness in cm	10	10
Kvp	66	54
Distance	40	40

Patient preparation

Remove clothing from part.

Palpation points

Lateral and medial epicondyles of humerus; acromion process of scapula.

Procedure

Place the patient in the supine position with the long axis of the humerus over the center line of the table. Rotate the arm internally so that a line through the humeral epicondyles is perpendicular to the film holder. Include the joint nearer to the injured site, and place the edge of the cassette 2 inches beyond this joint.

Central ray

Direct the central ray perpendicular through the shaft of the humerus to the center of the film holder.

Immobilization

Place a sandbag over the hand. Employ suspended respiration.

Right-left markers

Place the correct marker on the lateral side, center border of the film holder.

Technical tips

The distal humerus may best be demonstrated by seating the patient at the end of the table with his elbow extended on the tabletop and the upper arm in internal rotation.

Structures demonstrated

Lateral view of the upper two thirds or the lower two thirds of the humerus.

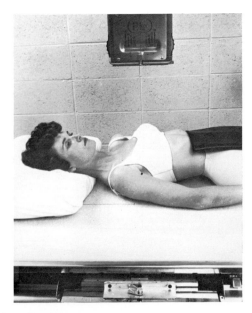

Fig. 10-15. Humerus—lateral position.

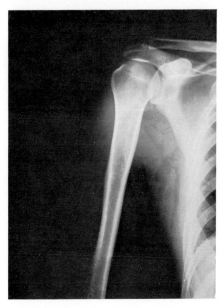

Fig. 10-16. Humerus—lateral view. (Courtesy Dr. E. I. L. Cilley, Dr. T. W. Crowell, Dr. R. E. Waud, and Dr. G. H. Hoffman.)

Toes

Toes—posterior (A-P) and oblique views (Figs. 10-17 and 10-18)

Film size—8″ × 10″   *Tabletop*
Cardboard   *Cone to cover*
Crosswise

Technique

Factors	Screen film cassette (par)	Screen film cardboard	No-screen film cardboard
Ma	100	100	100
Time	0.1	0.75	0.2
Mas	10	75	20
Thickness in cm	2	2	2
Kvp	40	56	50
Distance	40	40	40

Patient preparation

Remove shoes and socks from both feet.

Palpation points

Distal ends (heads) of metatarsal bones.

Procedure

Posterior (A-P)—Seat the patient on the table. Flex the knee, and instruct the patient to place the sole of the foot on the medial half of the film holder. Center the third toe to the center of this half of the film holder.

Oblique—From the posterior (A-P) position, rotate the foot internally 45 degrees. Center the third toe to the center of the lateral half of the film holder. Should the toes be superimposed, decrease the angle of rotation or separate the toes with small pieces of cotton, or both.

Central ray

Direct the central ray perpendicular to the long axis of the toe being examined and to the film holder.

Immobilization

Posterior (A-P)—Place a large sponge between the knees or use a compression band over the foot, or both.

Oblique—Rest the opposite leg on the table, and place a sponge between the knees or use a 45-degree wedge sponge under the sole of the foot, or both.

Right-left markers

Place the correct marker on the oblique view, center border of the film holder.

Technical tips

Patient strain and motion may be reduced by placing the patient in a chair on the floor or on top of the x-ray table.

Structures demonstrated

Posterior (A-P) and oblique views of the toes and distal metatarsals.

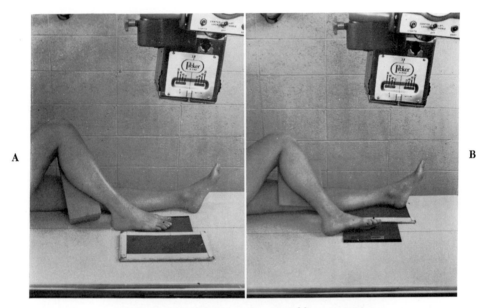

Fig. 10-17. Toe positions. **A,** Posterior (A-P) position. **B,** Oblique position.

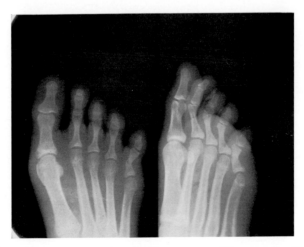

Fig. 10-18. Toe views. Posterior (A-P) and oblique views. (Courtesy Dr. E. I. L. Cilley, Dr. T. W. Crowell, Dr. R. E. Waud, and Dr. G. H. Hoffman.)

Foot

Foot—posterior (A-P) (dorsoplantar) and oblique views (Figs. 10-19 and 10-20)

Film size—10" × 12"   Tabletop
Cardboard   Cone to cover
Crosswise

Technique

Factors	Screen film cassette (par)	Screen film cardboard	No-screen film cardboard
Ma	100	100	100
Time	0.1	0.75	0.2
Mas	10	75	20
Thickness in cm	8	8	8
Kvp	54	66	68
Distance	40	40	40

Patient preparation

Remove shoes and socks from both feet.

Palpation point

Proximal end of third metatarsal.

Procedure

Posterior (A-P) (dorsoplantar)—Seat the patient on the table. Flex the knee, and instruct the patient to place the sole of the foot on the medial half of the film holder. Center the proximal end of the second metatarsal over the medial half of the film holder.

Oblique—From the posterior (A-P) position, rotate the foot internally 45 degrees. Center the proximal end of the fourth metatarsal over the lateral half of the film holder.

Central ray

Direct the central ray 15 degrees cephalad or perpendicular to the long axis of the metatarsal arch through the proximal end of the third metatarsal and to the center of each half of the film holder.

Immobilization

Posterior (A-P) (dorsoplantar)—Place a large sponge between the knees or use a compression band over the foot, or both.

Oblique—Rest the opposite leg on the table, and place a sponge between the knees or use a 45-degree wedge sponge under the sole of the foot, or both.

Right-left markers

Place the correct marker on the oblique view, center border of the film holder.

Technical tips

Patient strain and motion may be reduced by placing the patient in a chair on the floor or on top of the x-ray table.

Structures demonstrated

Posterior (A-P) (dorsoplantar) and oblique views of the tarsals, metatarsals, and phalanges.

Note:

Dorsoplantar and lateral *weight-bearing* views should be made when the request specifies pes-planus or pes-cavus radiographs. Dorsoplantar and lateral views should be made when the request specifies foreign body radiographs.

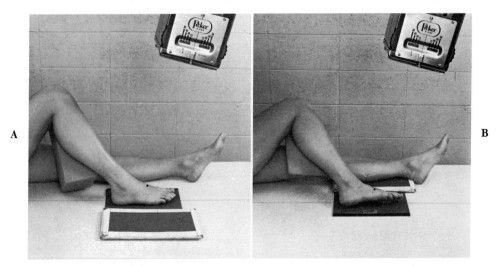

Fig. 10-19. Foot positions. **A,** Posterior (A-P) (dorsoplantar) position. **B,** Oblique position.

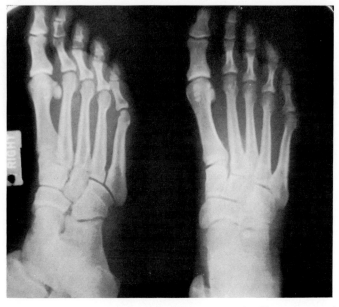

Fig. 10-20. Foot views. Posterior (A-P) (dorsoplantar) and oblique views. (Courtesy Dr. E. I. L. Cilley, Dr. T. W. Crowell, Dr. R. E. Waud, and Dr. G. H. Hoffman.)

Calcaneus (os calcis) heel

Calcaneus—plantodorsal (dorsal) and lateral views (Figs. 10-21 and 10-22)

Film size—8" × 10"   Tabletop
Cardboard   Cone to cover
Crosswise

Technique

Factors	Screen film cassette (par)	Screen film cardboard	No-screen film cardboard
Ma	100	100	100
Time	0.1	0.75	0.2
Mas	10	75	20
Thickness in cm	9	9	9
Kvp	58	76	70
Distance	40	40	40

Patient preparation

Remove shoes and socks from both feet.

Palpation points

Lateral and medial malleoli; calcaneal tuberosity.

Procedure

Plantodorsal (dorsal)—Seat the patient on the table. With the legs extended, center the heel being examined on the medial half of the film holder 2½ inches past the center line. Place a strip of gauze or rubber tubing around the ball of the foot, and instruct the patient to hold the flexed foot so that the plantar surface is perpendicular to the film surface.

Lateral—From the plantodorsal (dorsal) position, rotate the leg externally so that a line through both malleoli is perpendicular to the film surface. Cross the unaffected leg over the leg being examined. Center the midpart of the calcaneus to the center of the film holder with the long axis of the foot extending off the lateral side of the film holder.

Central ray

Plantodorsal (dorsal)—Direct the central ray 40 degrees cephalad through the calcaneus to the center of the film holder.

Lateral—Direct the central ray perpendicular to the calcaneus and to the center of the film holder.

Immobilization

Plantodorsal (dorsal)—Place heavy sandbags over the leg and gauze strip or rubber tubing.

Lateral—Place sandbags over the leg. Support the opposite knee with large sponges or sandbags.

Right-left markers

Place the correct marker on the lateral view, bottom center border of film holder.

Technical tips

A 45-degree internal oblique plantodorsal projection will demonstrate the talo-calcaneal articulation.

Structures demonstrated

Plantodorsal (dorsal)—An axial view of the calcaneus from the tuberosity to the sustentaculum tali.

Lateral—A lateral view of the body of the calcaneus.

Note:

Bilateral dorsoplantar projections may be made with the patient standing on the film holder or lying prone with the vertical film holder against the plantar surfaces of both feet.

A 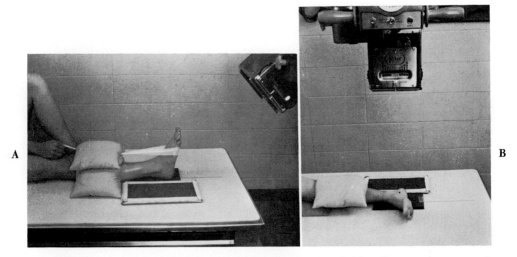 B

Fig. 10-21. Calcaneus (os calcis) heel positions. **A,** Plantodorsal (dorsal) position. **B,** Lateral position.

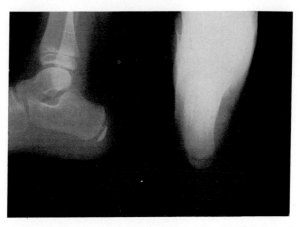

Fig. 10-22. Calcaneus (os calcis) views. Plantodorsal (dorsal) and lateral views. (Courtesy Dr. E. I. L. Cilley, Dr. T. W. Crowell, Dr. R. E. Waud, and Dr. G. H. Hoffman.)

Ankle

Ankle—posterior (A-P), internal oblique, and lateral views (Figs. 10-23 and 10-24)

> *Film size—10″ × 12″*   *Tabletop*
> *Cardboard*   *Cone to cover*
> *Crosswise*

Technique

Factors	Screen film cassette (*par*)	Screen film cardboard	No-screen film cardboard
Ma	100	100	100
Time	0.1	0.75	0.2
Mas	10	75	20
Thickness in cm	9	9	9
Kvp	58	76	70
Distance	40	40	40

Patient preparation

Remove shoes and socks from both feet.

Palpation points

Lateral and medial malleoli.

Procedure

Posterior (A-P)—Seat the patient on the table. With the leg extended, center the ankle mortise over the medial third of the film holder. The plantar surface of the foot is perpendicular to the film holder. Rotate the foot and ankle so that a line through both malleoli is parallel with the film surface.

Internal oblique—From the posterior (A-P) position, rotate the ankle internally so that a line through the malleoli forms a 45-degree angle with film surface.

Lateral—From the posterior (A-P) position, rotate the leg externally so that a line through the malleoli is perpendicular to the film surface. Cross the unaffected leg over the leg being examined. Center the lateral malleolus to the center of the film holder with the longer axis of the foot extending off the lateral side of the film holder.

Central ray

Direct the central ray perpendicular through the midportion of the ankle mortise in line with the tip of the medial malleolus to the center of each film division.

Immobilization

Place a radiolucent sponge beneath the knee. Place sandbags over the leg. Brace the plantar surface of the foot with a sponge and sandbag.

Right-left markers

Place the correct marker on the lateral view, bottom center border of the film holder.

Technical tips

For a true A-P position, the foot and ankle must be rotated internally 10-degrees.

Structures demonstrated

Posterior (A-P), internal oblique, and lateral views of the distal one third of the tibia and fibula, of the ankle mortise, and of the talus.

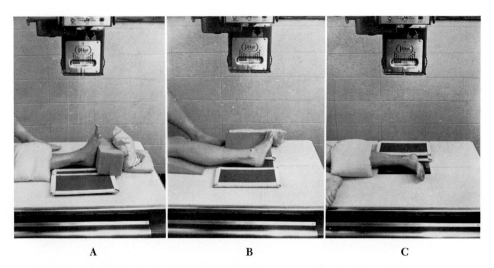

A   **B**   **C**

Fig. 10-23. Ankle positions. **A,** Posterior (A-P) position. **B,** Internal oblique position. **C,** Lateral position.

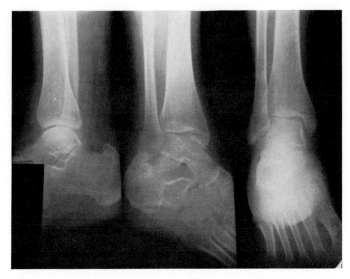

Fig. 10-24. Ankle views. Posterior (A-P), internal oblique, and lateral views. (Courtesy Dr. E. I. L. Cilley, Dr. T. W. Crowell, Dr. R. E. Waud, and Dr. G. H. Hoffman.)

Ankle—posterior (A-P) forced inversion and forced eversion views (Figs. 10-25 and
10-26)

Film size—8″ × 10″	*Tabletop*	
Cardboard	*Cone to cover*	
Crosswise		

Technique

Factors	Screen film cassette (par)	Screen film cardboard	No-screen film cardboard
Ma	100	100	100
Time	0.1	0.75	0.2
Mas	10	75	20
Thickness in cm	9	9	9
Kvp	58	76	70
Distance	40	40	40

Patient preparation

Remove shoes and socks from both feet.

Palpation points

Lateral and medial malleoli.

Procedure

Inversion—Seat the patient on the table. With the leg extended, center the
ankle mortise over the medial half of the film holder. The plantar surface of the
foot is perpendicular to the film holder. Rotate the ankle so that a line through
both malleoli is parallel with the film surface. Invert the foot as far as possible.
Place a strip of gauze around the ball of the foot and instruct the patient to hold
the foot forcibly in this position.

Eversion—From the posterior (A-P) inversion position evert the foot as far as
possible. Place a strip of gauze around the ball of the foot and instruct the patient to hold the foot forcibly in this position.

Central ray

Direct the central ray perpendicular through the midportion of the ankle
mortise in line with the tip of the medial malleolus to the center of each film
division.

Immobilization

Place a radiolucent sponge beneath the knee. Place heavy sandbags over the
leg. Brace the plantar surface of the foot with a sponge supported by a sandbag.

Right-left markers

Place the correct marker on the eversion view, lateral side, center border of
film holder.

Technical tips

Forced positions may be held in place by attaching a sandbag to the gauze sling
around the foot and allowing the sandbag to hang over the side of the table.

Structures demonstrated

Inversion—An unobstructed view of the external malleolus, and medial stress on the ankle mortise.

Eversion—Lateral stress on the ankle mortise.

Note:

Bilateral views should be made for comparison purposes.

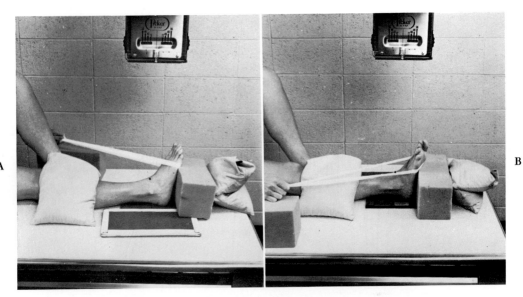

Fig. 10-25. Ankle positions. **A,** Forced inversion position. **B,** Forced eversion position.

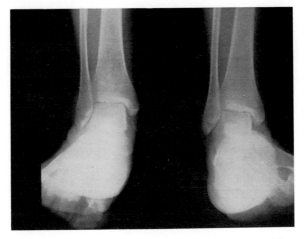

Fig. 10-26. Ankle views. Forced inversion and forced eversion views. (Courtesy Dr. E. I. L. Cilley, Dr. T. W. Crowell, Dr. R. E. Waud, and Dr. G. H. Hoffman.)

Leg
Leg—posterior (A-P) and lateral views (Figs. 10-27 and 10-28)

        Film size—14″ × 17″ or 7″ × 17″   *Tabletop*
        Cassette   *Cone to cover*
        Lengthwise

Technique

Factors	*Screen film cassette (par)*
Ma	100
Time	0.1
Mas	10
Thickness in cm	8
Kvp	56
Distance	40

Patient preparation

Remove shoes, socks, and any other garments from both legs.

Palpation points

Lateral and medial malleoli; lateral and medial epicondyles of the femur; apex of the patella.

Procedure

Posterior (A-P)—Place the patient in the supine position on the table. With the leg extended, center the shaft of the tibia over the medial half of the film holder. Include both ankle and knee joints on the film, if possible, or the joint nearer the injured site. Rotate the epicondyles of the femur so that a line through them is parallel with the film surface.

Lateral—From the posterior (A-P) position, rotate the leg externally so that a plane through both malleoli and both femoral epicondyles is perpendicular to the film surface. Cross the unaffected leg over the leg being examined. Center the anterior two thirds of the leg to the center of the lateral half of the film holder.

Central ray

Direct the central ray perpendicular through the long axis of the leg to the center of the film holder.

Immobilization

Place a sandbag against the foot and a large sponge under the flexed knee.

Right-left markers

Place the correct marker on the lateral view, lateral center border of the film holder.

Technical tips

In the lateral position, have the patient rest on his forearm to reduce strain and motion.

Structures demonstrated

Posterior (A-P) and lateral views of the tibia and fibula, and of the ankle or knee joints or both.

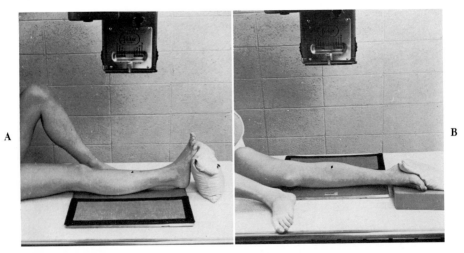

Fig. 10-27. Leg positions. **A,** Posterior (A-P) position. **B,** Lateral position.

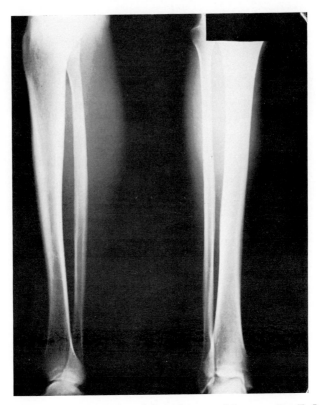

Fig. 10-28. Leg views. Posterior (A-P) and lateral views. (Courtesy Dr. E. I. L. Cilley, Dr. T. W. Crowell, Dr. R. E. Waud, and Dr. G. H. Hoffman.)

Knee

Knee—posterior (A-P) view (Figs. 10-29 and 10-30)

> *Film size—8″ × 10″*   *Tabletop*
> *Cassette*   *Cone to cover*
> *Lengthwise*

Technique

Factors	Screen film cassette (par)
Ma	100
Time	0.1
Mas	10
Thickness in cm	12
Kvp	62
Distance	40

Patient preparation

Remove both shoes and any garments around knee area. Provide a gown if necessary.

Palpation points

Lateral and medial epicondyles of femur; apex of patella; tibial tuberosity.

Procedure

Seat the patient on the table. With the legs extended, center the apex of the patella over the center of the film holder. Rotate the leg so that a line through both femoral epicondyles is parallel with the film surface.

Central ray

Direct the central ray 5 degrees caphalad to the center of the film holder.

Immobilization

Place sandbags on each side of the foot and on top of the leg.

Right-left markers

Place the correct marker on the lateral center border of the film holder.

Technical tips

The apex (bottom) of the patella is directly over the knee joint.

Structures demonstrated

Posterior (A-P) view of the knee joint, patella, and intercondylar eminence.

Note:

The patella or tibial tuberosity (for Osgood-Schlatter disease) is best demonstrated in P-A positions or 45-degree P-A (internal and external oblique positions.

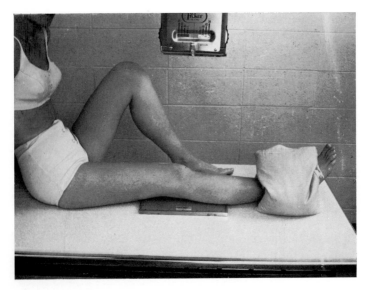

Fig. 10-29. Knee—posterior (A-P) position.

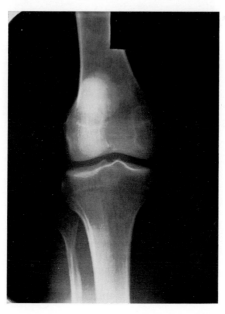

Fig. 10-30. Knee—posterior (A-P) view. (Courtesy Dr. E. I. L. Cilley, Dr. T. W. Crowell, Dr. R. E. Waud, and Dr. G. H. Hoffman.)

Knee—lateral view (Figs. 10-31 and 10-32)

> *Film size—8″ × 10″*   *Tabletop*
> *Cassette*   *Cone to cover*
> *Lengthwise*

Technique

Factors	Screen film cassette (par)
Ma	100
Time	0.1
Mas	10
Thickness in cm	10
Kvp	58
Distance	40

Patient preparation

Remove both shoes and any garments around the knee area. Provide a gown if necessary.

Palpation points

Lateral and medial epicondyles of the femur; apex of the patella; tibial tuberosity.

Procedure

Place the patient on the table with the side of the leg being examined down. Cross the opposite leg over the leg being examined. Flex the injured leg 45 degrees and center the midpart of the knee ½ inch below the medial epicondyle to the center of the film holder. The shaft of the femur should extend off the superior midcenter of the film holder. The shaft of the tibia should bisect the lower posterior angle of the film holder. Rotate the leg so that a line through both femoral epicondyles is perpendicular to the film surface.

Central ray

Direct the central ray perpendicular through the knee to the center of the film holder.

Immobilization

Place a wedge sponge or sandbag under the foot and a sandbag over the ankle and leg. Place a large sponge under the opposite knee for support.

Right-left markers

Center the correct marker on the inferior border of the film holder below the patella.

Technical tips

For correct superimposition of femoral condyles, keep the long axis of the femur and the tibia parallel with the film.

Structures demonstrated

Lateral view of the distal femur, patella, proximal tibia, and fibula.

Note:

For supine or prone patients, make lateral to medial projections on a vertical film holder placed between the patient's knees.

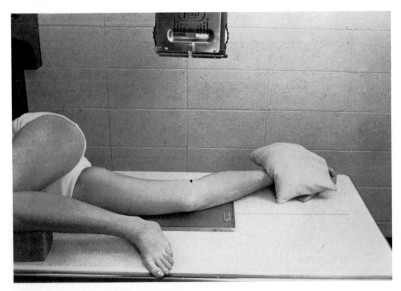

Fig. 10-31. Knee—lateral position.

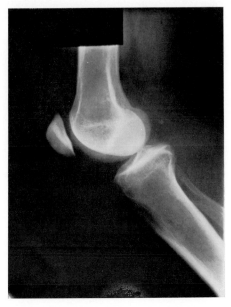

Fig. 10-32. Knee—lateral view. (Courtesy Dr. E. I. L. Cilley, Dr. T. W. Crowell, Dr. R. E. Waud, and Dr. G. H. Hoffman.)

Knee—notch (intercondylar) view (Figs. 10-33 and 10-34)

> *Film size—8″ × 10″*   *Tabletop*
> *Cassette*   *Extension cone*
> *Lengthwise*   *(fully extended)*

Technique

Factors	Screen film cassette (par)	Screen film cardboard	No-screen film cardboard
Ma	100	100	100
Time	0.1	0.75	0.2
Mas	10	75	20
Thickness in cm	13	13	13
Kvp	66	80	80
Distance	40	40	40

Patient preparation

Remove both shoes and any garments around the knee area. Provide a gown if necessary.

Palpation points

Lateral and medial epicondyles of the femur; apex of the patella.

Procedure

Place the patient on the table in the kneeling position with both feet extended over the end of the table. Center the apex of the patella to the center of the film holder. Position the body so that the long axis of both the femur and tibia are in the same plane. Instruct the patient to lean forward so the shaft of the femur will form a 25-degree angle with vertical.

Central ray

Direct the central ray perpendicular through the knee to the center of the film holder.

Immobilization

Place wedge sponges under both ankles and a sponge under the opposite knee to alleviate discomfort.

Right-left markers

The correct marker is burned in the superior center border of the film over the cone field after the exposure is made.

Technical tips

Place elderly patients in a kneeling position on a bench at the end of the table, with the thorax resting on the tabletop.

Structures demonstrated

Anterior (P-A) views of the intercondylar fossa, joint space between the femur and tibia, tibial plateau, and intercondylar eminence.

Note:

For supine patients, place a curved or flexible film holder beneath the posterior surface of the knee (flexed 115 degrees) and reverse the central ray angle through the notch to the film holder.

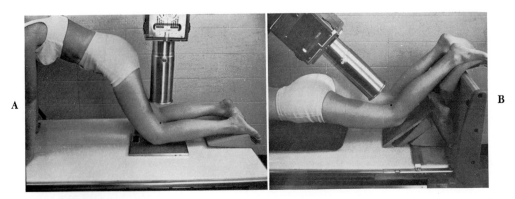

Fig. 10-33. Knee—notch (intercondylar) position. **A,** Normal notch position. **B,** Variation of normal notch position.

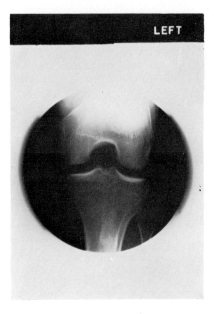

Fig. 10-34. Knee—notch (intercondylar) view. (Courtesy Dr. E. I. L. Cilley, Dr. T. W. Crowell, Dr. R. E. Waud, and Dr. G. H. Hoffman)

Knee—patella—tangential view (Figs. 10-35 and 10-36)

Film size—8″ × 10″	*Tabletop*
Cassette	*Extension cone*
Lengthwise	*(fully extended)*

Technique

Factors	Screen film cassette (par)	Screen film cardboard	No-screen film cardboard
Ma	100	100	100
Time	0.1	0.75	0.2
Mas	10	75	20
Thickness in cm	13	13	13
Kvp	66	80	80
Distance	40	40	40

Patient preparation

Remove both shoes and any garments around the knee area. Provide a gown if necessary.

Palpation points

Lateral and medial epicondyles of the femur; patellar body and apex.

Procedure

Place the patient in the prone position. Flex the knee slowly so that the long axis of the tibia forms a 60-degree angle with the femur. Center the cassette under the patella. Place a gauze strip around the ankle and extend the gauze over the shoulder; instruct the patient to hold the gauze securely.

Central ray

Direct the central ray 10 degrees cephalad through the patella to the the center of the film holder.

Immobilization

Place sandbags over the femur. Place a wedge sponge in the back of the knee to support the leg. The gauze strip around the ankle should complete the immobilization.

Right-left markers

The correct marker is burned in the superior center border of the film holder over the cone field after the exposure is made.

Technical tips

The long axis of the tibia is located in the anterior one third of the leg.

Structures demonstrated

Axial views of the patella and patellar surface of the femur.

Note:

For supine patients, have the patient support the film holder parallel with the femur over the anterior knee (flexed 60 degrees) and reverse the central ray angle through the patella to the film holder.

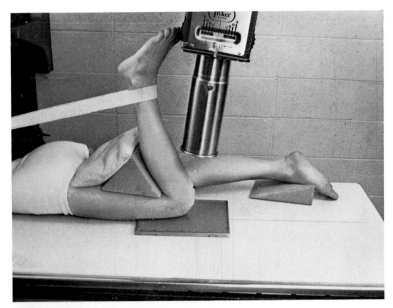

Fig. 10-35. Knee—patella, tangential position.

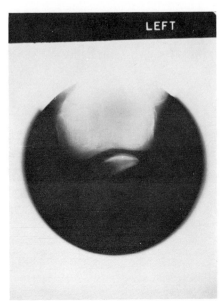

Fig. 10-36. Knee—patella, tangential view. (Courtesy Dr. E. I. L. Cilley, Dr. T. W. Crowell, Dr. R. E. Waud, and Dr. G. H. Hoffman.)

Femur

Femur—posterior (A-P) view (Figs. 10-37 and 10-38)

> Film size—14″ × 17″ or 7″ × 17″   Bucky
> Cassette   Cone to cover
> Lengthwise

Technique

Factors	Screen film cassette (par) Bucky	Screen film cassette (par) tabletop
Ma	100	100
Time	0.7	0.1
Mas	70	10
Thickness in cm	16	16
Kvp	66	64
Distance	40	40

Patient preparation

Remove shoes and garments from waist to knee. Provide a gown.

Palpation points

Lateral and medial epicondyles and greater trochanter of the femur; apex of the patella.

Procedure

Place the patient in the supine position with the legs fully extended. Center the long axis of the femur over the center line of the table. Rotate the leg so that a line through both femoral epicondyles is parallel with the film surface. Include the joint nearer to the injured site. For the upper femur, place the superior edge of the cassette 3 inches above the greater trochanter. For the lower femur, place the inferior edge of the cassette 2 inches below the apex of the patella.

Central ray

Direct the central ray perpendicular through the shaft of the femur to the center of the film holder.

Immobilization

Place sandbags on each side of the foot. Employ suspended expiration.

Right-left markers

Place the correct marker on the lateral center border of the film holder.

Technical tips

Keep the long axis of the femur parallel with the film by placing a radiolucent sponge beneath the posterior knee.

Structures demonstrated

Posterior (A-P) views of the femur, hip, and/or knee joints.

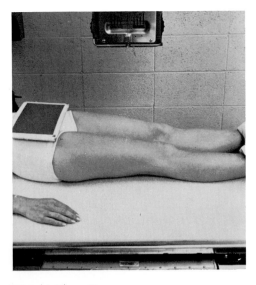

Fig. 10-37. Femur—posterior (A-P) position.

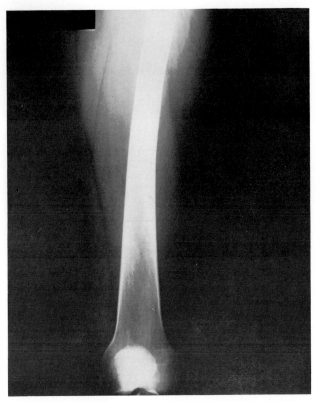

Fig. 10-38. Femur—posterior (A-P) view. (Courtesy Dr. E. I. L. Cilley, Dr. T. W. Crowell, Dr. R. E. Waud, and Dr. G. H. Hoffman.)

Femur—lateral view (Figs. 10-39 and 10-40)

> *Film size—14" × 17" or 7" × 17"*   *Bucky*
> *Cassette*   *Cone to cover*
> *Lengthwise*

Technique

Factors	Screen film cassette (par) Bucky	Screen film cassette (par) tabletop
Ma	100	100
Time	0.7	0.1
Mas	70	10
Thickness in cm	16	16
Kvp	66	64
Distance	40	40

Patient preparation

Remove shoes and garments from waist to knee. Provide a gown.

Palpation points

Lateral and medial epicondyles and greater trochanter of the femur; apex of the patella.

Procedure

Place the patient in a lateral recumbent position on the side being examined. Flex the opposite knee and cross it over the affected leg as far as possible. Center the long axis of the femur over the center line of the table. Rotate the body so that a line through both femoral epicondyles is perpendicular to the film surface. Place the inferior edge of the cassette 2 inches below the apex of the patella.

Central ray

Direct the central ray perpendicular through the shaft of the femur to the center of the film holder.

Immobilization

Place a sponge under the foot, and sandbags on the leg of the affected side. Place a large sponge under the opposite knee for support.

Right-left markers

Place the correct marker on the anterior center border of the film holder.

Technical tips

Adjust technique as necessary to compensate for an increased thickness of the proximal thigh.

Structures demonstrated

Lateral views of the lower two thirds of the femur, knee joint, and patella.

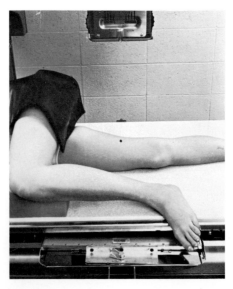

Fig. 10-39. Femur—lateral position.

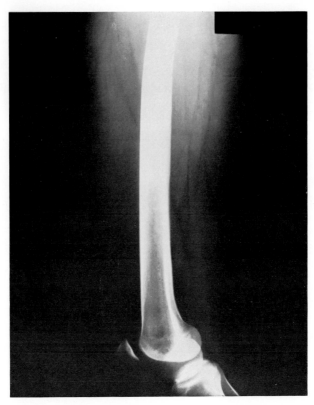

Fig. 10-40. Femur—lateral view. (Courtesy Dr. E. I. L. Cilley, Dr. T. W. Crowell, Dr. R. E. Waud, and Dr. G. H. Hoffman.)

Chapter 11

Bones of the trunk

Vertebral column

The vertebral column consists of twenty-four true vertebrae and nine other segments. It is divided into five sections: the *cervical*, seven vertebrae, the first of which is called the *atlas* and the second the *axis;* the *thoracic*, twelve vertebrae; the *lumbar*, five vertebrae; the *sacrum*, five segments that are fused together; and the *coccyx*, from three to five segments, with an average of four. A lateral projection of the vertebral column demonstrates four distinct curves: the cervical, anteriorly convex; the thoracic, anteriorly concave; the lumbar, anteriorly convex; and the sacrum and coccyx, anteriorly concave. (See Fig. 11-1.)

Since the x-rays radiate from the target in an arc limited in degrees by the tube port and the cone or diaphragm, it is often useful to take advantage of the natural spinal curvatures for radiography. Since the anterior curvatures of the thoracic spine and sacrococcygeal region are concave, a posterior projection permits the x-rays to pass between the vertebral bodies and demonstrate the intervertebral spaces. Because the anterior curvatures of the cervical and lumbar regions are convex, the best separation of the vertebral bodies in these regions results from anterior projections. It is necessary either to obtain prior permission to change routine or to inform the physician who reads the radiographs of any changes from routine in the positions used.

Common aspects of all vertebrae

Two distinct portions are found in each vertebra: anteriorly, the *body*, and posteriorly, the *neural*, or vertebral, *arch*. These parts enclose the *spinal foramen.** The neural arch is composed of the two *pedicles* and the two *laminae*. Seven processes extend from the neural arch: four articular, two transverse, and one spinous. One of the functions of the vertebrae is the formation of a column that supports the entire body. Since each vertebra articulates closely with the one immediately above and the one immediately below it, the spinal foramina join together to form the *spinal canal*, which protects the spinal cord *(medulla spinalis);* this is another function of the spine. The spinal nerves and branches, along with the nutrient vessels, pass through the *intervertebral foramina*, which are bilateral between each two vertebrae.

Body. The body is round and is the largest single part. The superior and inferior surfaces are flat and rough, and their margins form a distinct rim.

---

*The spinal foramen is also called the vertebral foramen.

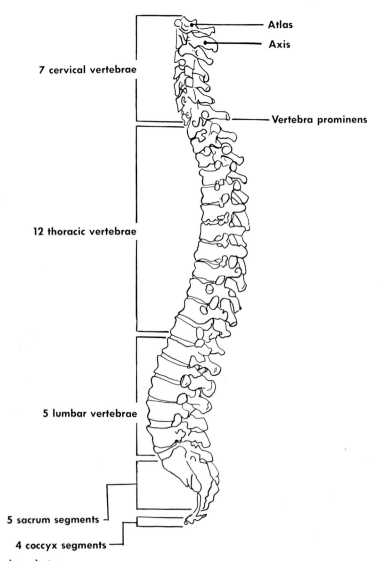

7 cervical vertebrae

Atlas

Axis

Vertebra prominens

12 thoracic vertebrae

5 lumbar vertebrae

5 sacrum segments

4 coccyx segments

Fig. 11-1. Spine, lateral view.

Pedicles. There are two strong pedicles located bilaterally and posteriorly on each body. They project from the junction of the posterior and lateral surfaces. The *vertebral notches* are the depressions that are superior and inferior to the pedicles. The intervertebral foramen is formed by the inferior vertebral notch of the body of the vertebra above joining the superior vertebral notch of the body of the vertebra below.

Laminae. The laminae extend posteriorly and medially from the pedicles. The spinal foramen is closed posteriorly by their midline fusion.

Processes. There are seven processes common to all typical vertebral bodies.

Spinous process. The spinous process, which can be palpated, projects posteriorly and inferiorly from the fusion of the laminae.

Articular processes. The pedicles join the laminae bilaterally to form parts of the neural arch. From these junctions extend the two superior and two inferior articular processes. The superior articular surfaces extend posteriorly and the inferior articular surfaces extend anteriorly. The superior facet of the body of the vertebra below articulates with the inferior facet of the body of the vertebra above.

Transverse processes. The juncture of the laminae with the pedicles is below the base of the superior articular process and above the base of the inferior articular process. From this site extend the transverse processes.

Cervical vertebrae

The cervical vertebrae are quite small and are the only vertebrae that contain a foramen in each transverse process (called *transverse foramina*). There is uniqueness in the structure of three of the cervical vertebrae, the first, second, and seventh. The second through the seventh have two superior and two inferior articular facets, one spinous process, and two transverse processes.

First cervical vertebra (atlas). The head rotates upon the ring-shaped atlas (first cervical vertebra), which has no body. In prenatal life the body of the first cervical vertebra fuses with that of the second (axis), forming a superior projection *(odontoid process)* of the axis. The first cervical vertebra has no spinous process. Two lateral masses separate its anterior and posterior arches. In the center of the posterior margin of the anterior arch there is an articular surface with which the odontoid process (dens) articulates. The posterior arch presents a posterior tubercle instead of a spinous process. The superior articular facets articulate with the occipital condyles, and the inferior articular facets articulate with the superior articular facets of the axis. (See Fig. 11-2.)

Second cervical vertebra (axis). The axis is unique in that it supports the odontoid process, which enables rotation of the atlas. (See Fig. 11-3.)

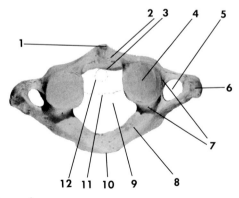

Fig. 11-2. Atlas, superior surface.

1. Anterior tubercle	7. Lateral mass
2. Anterior arch	8. Posterior arch
3. Articulation for odontoid process	9. Vertebral foramen
4. Superior articular facet	10. Posterior tubercle
5. Transverse foramen	11. Site of transverse atlantal ligament
6. Transverse process	12. Outline of odontoid process

Seventh cervical vertebra. The most prominent spinous process of all the sections is on the seventh cervical vertebra. For this reason this vertebra is called the *vertebra prominens.* The posterior end of the spinous process of the seventh cervical vertebra is usually bifurcated, while this condition is nonexistent in the spinous processes of the other cervical vertebra. The transverse processes are larger in this vertebra than in the other cervical vertebrae. (See Fig. 11-4.)

Thoracic vertebrae

The thoracic vertebrae are larger than the cervical vertebrae. They become progressively larger from the first through the twelfth. The *costal* (rib) *facets* are

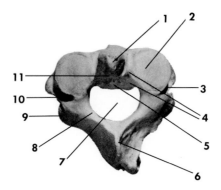

Fig. 11-3. Axis, posterosuperior surface.

1. Odontoid process
2. Superior articular surface (facet)
3. Transverse foramen
4. Attachment for alar ligaments
5. Body
6. Spinous process
7. Vertebral foramen
8. Lamina
9. Transverse process
10. Transverse foramen
11. Articulation for transverse ligament of atlas

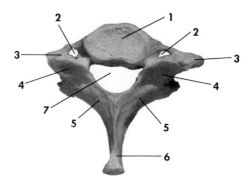

Fig 11-4. Vertebra prominens, superior surface.

1. Body
2. Transverse foramen
3. Transverse process
4. Superior articular facet
5. Lamina
6. Spinous process
7. Vertebral foramen

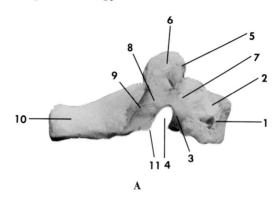

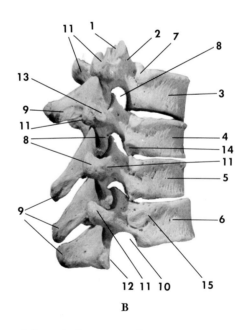

Fig. 11-5. Thoracic vertebrae, lateral surfaces.

A, First thoracic vertebra

1. Body
2. Costovertebral facet
3. Lower costal facet
4. Inferior vertebral notch
5. Superior articular facet
6. Superior articular process

7. Pedicle
8. Costotransverse facet
9. Transverse process
10. Spinous process
11. Inferior articular facet

B, Eighth, ninth, tenth, and eleventh thoracic vertebrae.

1. Superior articular facet
2. Superior articular process
3. Body of T-8
4. Body of T-9
5. Body of T-10
6. Body of T-11
7. Upper costal facet
8. Intervertebral foramen

9. Spinous process
10. Inferior vertebral notch
11. Transverse process
12. Inferior articular facet
13. Costotransverse facet
14. Lower costal facet
15. Costovertebral facet

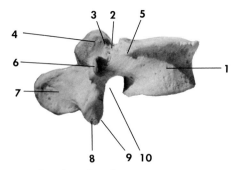

Fig. 11-6. Fourth lumbar vertebra, lateral surface.

1. Body
2. Superior vertebral notch
3. Superior articular facet
4. Superior articular process
5. Pedicle

6. Transverse process
7. Spinous process
8. Inferior articular process
9. Inferior articular facet
10. Inferior vertebral notch

found only on these vertebrae. From the first through the tenth there are additional facets that articulate with the rib tubercles. The differences of articulation in the thoracic vertebral bodies are as follows:

1. The first pair of ribs articulates with the costotransverse facet and the costovertebral facet of the first thoracic vertebra. The second pair of ribs articulates with the costotransverse facet and the upper costal facet of the second thoracic vertebra and the lower costal facet of the first.
2. The third pair of ribs articulates with the costotransverse facet and the upper costal facet of the third thoracic vertebra and the lower costal facet of the second.
3. The first through the eighth thoracic vertebrae have two rib articulations on each side of each vertebra.
4. The ninth and tenth thoracic vertebrae are slightly different in that the ninth pair of ribs articulates with a costotransverse facet and a costovertebral facet of the ninth thoracic vertebra, and the tenth pair of ribs articulates with a costotransverse facet and a costovertebral facet of the tenth thoracic vertebra. The eleventh and twelfth thoracic vertebra have no costotransverse facets, only costovertebral facets on each side.

Throughout the vertebral column the superior articular facets of a body articulate with the inferior articular facets of the body above. This type of articulation is a true *apophyseal articulation;* an apophysis is an outgrowth (process) that has never been entirely separated from a bone. Each vertebral body (centrum) articulates with the intervertebral disks, the spongelike fibrocartilages located between each two vertebral bodies. (See Fig. 11-5.)

Lumbar vertebrae

The lumbar vertebrae are remarkably larger than the thoracic. The transverse processes are more prominent radiographically, although they are longer and more slender than are those of the other sections. The processes of the first three lumbar vertebrae are truly horizontal, while those of the last two are inclined somewhat superiorly. The thickness of the fifth lumbar vertebra (anteriorly) accounts for the prominence of the *lumbosacral articulation*. Its spinous process is smaller and its transverse processes are thicker. The inferior articular facets are spaced farther apart. The fifth lumbar body frequently presents a condition termed spina bifida occulta. The articulations of the lumbar vertebrae are the same as the thoracic except that there are no rib articulations. (See Fig. 11-6.) The one very important articulation, called the lumbosacral joint, is that of the last lumbar vertebra with the sacrum.

Sacrum and coccyx

In very young children the sacrum and coccyx (nine segments) are distinct and separate. The proximal five fuse and constitute the sacrum. The distal four, which do not usually fuse, constitute the coccyx. At times the coccyx may consist of three or five segments.

Sacrum. The sacrum is large and resembles a triangle whose base is proximal and apex distal. It is inferior to the fifth lumbar vertebra, between the ilia. It forms the superior and posterior parts of the pelvic cavity. Superiorly it articulates with the inferior surface of the last (usually fifth) lumbar vertebra, forming the lumbosacral joint. Inferiorly it articulates with the coccyx, forming the sacrococcygeal joint. Bilaterally its articulations form the right and left *sacroiliac joints*. In radiographic examinations the sacrum and coccyx are considered as parts of the pelvis and not true vertebrae. Anatomically the sacrum and coccyx are considered as parts of the vertebral column. The first sacral segment has articular facets that

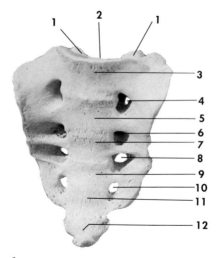

Fig. 11-7. Sacrum, dorsal surface.

1. Articular facet of S-1	7. Body of third sacral segment
2. Articulates with last lumbar vertebra	8. Third posterior sacral foramen
3. Body of first sacral segment	9. Body of fourth sacral segment
4. First posterior sacral foramen	10. Fourth posterior sacral foramen
5. Body of second sacral segment	11. Body of fifth sacral segment
6. Second posterior sacral foramen	12. First coccygeal segment

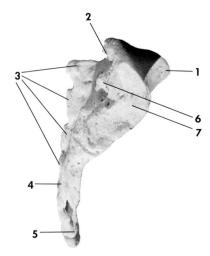

Fig. 11-8. Sacrum and coccyx, lateral surface.

1. Body of first sacral segment
2. Articular facet
3. Medial sacral crest
4. Cornu of sacrum

5. Coccyx
6. Sacral tuberosity
7. Articular surface (for ilium)

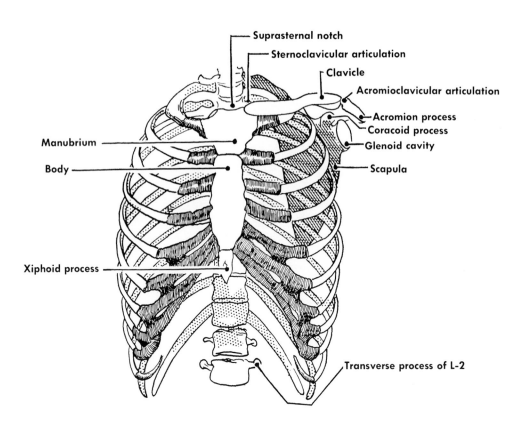

Fig. 11-9. Thoracic cage, anterior view.

articulate with the inferior articular facets of the last lumbar vertebra. The concave pelvic surface of the sacrum presents four transverse ridges that are in line with the early articulations of the five segments. The anterior sacral foramina are bilateral at the ends of these ridges. The spinal canal exists in most of the sacrum and contains the sacral nerves. The walls of the spinal canal contain the anterior and posterior sacral foramina. (See Fig. 11-7.)

Coccyx. None of the coccygeal segments has pedicles, laminae, or spinous processes. The proximal segment is the largest of these segments and is usually separate. The remaining segments become progressively smaller in size and are frequently fused. The apex of the coccyx is rounded, sometimes bifid, and frequently displaced to either side. (See Fig. 11-8.)

Thoracic cage

Radiographically the bones of the thoracic cage present essentially the same, or at least similar, problems in penetration. These bones include the clavicles, sternum, scapulae, and ribs. (See Fig. 11-9.)

Clavicle

The anterosuperior portion of the shoulder girdle is formed by the clavicle. This bone is shaped somewhat like a shallow S. It is slightly superior to the first rib anteriorly and is very nearly horizontal. It is easily palpated. The clavicle extends from the sternum, medially, to the acromion process of the scapula, laterally. As previously mentioned, it presents two curves: convex anteriorly and medially and concave anteriorly and laterally. It forms the *sternoclavicular articulation,* or joint, in its articulation with the manubrium of the sternum, and the *acromioclavicular articulation,* or joint, in its articulation with the acromion process of the scapula. In addition to the medial articulation with the sternum, it articulates medially and inferiorly with the cartilage of the first rib. Cancellous tissue makes up most of the clavicle. It is the last bone of the body to ossify. It is ossified from two centers, a medial and a lateral for the body, and one center for the sternal end. The first two centers are primary, and the latter is secondary. The clavicle is not completely ossified until about the twenty-fifth year of life.

Sternum

The sternum, or breastbone, consists of three parts: proximally, the *manubrium,* or handle; medially, the *body* or gladiolus; and distally, the *xiphoid process,* or ensiform cartilage. It lies between the anterior ends of the first seven ribs in the anterior wall of the thoracic cavity. It is thin and flat and is composed chiefly of cancellous tissue. True bone forms the outer layer. The manubrium is the thickest part of the sternum. The xiphoid process does not completely ossify and is usually entirely cartilaginous until late in life. Superiorly on the manubrium and between the sternoclavicular articulations is the *sternal notch.* In addition to the articulations with the clavicles, the manubrium has five other articular surfaces: inferiorly, one for the body; bilaterally on each side and inferior to the sternoclaviculars, two for the first costal cartilages; bilaterally on each side and inferiorly, two for the second costal cartilages. The body articulates superiorly with the manubrium and inferiorly with the xiphoid process. The second rib articulates in the angle formed by the junction of the body and manubrium. The body articulates with the second through the seventh ribs on both sides. These articulations are with the costal cartilages. The xiphoid process articulates superiorly with the body and slightly with the seventh rib cartilage on each side. It usually ends in a rather sharp point but may be bifid or angled to either side.

Scapula

The scapula, or shoulder blade, is located posteriorly, superiorly, and laterally in relation to the thoracic cage. Together with the clavicle, it forms the *shoulder girdle*. The scapula is a flat bone. The three borders with the three angles form a triangle. The *spine* of the scapula is on the posterior surface and extends obliquely upward from the junction of the proximal and mid-thirds of the vertebral border and across the lateral angle. The scapula has a base, which is the superior border, and an apex, which is inferior to the body. The three borders are as follows: the vertebral, or medial; axillary, or lateral; and superior, or base. The three angles are as follows: the medial, at the junction of the vertebral and superior borders; the inferior (apex), at the junction of the vertebral and axillary borders; and the lateral (head of the scapula), at the junction of the axillary and superior borders. The lateral angle contains a shallow fossa called the *glenoid cavity*, which is the articular surface for the head of the humerus. The spine of the scapula extends beyond the lateral angle and curves forward over the glenoid cavity, terminating in a process called the *acromion*. The acromion process articulates with the lateral end of the clavicle. The *coracoid process* is quite thick and is attached to the neck of the scapula. It extends in a generally ventral or anterior direction from the scapula.

Ribs

There are usually twelve pairs of ribs; however, there may be an additional pair of ribs, either on the last cervical body or on the first lumbar body. Sometimes there are only eleven pairs. The first seven pairs articulate with the sternum and vertebral column; these are called *true ribs*. The eighth, ninth, and tenth pairs articulate posteriorly with the vertebral column and anteriorly with the cartilage of the rib above; the latter are called *false ribs*. The eleventh and twelfth pairs are not attached anteriorly and are the *floating* or vertebral, *ribs*. Radiographically the ribs must be considered in two groups: those above the diaphragm and those below the diaphragm. Each rib has a posterior, or vertebral end, and an anterior, or sternal end, which are separated by the body. The major articulation of each rib is with the thoracic vertebra of the same number. In addition to a head, each rib has a neck and a tubercle. A rib extends obliquely downward to the midaxillary line, from which point it continues downward and anteriorly to its anterior (sternal) articulation. The spaces between each two ribs are called the intercostal spaces.

Pelvis

Anatomically the pelvis consists of two bones, the pelvic (innominate) bones. Each pelvic bone is composed of three bones that are solidly fused: the *ilium,*

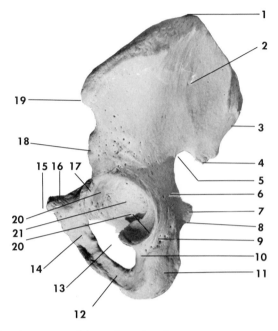

Fig. 11-10. Left pelvic (innominate) bone, lateral surface.

1. Crest of ilium
2. Wing (ala) of ilium
3. Posterior superior spine
4. Posterior inferior spine
5. Greater sciatic notch
6. Body of ilium
7. Ischial spine
8. Lesser sciatic notch
9. Body of ischium
10. Descending ramus of ischium
11. Ischial tuberosity

12. Ascending ramus of ischium
13. Obturator foramen
14. Posterior ramus of pubis
15. Symphysis pubis
16. Anterior ramus of pubis
17. Body of pubis
18. Anterior inferior spine
19. Anterior superior spine
20. Acetabulum
21. Articular ring of acetabulum

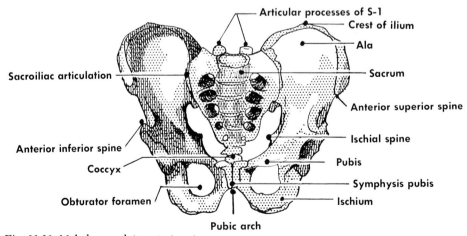

Fig. 11-11. Male bony pelvis, anterior view.

the *ischium,* and the *pubis.* They are fused in the *acetabulum* (hip socket), which is the articular fossa for the head of the femur. (See Figs. 11-10 and 11-11.)

Ilium

The ilium is composed of a body and a wing (ala). The body is inferior, near the acetabulum. The wing is quite large and extends upward, laterally and medially. It forms the lateral boundary of the pelvis and derives its name from its relation with the flank. In general outline the crest of the ilium is convex and rough. The thickened anterior and posterior parts terminate in the *anterior* and *posterior superior iliac spines.* The *anterior* and *posterior inferior iliac spines* are separated from the superior iliac spines by a distinct notch. The anterior superior iliac spine is a very important landmark radiographically.

Ischium

The ischium is the most inferior and the strongest bone of the pelvis. It extends inferiorly from the acetabulum, forming a large tuberosity, and then continues and curves anteriorly, where it forms, with the pubis, the *obturator foramen.* The ischium consists of a *body,* a *superior ramus,* and an *inferior ramus.* The superior and inferior rami join below the obturator foramen. On the inferior surface of this junction is the *ischial tuberosity.* The superior ramus descends posteriorly from the acetabulum to its junction with the inferior ramus, while the inferior ramus ascends anteriorly from this junction. The *ischial spine,* an important radiographic landmark in posterior projections of the pelvis, projects medially from the posterior border of the body.

Pubis

The pubis lies medially and inferiorly to the acetabulum. It articulates with the opposite pubis in the midsagittal plane, forming the *symphysis pubis.* It forms the anterior portion of the pelvis. The pubis consists of a body and two rami. From its junction with the inferior ramus of the ischium, the *inferior ramus* of the pubis ascends to its junction with the *superior ramus.*

Acetabulum

The acetabulum is formed by the fusion of the bodies of the ilium, ischium, and pubis. The pubis forms only one fifth, while the remainder is formed equally by the ilium and the ischium. The pubis is medial, the ilium is superior, and the ischium is inferior.

Obturator foramen

The obturator foramen is bounded as follows: superiorly by the superior ramus of the pubis; medially and anteriorly, by the union of the superior and inferior rami of the pubis; laterally and posteriorly, by the superior ramus of the ischium; and inferiorly, by the inferior rami of the ischium and pubis.

REFERENCES

Anthony, Catherine Parker: Textbook of anatomy and physiology, St. Louis, 1967, The C. V. Mosby Co.
Best, C. H., and Taylor, N. B.: The living body, New York, 1952, Henry Holt & Co., Inc.
Best, C. H., and Taylor, N. B.: The human body, New York, 1956, Henry Holt & Co., Inc.

De Coursey, Russell Myles: The human organism, New York, 1955, McGraw-Hill Book Co.

Goss, Charles M.: Gray's anatomy, ed. 28, Philadelphia, 1966, Lea & Febiger.

Greisheimer, Esther M.: Physiology and anatomy, Philadelphia, 1950, J. B. Lippincott Co.

Kimber, Diana Clifford, and Gray, Carolyn E.: Textbook of anatomy and physiology, New York, 1928, The Macmillan Co.

Meschan, Isadore: Normal radiographic anatomy, Philadelphia, 1951, W. B. Saunders Co.

Chapter 12

Positioning for the trunk

Routine

The routine steps are as follows:

1. Know the desired position.
2. Select all factors except kilovoltage.
3. Conduct the patient into the radiographic room. If cooperation of the patient is possible, have him assume the desired position.
4. After deciding what size film to use, place the film in the Bucky tray. Use proper identification and an R or L to denote the right or left side.
5. If possible, explain to the patient what is going to be done.
6. Use the center of the cone or tube as a guide to center the patient crosswise on the table.
7. Center the film holder or the tube (the selection depends upon the radiographic position) to the part being radiographed.
8. If the patient is centered with the tube, then center the film holder to the tube. If the film holder is centered to the patient, then center the tube to the center of the film holder.
9. Measure the patient for the thickness of the part, and, from the technique chart, determine the kilovoltage and select the proper kilovoltage on the control panel.
10. Close the primary switch, and check the line voltage.
11. Double check the Bucky switch.
12. Give the patient proper breathing instructions.
13. *Observe movement of the patient until the moment that the exposure is made.*
14. During the exposure, ascertain that the machine is delivering the desired milliamperage by watching the milliampere meter.
15. Instruct the patient to resume normal breathing.

If another view is required, select the proper factors on the control panel at this time, remove the exposed film (in the cassette), and replace with the proper-sized film and film holder for the next exposure. Then repeat the same routine steps. The starting factors stated for all the following techniques are for a 12:1 grid when a Bucky is used.

Cervical spine
Cervical spine—posterior (A-P) view (Figs. 12-1 and 12-2)

Film size—8″ × 10″   Bucky
Cassette   Cone to cover
Lengthwise

Technique

Factors	Screen film cassette (par) Bucky
Ma	100
Time	0.5
Mas	50
Thickness in cm	14
Kvp	62
Distance	40

Patient preparation

Remove all garments down to the shoulders. Remove dentures, hairpins, and jewelry around the cervical area. Provide a gown for female patients.

Palpation points

Angle of the mandible; thyroid cartilage; vertebra prominens.

Procedure

Place the patient in the supine position with the midline of the body over the center line of the table. The midsagittal plane of the head is perpendicular to the tabletop. Elevate the chin so that a line from the upper occlusal plane to the base of the occiput is perpendicular to the tabletop.

Central ray

Direct the central ray 15 degrees cephalad through the thyroid cartilage to the center of the film holder.

Immobilization

If necessary, brace both sides of the cranium with sandbags. Place sponges under the knees. Employ suspended expiration.

Right-left markers

Place the R marker on the right side, center border of the film holder.

Technical tips

Decrease the central ray angle to demonstrate the upper intervertebral spaces. Increase the central ray angle to demonstrate the lower intervertebral spaces.

Structures demonstrated

Posterior (A-P) views of the lower five cervical bodies, the corresponding intervertebral spaces, the transverse processes, the interpedicular spaces, and the upper two or three thoracic bodies.

Note:

To demonstrate cervical ribs, direct the central ray perpendicular through the seventh cervical vertebra to the center of a 10″ × 12″ film holder.

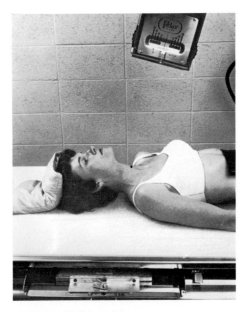

Fig. 12-1. Cervical spine—posterior (A-P) position.

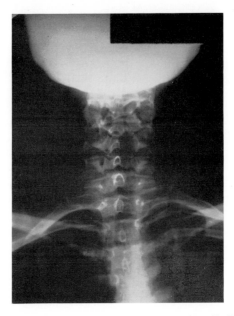

Fig. 12-2. Cervical spine—posterior (A-P) view. (Courtesy Dr. E. I. L. Cilley, Dr. T. W. Crowell, Dr. R. E. Waud, and Dr. G. H. Hoffman.)

Cervical spine—posterior (A-P) atlas and axis (open-mouth) view (Figs. 12-3 and 12-4)

Film size—8″ × 10″   *Bucky*
Cassette   *Extension cone*
Lengthwise   *(fully extended)*

Technique

Factors	Screen film cassette (par) Bucky
Ma	100
Time	0.5
Mas	50
Thickness in cm	14
Kvp	66
Distance	40

Patient preparation

Remove dentures, and hairpins over the occipital area.

Palpation point

Base of occiput.

Procedure

Place the patient in the supine position with the midline of the body over the center line of the table. The midsagittal plane of the head is perpendicular to the tabletop. Elevate the chin so that a line from the upper occlusal plane to the base of the occiput is perpendicular to the tabletop. Insert a sterile 1½-inch cork between the patient's jaws.

Central ray

Direct the central ray ½ inch inferior to and parallel with the upper occlusal plane to the center of the film holder.

Immobilization

Place sandbags against the vertex of the cranium. Employ suspended expiration.

Right-left markers

Burn the R marker in the superior border of the right side of the film holder above the cone field after the exposure is made.

Technical tips

For patients with short stocky necks, elevate the occiput slightly with a radiolucent sponge to aid in vertical alignment.

Structures demonstrated

Posterior (A-P) views of the atlas and axis through the open mouth.

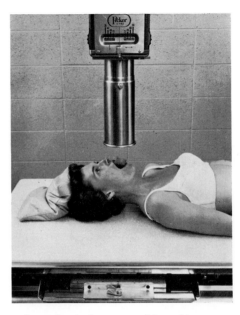

Fig. 12-3. Cervical spine—atlas and axis (open-mouth) position.

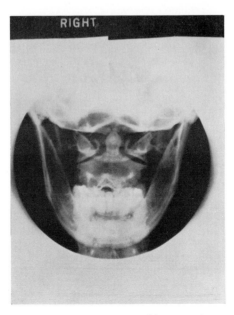

Fig. 12-4. Cervical spine—atlas and axis (open-mouth) view. (Courtesy Dr. E. I. L. Cilley, Dr. T. W. Crowell, Dr. R. E. Waud, and Dr. G. H. Hoffman.)

Cervical spine—lateral view (Figs. 12-5 and 12-6)

> *Film size—10″ × 12″*   *Erect film holder*
> *Cassette*   *Cone to cover*
> *Lengthwise*

Technique

Factors	Screen film cassette (par)
Ma	100
Time	0.3
Mas	30
Thickness in cm	12
Kvp	66
Distance	72

Patient preparation

Remove all garments down to the shoulders. Remove dentures, hairpins, and jewelry around the cervical area. Provide a gown for female patients.

Palpation points

Angle of the mandible; thyroid cartilage; vertebra prominens.

Procedure

Place the patient in a lateral position, either sitting or standing, with one shoulder against an erect film holder. Have the patient keep his back straight and shoulders relaxed, then place a sandbag in each hand to hold the shoulders down. The midsagittal plane of the head and body is parallel with the film surface. Elevate the chin, and place the top of the cassette 2 inches above the external auditory meatus.

Central ray

Direct the central ray perpendicular through the cervical spine to the center of the film holder.

Immobilization

Place a radiolucent sponge between the head and the film holder. Use a compression band if necessary. Employ suspended expiration.

Right-left markers

Place the correct marker on the posterior center border of the film holder.

Technical tips

Because the patient will always move slightly after suspending respiration, delay the exposure approximately 2 seconds.

Structures demonstrated

Lateral views of the cervical bodies, interspaces, lower apophyseal articulations, and spinous processes.

Note:

For supine patients, elevate the head and place a vertical film holder parallel with the cervical spine. If possible, use a 72-inch focal-film distance to compensate for increased object-film distance.

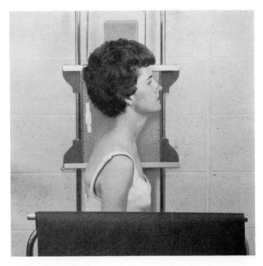

Fig. 12-5. Cervical spine—lateral position.

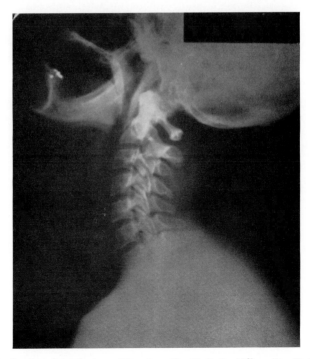

Fig. 12-6. Cervical spine—lateral view. (Courtesy Dr. E. I. L. Cilley, Dr. T. W. Crowell, Dr. R. E. Waud, and Dr. G. H. Hoffman.)

Cervical spine—posteroanterior-oblique (L.A.O.-R.A.O.) view (Figs. 12-7 and 12-8)

> *Film size*—*8″ × 10″*   *Bucky*
> *Cassette*   *Cone to cover*
> *Lengthwise*

Technique

Factors	Screen film cassette (par)
Ma	100
Time	0.6
Mas	60
Thickness in cm	14
Kvp	66
Distance	40

Patient preparation

Remove all garments down to the shoulders. Remove dentures, hairpins, and jewelry around the cervical area. Provide a gown for female patients.

Palpation points

Base of occiput; vertebra prominens.

Procedure

Place the patient in the prone position. Elevate the side opposite the one being examined so that the midsagittal plane of the head and body forms a 45-degree angle with the tabletop. Flex the knee and elbow of the elevated side for support. Align the long axis of the spine over the center line of the table.

Central ray

Direct the central ray 15 degree caudad through the fourth cervical vertebra to the center of the film holder.

Immobilization

Place wedge sponges under the head and flexed knee. A compression band may be used across the patient's head for additional support. Employ suspended expiration.

Right-left markers

Place the correct marker on the posterior center border of the film holder.

Technical tips

Extend the neck to eliminate the possibility of superimposing the mandibular angle over the vertebral bodies.

Structures demonstrated

Oblique view of the cervical spine, which demonstrates the intervertebral foramina of the side nearest the film; oblique view of the vertebral bodies.

Note:

Both oblique views are usually made for comparison. Erect patients may be positioned 45 degrees right posterior oblique and 45 degrees left posterior oblique with a 15-degree cephalad angle and a 72-inch focal-film distance to compensate for the increased object-film distance.

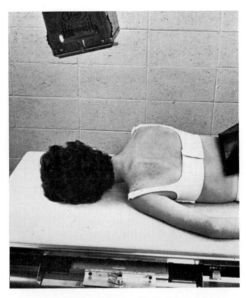

Fig. 12-7. Cervical spine—posteroanterior-oblique (L.A.O.) position.

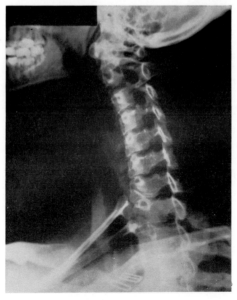

Fig. 12-8. Cervical spine—posteroanterior-oblique (L.A.O.) view. (Courtesy Dr. E. I. L. Cilley, Dr. T. W. Crowell, Dr. R. E. Waud, and Dr. G. H. Hoffman.)

Thoracic spine

Thoracic spine—posterior (A-P) view (Figs. 12-9 and 12-10)

Film size—14" × 17" or 7" × 17"   *Bucky*
Cassette   *Cone to cover*
Lengthwise

Technique

Factors	Screen film cassette (par)
Ma	100
Time	1.0
Mas	100
Thickness in cm	20
Kvp	66
Distance	40

Patient preparation

Remove all garments down to the waist. Provide a gown for female patients.

Palpation point

Vertebra prominens.

Procedure

Place the patient in the supine position. Center the midline of the body over the center line of the table. Extend the arms at the sides of the body. Grasp the patient by the ankles and pull gently to straighten the spine. Place the top of the cassette 3 inches above the vertebra prominens (spinous process of the seventh cervical vertebra).

Central ray

Direct the central ray perpendicular through the long axis of the thoracic spine to the center of the film holder.

Immobilization

Place large sponges or sandbags under both knees for comfort. Employ suspended inspiration.

Right-left markers

Place the R marker on the right lateral center border of the film holder.

Technical tips

For uniform radiographic density, use $\frac{1}{10}$ mm added copper filter internally plus an increase of 10 kvp.

Structures demonstrated

Posterior (A-P) views of the thoracic bodies, the corresponding interpedicular spaces, and generally of the intervertebral spaces.

Note:

The *heel effect* is most effective in this view. Position the patient with his head at the anode end of the x-ray tube.

For posture radiographs, place the patient in the anteroposterior erect position with the body weight distributed equally on both feet.

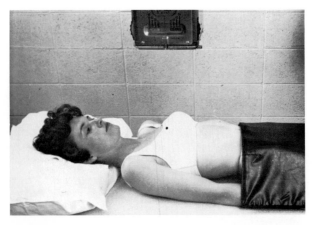

Fig. 12-9. Thoracic spine—posterior (A-P) position.

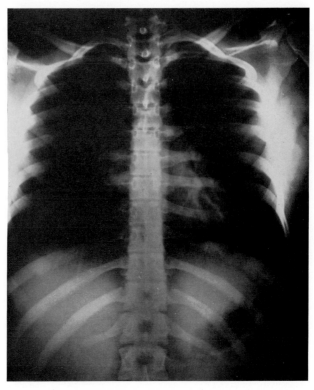

Fig. 12-10. Thoracic spine—posterior (A-P) view. (Courtesy Dr. E. I. L. Cilley, Dr. T. W. Crowell, Dr. R. E. Waud, and Dr. G. H. Hoffman.)

Thoracic spine—lateral view (Figs. 12-11 and 12-12)

> *Film size—14" × 17" or 7" × 17"*   *Bucky*
> *Cassette*   *Cone to cover*
> *Lengthwise*

Technique

Factors	Screen film cassette (par)
Ma	100
Time	1.0
Mas	100
Thickness in cm	32
Kvp	70
Distance	40

Patient preparation

Remove all garments down to the waist. Provide a gown for female patients.

Palpation points

Vertebra prominens; spinous processes of the thoracic vertebrae.

Procedure

Place the patient in a lateral recumbent position. Flex the hips and knees for support. Center the midaxillary plane of the body over the center line of the table. Flex the bottom elbow and place the forearm under the pillow. Flex the top elbow and place the forearm above the head with the hand grasping the edge of the table. Rotate the body into the true lateral position.

Central ray

Direct the central ray perpendicular to the long axis of the spine and through the sixth thoracic body to the center of the film holder.

Immobilization

Place a sponge or sandbag between the knees. Place a compression band over the pelvis. Employ suspended inspiration.

Right-left markers

Place the correct marker on the anterior center border of the film holder.

Technical tips

A slight lateral concavity or "sagging" of the thoracic spine is beneficial in demonstrating intervertebral spaces.

Structures demonstrated

Lateral views of the thoracic bodies, the corresponding interspaces, and intervertebral foramina.

Note:

The upper three thoracic vertebrae are not demonstrated in this view.

To better demonstrate the upper lateral thoracic vertebrae, employ the rapid, shallow breathing technique with low milliamperage for a longer time (25 ma for 6 seconds).

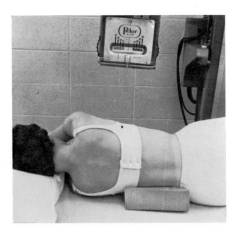

Fig. 12-11. Thoracic spine—lateral position.

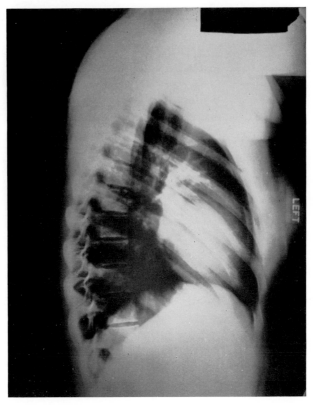

Fig. 12-12. Thoracic spine—lateral view. (Courtesy Dr. E. I. L. Cilley, Dr. T. W. Crowell, Dr. R. E. Waud, and Dr. G. H. Hoffman.)

Thoracic spine—upper oblique view (Figs. 12-13 and 12-14)

> *Film size—10″ × 12″*   *Bucky*
> *Cassette*   *Cone to cover*
> *Lengthwise*

Technique

Factors	Screen film cassette (par)
Ma	100
Time	0.6
Mas	60
Thickness in cm	30
Kvp	78
Distance	40

Patient preparation

Remove all garments down to the waist. Provide a gown for female patients.

Palpation points

Manubrium; vertebra prominens.

Procedure

Place the patient in a lateral position, either sitting or standing, with one shoulder against an erect Bucky. The midsagittal plane of the head and body is parallel with the film surface. Flex the elbow nearer to the film; at the same time raise the arm and rotate that shoulder anteriorly as far as possible without rotating the thorax. Place the opposite hand on the hip; relax this shoulder and rotate it posteriorly as far as possible. Center the midportion of the cervico-thoracic spine over the center line of the Bucky.

Central ray

Direct the central ray perpendicular through a point at the level of the manubrium to the center of the film holder.

Immobilization

Place a large sponge between the patient's head and the film holder. A compression band may be employed around the abdomen. Employ suspended expiration.

Right-left markers

Place the correct marker on the anterior center border of the film holder.

Technical tips

For uniform radiographic density, use $\frac{1}{10}$ mm added copper filter internally plus an increase of 10 kvp.

Structures demonstrated

Semilateral view of the upper thoracic and lower cervical vertebrae between the humeral heads; this view demonstrates the apophyseal articulations and the intervertebral spaces.

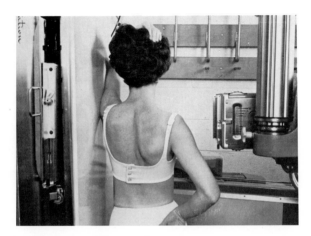

Fig. 12-13. Thoracic spine—upper oblique position.

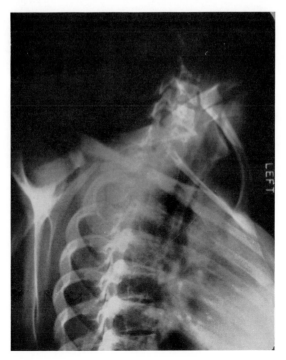

Fig. 12-14. Thoracic spine—upper oblique view. (Courtesy Dr. E. I. L. Cilley, Dr. T. W. Crowell, Dr. R. E. Waud, and Dr. G. H. Hoffman.)

Lumbar spine
Lumbar spine—posterior (A-P) view (Figs. 12-15 and 12-16)

Film size—14″ × 17″	*Bucky*
Cassette	*Cone to cover*
Lengthwise	

Technique

Factors	Screen film cassette (par)
Ma	100
Time	1.0
Mas	100
Thickness in cm	20
Kvp	66
Distance	40

Patient preparation

Remove all clothing except shoes and socks. Provide a gown for the patient.

Palpation point

Crest of ilium.

Procedure

Place the patient in the supine position with the midline of the body over the center line of the table. Grasp the patient by the ankles and pull gently to straighten the spine. Flex both knees a minimum of 6 inches and support them with sponges. Rotate the ankles internally into a true posterior (A-P) position. Center the film holder to the crest of the ilium.

Central ray

Direct the central ray perpendicular to the center of the film holder.

Immobilization

Place sandbags on the lateral sides of the ankles. A compression band may be used across large abdomens. Employ suspended expiration.

Right-left markers

Place the *R* marker on the right lateral center border of the film holder.

Technical tips

Increased knee flexion will aid in relaxation of the normal lumbar curve.

Structures demonstrated

Posterior (A-P) views of the lumbar bodies, the associated interspaces, the interpedicular spaces, the laminae, the transverse processes, the pelvis, and femoral heads; axial views of the spinous processes.

Note:

For thin patients, a posteroanterior projection will better demonstrate the intervertebral spaces.

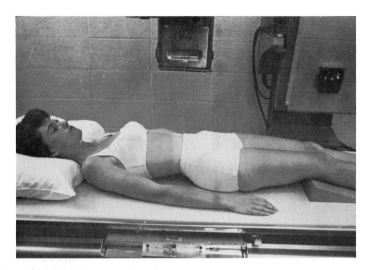

Fig. 12-15. Lumbar spine—posterior (A-P) position.

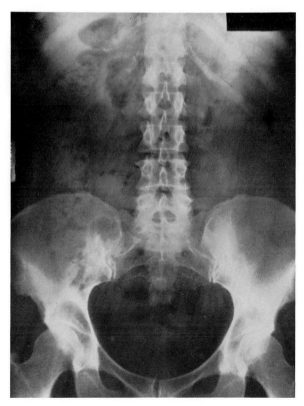

Fig. 12-16. Lumbar spine—posterior (A-P) view. (Courtesy Dr. E. I. L. Cilley, Dr. T. W. Crowell, Dr. R. E. Waud, and Dr. G. H. Hoffman.)

Lumbar spine—upper lateral view (Figs. 12-17 and 12-18)

> *Film size—10″ × 12″*   *Bucky*
> *Cassette*   *Cone to cover*
> *Lengthwise*

Technique

Factors	Screen film cassette (par)
Ma	100
Time	2.75
Mas	275
Thickness in cm	28
Kvp	76
Distance	40

Patient preparation

Remove all clothing except shoes and socks. Provide a gown for the patient.

Palpation points

Crest of the ilium; spinous processes of the lumbar vertebrae.

Procedure

Place the patient in the lateral recumbent position. Flex the hips and knees for support. Align the long axis of the spine over the center line of the table (4 inches anterior to the posterior surface). Flex the bottom elbow and place the forearm under the pillow. Flex the top elbow and place the forearm above the head with the hand grasping the edge of the table. Rotate the body into a true lateral position.

Central ray

Direct the central ray perpendicular through a point 4 inches superior to the crest of the ilium to the center of the film holder.

Immobilization

Place a sponge or sandbag between the knees. Place a compression band over the pelvis. Employ suspended expiration.

Right-left markers

Place the correct marker on the anterior center border of the film holder.

Technical tips

A slight lateral concavity or "sagging" of the lumbar spine is beneficial in demonstrating intervertebral spaces. Excessive sagging will produce "wedging" of the vertebral bodies and decrease diagnostic quality.

Structures demonstrated

Lateral views of the lower thoracic and the lumbar bodies, the corresponding interspaces, the intervertebral foramina, and the spinous processes.

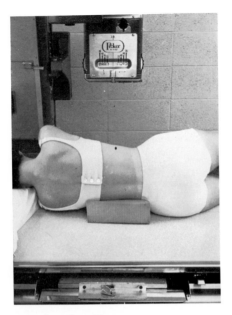

Fig. 12-17. Lumbar spine—upper lateral position.

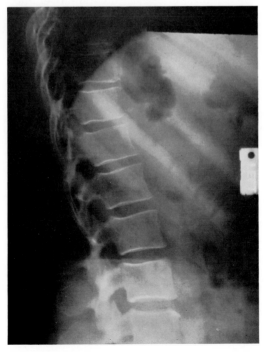

Fig. 12-18. Lumbar spine—upper lateral view. (Courtesy Dr. E. I. L. Cilley, Dr. T. W. Crowell, Dr. R. E. Waud, and Dr. G. H. Hoffman.)

Lumbar spine—lateral lumbosacral view (Figs. 12-19 and 12-20)

> *Film size—10″ × 12″*   *Bucky*
> *Cassette*   *Cone to cover*
> *Lengthwise*

Technique

Factors	Screen film cassette (par)
Ma	100
Time	3.0
Mas	300
Thickness in cm	32
Kvp	82
Distance	40

Patient preparation

Remove all clothing except shoes and socks. Provide a gown for the patient.

Palpation points

Crest of the ilium; spinous processes of the lumbar vertebrae.

Procedure

Place the patient in the lateral recumbent position. Flex the hips and knees for support. Align the long axis of the spine over the center line of the table (4 inches anterior to the posterior surface). Flex the bottom elbow and place the forearm under the pillow. Flex the top elbow and place the forearm above the head with the hand grasping the edge of the table. Rotate the body into a true lateral position.

Central ray

Direct the central ray perpendicular 1½ inches inferior to and parallel with a line between the crests of the ilia, through the lumbosacral junction to the center of the film holder.

Immobilization

Place a sponge or sandbag between the knees. Place a compression band over the pelvis. Employ suspended expiration.

Right-left markers

Place the correct marker on the anterior center border of the film holder.

Technical tips

Most patients will require a caudad central ray angle for this view.

Structures demonstrated

Lateral views of the lumbar bodies, the lumbar interspaces, the intervertebral foramina, the spinous processes, the lumbosacral junction, and the sacrum.

Note:

For suspected spondylolisthesis, make an erect lateral view utilizing the above procedure. Sacral depressions are unreliable landmarks for consistent accuracy.

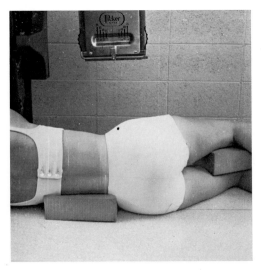

Fig. 12-19. Lumbar spine–lumbosacral region, lateral position.

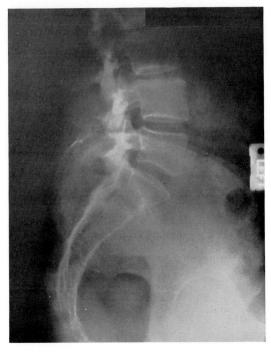

Fig. 12-20. Lumbar spine–lumbosacral region, lateral view. (Courtesy Dr. E. I. L. Cilley, Dr. T. W. Crowell, Dr. R. E. Waud, and Dr. G. H. Hoffman.)

Lumbar spine—anterior (P-A) oblique (L.A.O.-R.A.O.) view (Figs. 12-21 and 12-22)

> *Film size—10″ × 12″*   *Bucky*
> *Cassette*   *Cone to cover*
> *Lengthwise*

Technique

Factors	Screen film cassette (par)
Ma	100
Time	1.5
Mas	150
Thickness in cm	28
Kvp	74
Distance	40

Patient preparation

Remove all clothing except shoes and socks. Provide a gown for the patient.

Palpation points

Crest of the ilium; spinous processes of the lumbar vertebrae.

Procedure

Place the patient in the prone position. Elevate the side being examined so that the midsagittal plane of the body forms a 35-degree angle with the tabletop. Flex the knee and elbow of the elevated side for support. Center a line on the elevated side that is 1 inch lateral to the long axis of the spine over the center line of the table. Center the film holder to the top of the iliac crest.

Central ray

Direct the central ray perpendicular to the center of the film holder.

Immobilization

Place a wedge sponge under the flexed knee. Employ suspended expiration.

Right-left markers

Place the correct marker on the elevated side, lateral center border of the film holder.

Technical tips

Reduce the body rotation 10 degrees if the lower apophyseal joints are non-visualized.

Structures demonstrated

Oblique view of the lumbar vertebrae demonstrating the apophyseal joints of the elevated side.

Note:

Both oblique views are usually made for comparison.

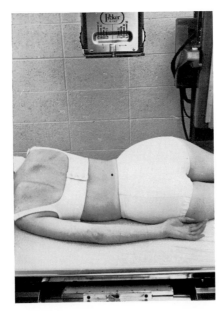

Fig. 12-21. Lumbar spine—left anterior oblique (L.A.O.) position.

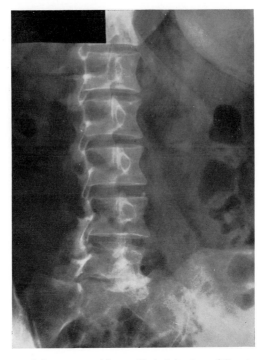

Fig. 12-22. Lumbar spine—left anterior oblique (L.A.O.) view. (Courtesy Dr. E. I. L. Cilley, Dr. T. W. Crowell, Dr. R. E. Waud, and Dr. G. H. Hoffman.)

Lumbar spine—posterior (A-P) lumbosacral articulation view (Figs. 12-23 and 12-24)

Film size—8″ × 10″	*Bucky*
Cassette	*Extension cone*
Lengthwise	*(fully extended)*

Technique

Factors	Screen film cassette (par)
Ma	100
Time	1.25
Mas	125
Thickness in cm	22
Kvp	70
Distance	40

Patient preparation

Remove all garments from the waist down. Provide a gown for the patient.

Palpation point

Symphysis pubis.

Procedure

Place the patient in the supine position with the midline of the body over the center line of the table. Grasp the patient by the ankles and pull gently to straighten the spine. Flex the knees 90 degrees, placing the feet flat on the table. Brace the feet with sandbags.

Central ray

Direct the central ray 15 degrees cephalad to enter a point 4 inches above the symphysis pubis, through the lumbosacral spine to the center of the film holder.

Immobilization

Place sandbags on the lateral sides of the ankles. A compression band may be used across large abdomens. Employ suspended expiration.

Right-left markers

Burn the R marker in the superior border of the right side of the film holder above the cone field after the exposure is made.

Technical tips

To assist in palpation, the symphysis pubis is in the transverse line with the greater trochanter of the femur.

Structures demonstrated

Posterior (A-P) views of the lumbosacral structures and interspaces.

Note:

The degree of central ray angulation will be governed somewhat by the physical stature and sex of the patient.

For prone patients, reverse the central ray angle, centering to the spinous process of the fifth lumbar vertebra.

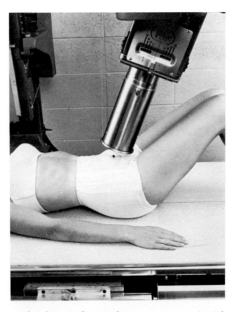

Fig. 12-23. Lumbar spine—lumbosacral articulation, posterior (A-P) position.

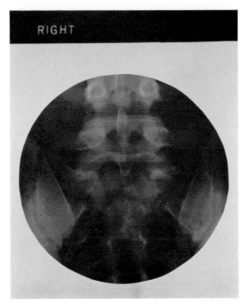

Fig. 12-24. Lumbar spine—lumbosacral articulation, posterior (A-P) view. (Courtesy Dr. E. I. L. Cilley, Dr. T. W. Crowell, Dr. R. E. Waud, and Dr. G. H. Hoffman.)

Pelvis
Pelvis—posterior (A-P) view (Figs. 12-25 and 12-26)

Film size—14″ × 17″	*Bucky*
Cassette	*Cone to cover*
Crosswise	

Technique

Factors	Screen film cassette (par)
Ma	100
Time	1.0
Mas	100
Thickness in cm	20
Kvp	66
Distance	40

Patient preparation

Remove all clothing from the waist down except shoes and socks. Provide a gown for the patient.

Palpation points

Symphysis pubis; crest of the ilium; greater trochanter of the femur.

Procedure

Place the patient in the supine position with the midline of the body over the center line of the table. Grasp the patient by the ankles and pull gently to straighten the spine. Flex the knees approximately 6 inches and support them with sponges. Rotate the ankles internally into a true posterior (A-P) position. Center a point midway between the crest of the ilium and the greater trochanter to the center of the film holder.

Central ray

Direct the central ray perpendicular to the center of the film holder.

Immobilization

Place sandbags on the lateral sides of the ankles. A compression band may be used across large abdomens. Employ suspended expiration.

Right-left markers

Place the *R* marker on the right lateral center border of the film holder.

Technical tips

To assist in palpation, the symphysis pubis is in the transverse line with the greater trochanter of the femur.

Structures demonstrated

Posterior (A-P) views of the pelvic girdle and the head, neck, and trochanters of each femur.

Note:

To better demonstrate the symphysis pubis, make an anterior (P-A) view of the pelvis.

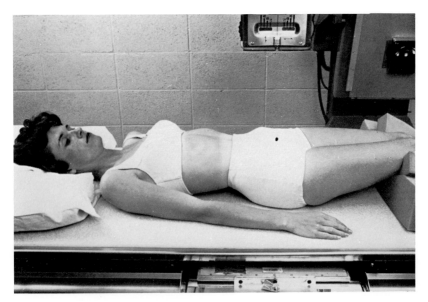

Fig. 12-25. Pelvis—posterior (A-P) position.

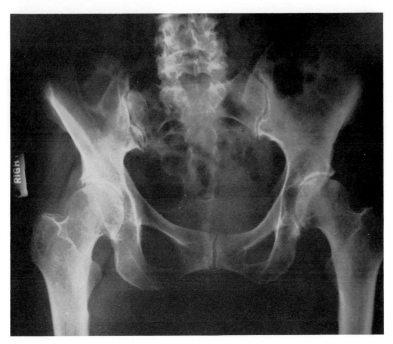

Fig. 12-26. Pelvis—posterior (A-P) view. (Courtesy Dr. E. I. L. Cilley, Dr. T. W. Crowell, Dr. R. E. Waud, and Dr. G. H. Hoffman.)

Sacrum

Sacrum—posterior (A-P) view (Figs. 12-27 and 12-28)

> *Film size—10″ × 12″*   *Bucky*
> *Cassette*   *Cone to cover*
> *Lengthwise*

Technique

Factors	Screen film cassette (par)
Ma	100
Time	1.0
Mas	100
Thickness in cm	20
Kvp	66
Distance	40

Patient preparation

Remove all clothing from the waist down except shoes and socks. Provide a gown for the patient.

Palpation points

Symphysis pubis; anterior superior iliac spinous processes; greater trochanter of the femur.

Procedure

Place the patient in the supine position with the midline of the body over the center line of the table. Grasp the patient by the ankles and pull gently to straighten the spine. Flex the knees approximately 6 inches and support them with sponges.

Central ray

Direct the central ray 15 degrees cephalad to enter a point 2½ inches above the symphysis pubis, to the center of the film holder.

Immobilization

A compression band may be used across large abdomens. Employ suspended expiration.

Right-left markers

Place the R marker on the right lateral center border of the film holder.

Technical tips

Improved radiographic quality results when the patient is requested to void his urine prior to the examination.

Structures demonstrated

Posterior (A-P) views of the sacrum, the lumbosacral junction, and the sacro-iliac joints.

Note:

For prone patients, angle the central ray 15 degrees caudad, centering to a point 3 inches inferior to a line connecting the iliac crests.

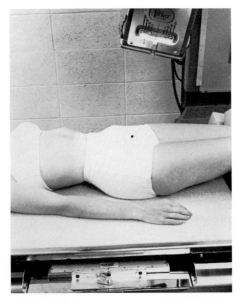

Fig. 12-27. Sacrum—posterior (A-P) position.

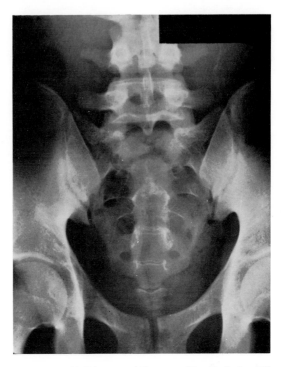

Fig. 12-28. Sacrum—posterior (A-P) view. (Courtesy Dr. E. I. L. Cilley, Dr. T. W. Crowell, Dr. R. E. Waud, and Dr. G. H. Hoffman.)

Sacrum—lateral view (Figs. 12-29 and 12-30)

> *Film size—10″ × 12″*   *Bucky*
> *Cassette*   *Cone to cover*
> *Lengthwise*

Technique

Factors	Screen film cassette (par)
Ma	100
Time	2.5
Mas	250
Thickness in cm	30
Kvp	80
Distance	40

Patient preparation

Remove all clothing from the waist down except shoes and socks. Provide a gown for the patient.

Palpation points

Anterior superior iliac spines.

Procedure

Place the patient in a lateral recumbent position. Flex the hips and knees for support. Align the long axis of the sacrum over the center line of the table (2 inches anterior to the posterior surface). Flex the bottom elbow and place the forearm under the pillow. Flex the top elbow and place the forearm above the head with the hand grasping the edge of the table. Rotate the body into a true lateral position. Center the film holder to the level of the anterior superior iliac spines.

Central ray

Direct the central ray perpendicular to the center of the film holder.

Immobilization

Place sponges or sandbags between the knees and ankles. Place a compression band over the pelvis. Employ suspended expiration.

Right-left markers

Place the correct marker on the anterior center border of the film holder.

Technical tips

For uniform radiographic density, use an aluminum wedge filter or $\frac{1}{10}$ mm added copper filter internally plus an increase of 10 kvp.

Structures demonstrated

Lateral views of the sacrum and coccyx, and of the lumbosacral junction.

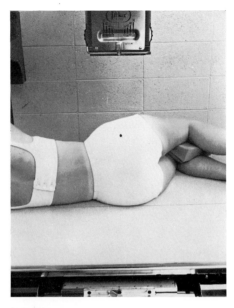

Fig. 12-29. Sacrum—lateral position.

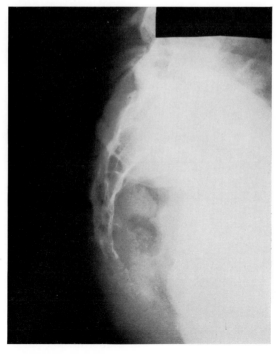

Fig. 12-30. Sacrum—lateral view. (Courtesy Dr. E. I. L. Cilley, Dr. T. W. Crowell, Dr. R. E. Waud, and Dr. G. H. Hoffman.)

Coccyx

Coccyx–posterior (A-P) view (Figs. 12-31 and 12-32)

Film size—8″ × 10″	*Bucky*
Cassette	*Extension cone*
Lengthwise	*(fully extended)*

Technique

Factors	Screen film cassette (par)
Ma	100
Time	1.0
Mas	100
Thickness in cm	22
Kvp	70
Distance	40

Patient preparation

Remove all clothing from the waist down except shoes and socks. Provide a gown for the patient.

Palpation points

Symphysis pubis; greater trochanter of the femur.

Procedure

Place the patient in the supine position with the midline of the body over the center line of the table. Grasp the patient by the ankles and pull gently to straighten the spine. Flex the knees approximately 6 inches and support them with sponges.

Central ray

Direct the central ray 15 degrees caudad to enter a point 2½ inches above the symphysis pubis, to the center of the film holder.

Immobilization

A compression band may be used across large abdomens. Employ suspended expiration.

Right-left markers

Burn the R marker in the superior border of the right side of the film holder above the cone field after the exposure is made.

Technical tips

Improved radiographic quality results when the patient is requested to void urine and evacuate any intestinal contents prior to the examination.

Structures demonstrated

Posterior (A-P) view of the coccyx.

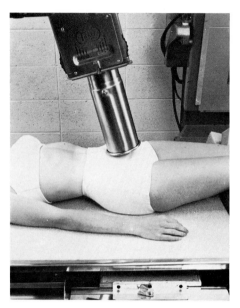

Fig. 12-31. Coccyx—posterior (A-P) position.

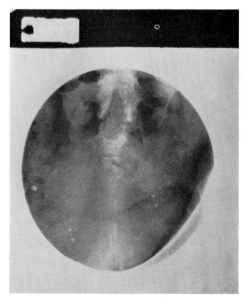

Fig. 12-32. Coccyx—posterior (A-P) view. (Courtesy Dr. E. I. L. Cilley, Dr. T. W. Crowell, Dr. R. E. Waud, and Dr. G. H. Hoffman.)

Coccyx—lateral view (Figs. 12-33 and 12-34)

Film size—8″ × 10″	*Bucky*
Cassette	*Extension cone*
Lengthwise	*(fully extended)*

Technique

Factors	Screen film cassette (par)
Ma	100
Time	2.5
Mas	250
Thickness in cm	30
Kvp	80
Distance	40

Patient preparation

Remove all clothing from the waist down except shoes and socks. Provide a gown for the patient.

Palpation points

Posterior surface of the coccyx; greater trochanter of the femur.

Procedure

Place the patient in a lateral recumbent position. Flex the hips and knees for support. Align the long axis of the sacrum and coccyx over the center line of the table (2 inches anterior to the posterior surface of the sacrum). Flex the bottom elbow and place the forearm under the pillow. Flex the top elbow and place the forearm above the head with the hand grasping the edge of the table. Rotate the body into a true lateral position.

Central ray

Direct the central ray perpendicular through a point 1 inch superior to the greater trochanter to the center of the film holder.

Immobilization

Place sponges or sandbags between the knees and ankles. Place a compression band over the pelvis. Employ suspended expiration.

Right-left markers

Burn the left or right marker in the superior center border of the film after the exposure is made.

Technical tips

Use the smallest cone possible and a minimum distance of 40 inches to compensate for the increased object-film distance.

Structures demonstrated

Lateral views of the coccyx and lower sacrum.

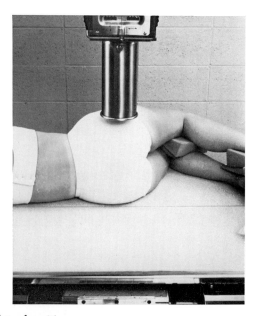

Fig. 12-33. Coccyx—lateral position.

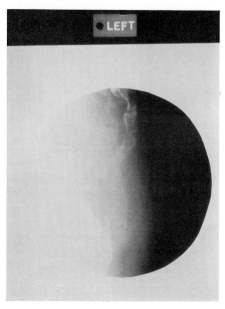

Fig. 12-34. Coccyx—lateral view. (Courtesy Dr. E. I. L. Cilley, Dr. T. W. Crowell, Dr. R. E. Waud, and Dr. G. H. Hoffman.)

Hip

Hip—posterior (A-P) (unilateral) view (Figs. 12-35 and 12-36)

> *Film size—10″ × 12″*   *Bucky*
> *Cassette*   *Cone to cover*
> *Lengthwise*

Technique

Factors	Screen film cassette (*par*)
Ma	100
Time	1.0
Mas	100
Thickness in cm	20
Kvp	66
Distance	40

Patient preparation

Remove all clothing from the waist down except shoes and socks. Provide a gown for the patient.

Palpation points

Symphysis pubis; anterior superior iliac spine.

Procedure

Place the patient in the supine position. Locate the hip joint as follows: at right angles bisect a line between the anterior superior iliac spine and the symphysis pubis; select a point on the bisecting line 2 inches inferior to the first line; center this point over the center line of the table. Rotate the ankles internally into a true posterior (A-P) position.

Central ray

Direct the central ray perpendicular through the located point to the center of the film holder.

Immobilization

Place sandbags on each side of the foot and ankle. Employ suspended expiration.

Right-left markers

Place the correct marker in the superior lateral border of the film holder.

Technical tips

To locate the femoral head and neck, select points 2½ inches and 3 inches, respectively, inferior to the bisected line.

Structures demonstrated

Posterior (A-P) views of the femoral head, anatomic and surgical necks, and trochanters, all in relationship to the acetabulum.

Note:

For children under 12 years of age, the radiographic request may be for views of both hips for comparison; this examination should be performed employing a single exposure on a film of suitable size placed crosswise with the pelvis. *Be sure to employ gonadal protection.*

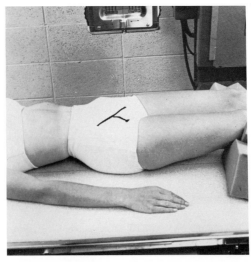

Fig. 12-35. Hip—posterior (A-P) position.

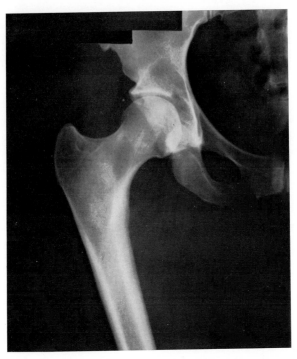

Fig. 12-36. Hip—posterior (A-P) view. (Courtesy Dr. E. I. L. Cilley, Dr. T. W. Crowell, Dr. R. E. Waud, and Dr. G. H. Hoffman.)

Hip—lateral (unilateral) "frog" view (Figs. 12-37 and 12-38)

> *Film size—10″ × 12″*   *Bucky*
> *Cassette*   *Cone to cover*
> *Crosswise*

Technique

Factors	Screen film cassette (par)
Ma	100
Time	1.0
Mas	100
Thickness in cm	20
Kvp	66
Distance	40

Patient preparation

Remove all clothing from the waist down except shoes and socks. Provide a gown for the patient.

Palpation points

Symphysis pubis; anterior superior iliac spine.

Procedure

Place the patient in the supine position. Locate the hip joint as follows: at right angles bisect a line between the anterior superior iliac spine and the symphysis pubis; select a point on the bisecting line 2 inches inferior to the first line; center this point over the center line of the table. Flex the knee 90 degrees, and abduct it as far as possible, turning the foot on its lateral side.

Central ray

Direct the central ray perpendicular through the located point to the center of the film holder.

Immobilization

Place a sponge or sandbag under the lateral side of the flexed knee, and a heavy sandbag on top of the foot. Employ suspended expiration.

Right-left markers

Place the correct marker in the superior lateral border of the film holder.

Technical tips

A reduction in technique from the anteroposterior hip view is usually necessary for this view.

Structures demonstrated

Lateral views of the femoral head, anatomic and surgical necks, and the trochanters in relationship to the acetabulum.

Note:

For children under 12 years of age, the radiographic request may be for views of both hips for comparison; this examination should be performed employing a single exposure on a film of suitable size placed crosswise with the pelvis, and with both hips in the position described above (frog position). *Be sure to employ gonadal protection.*

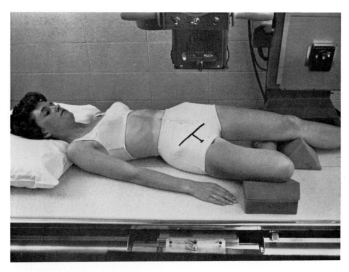

Fig. 12-37. Hip—unilateral (frog) position.

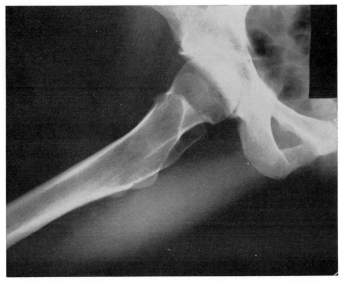

Fig. 12-38. Hip—unilateral (frog) view. (Courtesy Dr. E. I. L. Cilley, Dr. T. W. Crowell, Dr. R. E. Waud, and Dr. G. H. Hoffman.)

Hip—translateral view (Figs. 12-39 and 12-40)

Film size—8″ × 10″	*Grid cassette*
Cassette	*Extension cone*
Lengthwise	*(fully extended)*

Technique

Factors	Screen film cassette (par)
Ma	100
Time	1.75
Mas	175
Thickness in cm	22
Kvp	68
Distance	40

Patient preparation

Remove all clothing from the waist down. Provide a gown for the patient.

Palpation points

Symphysis pubis; anterior superior iliac spine; iliac crest.

Procedure

Place the patient in the supine position on a cushion or pillows to elevate the body. Fully extend the leg to be examined; rotate the ankle internally into a true posterior (A-P) position. Flex the opposite knee to form an arch, and place the foot on an elevated support. Place the cassette on edge and brace its superior edge against the body above the crest of the ilium with a sandbag. The cassette face is parallel with a perpendicular plane that bisects a line between the anterior superior iliac spine and the symphysis pubis.

Central ray

In a horizontal plane direct the central ray perpendicular under the flexed knee through the greater trochanter to the center of the film holder.

Immobilization

Place sandbags on each side of the foot. Employ suspended expiration.

Right-left markers

Burn the correct marker in the superior center border of the film holder above the cone field after the exposure is made.

Technical tips

If the patient cannot flex the opposite knee, have him abduct that thigh and hang the leg over the table edge.

Structures demonstrated

Lateral views of the femoral head, anatomic neck, and trochanters. This examination results in minimum discomfort to the patient.

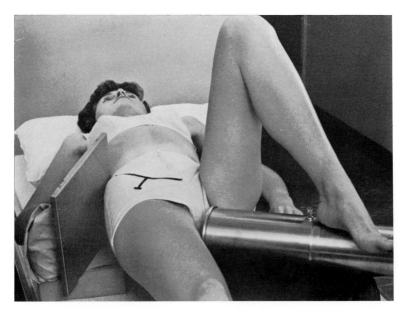

Fig. 12-39. Hip—translateral position.

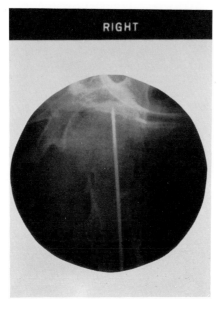

Fig. 12-40. Hip—translateral view. (Courtesy Dr. E. I. L. Cilley, Dr. T. W. Crowell, Dr. R. E. Waud, and Dr. G. H. Hoffman.)

Shoulder
Shoulder—posterior (A-P) view, external rotation (Figs. 12-41 and 12-42)

> *Film size—10″ × 12″*   *Bucky*
> *Cassette*   *Cone to cover*
> *Crosswise*

Technique

Factors	Screen film cassette (par) Bucky	Screen film cassette (par) tabletop
Ma	100	100
Time	0.2	0.1
Mas	20	10
Thickness in cm	14	14
Kvp	74	64
Distance	40	40

Patient preparation

Remove all garments down to the waist. Provide a gown for female patients.

Palpation points

Coracoid process of the scapula; humeral epicondyles.

Procedure

Place the patient in the supine position. Center the coracoid process over the center line of the table. Elevate the opposite shoulder 6 inches and support it with a sandbag. Rotate the entire arm externally so that a line through the humeral epicondyles is parallel with the tabletop.

Central ray

Direct the central ray perpendicular through the coracoid process to the center of the film holder.

Immobilization

Place one sandbag under, and a second on top of, the hand. Employ suspended expiration.

Right-left markers

Place the correct marker on the superior center border of the film holder.

Technical tips

The external rotation view will demonstrate the humeral head projected medially.

Structures demonstrated

Posterior (A-P) views of the bony structures of the shoulder in the true anatomic position.

Note:

Both internal and external rotation views of the shoulder should be made in routine examinations, particularly on patients with suspected bursitis.

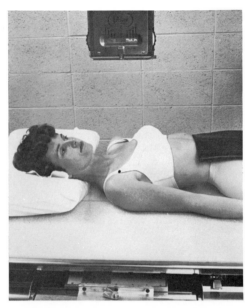

Fig. 12-41. Shoulder—posterior (A-P) position, external rotation.

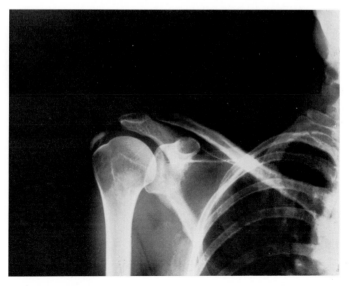

Fig. 12-42. Shoulder—posterior (A-P) view, external rotation. (Courtesy Dr. E. I. L. Cilley, Dr. T. W. Crowell, Dr. R. E. Waud, and Dr. G. H. Hoffman.)

Shoulder—posterior (A-P) view, internal rotation (Figs. 12-43 and 12-44)

Film size—10″ × 12″   *Bucky*
Cassette   *Cone to cover*
Crosswise

Technique

Factors	Screen film cassette (par) Bucky	Screen film cassette (par) tabletop
Ma	100	100
Time	0.2	0.1
Mas	20	10
Thickness in cm	14	14
Kvp	74	64
Distance	40	40

Patient preparation

Remove all garments down to the waist. Provide a gown for female patients.

Palpation points

Coracoid process of the scapula; humeral epicondyles.

Procedure

Place the patient in the supine position. Center the coracoid process over the center line of the table. Elevate the opposite shoulder 6 inches and support it with a sandbag. Rotate the entire arm internally so that a line through the humeral epicondyles is perpendicular to the tabletop.

Central ray

Direct the central ray perpendicular through the coracoid process to the center of the film holder.

Immobilization

Place a sandbag on top of the hand. Employ suspended expiration.

Right-left markers

Place the correct marker on the superior center border of the film holder.

Technical tips

The internal rotation view will demonstrate the humeral head projected posteriorly.

Structures demonstrated

Posterior (A-P) views of the bony structures of the shoulder and of the lateral humerus in relationship to the glenoid cavity.

Note:

Both internal and external rotation views of the shoulder should be made in routine examinations, particularly on patients with suspected bursitis.

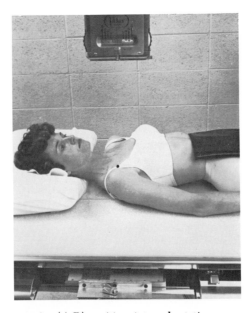

Fig. 12-43. Shoulder—posterior (A-P) position, internal rotation.

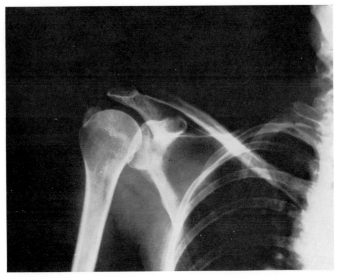

Fig. 12-44. Shoulder—posterior (A-P) view, internal rotation. (Courtesy Dr. E. I. L. Cilley, Dr. T. W. Crowell, Dr. R. E. Waud, and Dr. G. H. Hoffman.)

Shoulder—lateral view through the thorax (Figs. 12-45 and 12-46)

Film size—10″ × 12″　　　　　*Bucky (erect)*
Cassette　　　　　　　　　　*Cone to cover*
Lengthwise　　　　　　　　　*(Rapid shallow*
　　　　　　　　　　　　　　　breathing technique)

Technique

Factors	Screen film cassette (par)
Ma	25
Time	6
Mas	150
Thickness in cm	32
Kvp	78
Distance	40

Patient preparation

Remove all garments down to the waist. Provide a gown for female patients.

Palpation points

Greater tubercle and surgical neck of the humerus; sternum; spinous processes of the thoracic vertebrae.

Procedure

Place the patient in the erect position, either sitting or standing, with the shoulder being examined against the erect Bucky or grid. Flex this elbow, and rest the palm of the hand against the anterior chest. Place the opposite forearm on top of the head. Rotate the body so that the humerus being radiographed is midway between the sternum and the vertebral column.

Central ray

Direct the central ray 10 degrees cephalad through the surgical neck of the humerus to the center of the film holder.

Immobilization

Use a compression band around the thorax. Employ rapid shallow breathing during the radiographic exposure.

Right-left markers

Place the correct marker on the anterior side, center border of the film holder.

Technical tips

In this position the surgical neck of the humerus is on the same plane as the spinous process of the fourth thoracic vertebra.

Structures demonstrated

Lateral views of the humeral head, neck, and the upper one third of the shaft projected through the thorax.

Note:

This view should be made for all patients with suspected fractures, immobilized fractures, or hanging casts involving the proximal humerus.

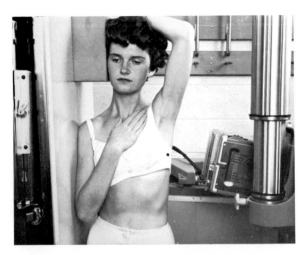

Fig. 12-45. Shoulder—lateral (through the thorax) position.

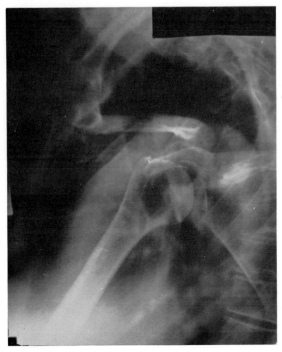

Fig. 12-46. Shoulder—lateral (through the thorax) view. (Courtesy Dr. E. I. L. Cilley, Dr. T. W. Crowell, Dr. R. E. Waud, and Dr. G. H. Hoffman.)

Clavicle
Clavicle—anterior (P-A) view (Figs. 12-47 and 12-48)

> *Film size—10″ × 12″*   *Bucky*
> *Cassette*   *Cone to cover*
> *Crosswise*

Technique

Factors	Screen film cassette (par) Bucky	Screen film cassette (par) tabletop
Ma	100	100
Time	0.2	0.1
Mas	20	10
Thickness in cm	14	14
Kvp	74	64
Distance	40	40

Patient preparation
Remove all garments down to the waist. Provide a gown for female patients.

Palpation points
Acromioclavicular articulation; sternoclavicular articulation; shaft of the clavicle.

Procedure
Place the patient in the prone or anterior (P-A) erect position with the arms extended down the body. Extend the chin and rest it on the table. Center the midshaft of the clavicle over the center line of the table.

Central ray
Direct the central ray 10 degrees caudad through the clavicle to the center of the film holder.

Immobilization
A compression band may be used across the chest. Employ suspended expiration.

Right-left markers
Place the correct marker on the superior center border of the film holder.

Technical tips
To better demonstrate the sternal end of the clavicle, elevate the side being examined 5 to 10 degrees.

Structures demonstrated
Anterior (P-A) view of the entire clavicle.

Note:
For supine patients, angle the central ray 10 degrees cephalad.

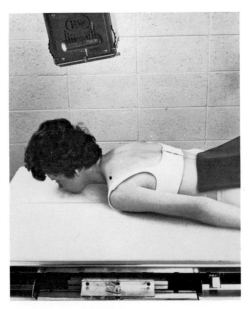

Fig. 12-47. Clavicle—anterior (P-A) position.

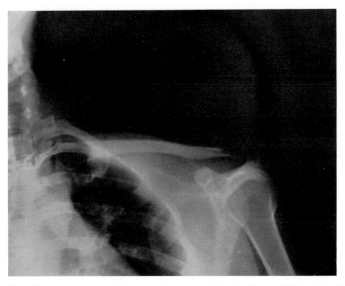

Fig. 12-48. Clavicle—anterior (A-P) view. (Courtesy Dr. E. I. L. Cilley, Dr. T. W. Crowell, Dr. R. E. Waud, and Dr. G. H. Hoffman.)

Clavicle—anterior (P-A) view, sternoclavicular articulations (Figs. 12-49 and 12-50)

    Film size—8″ × 10″   *Bucky*
    Cassette   *Cone to cover*
    Crosswise

Technique

Factors	*Screen film cassette (par)*
Ma	100
Time	0.6
Mas	60
Thickness in cm	21
Kvp	78
Distance	40

Patient preparation

Remove all garments down to the waist. Provide a gown for female patients.

Palpation points

Sternoclavicular articulations; shaft of the clavicle; manubrium.

Procedure

Place the patient in the prone or anterior (P-A) erect position with the arms extended down the body. Extend the chin and rest it on the table. Center the midsagittal plane of the body over the center line of the table.

Central ray

Direct the central ray perpendicular through the third thoracic vertebra to the center of the film.

Immobilization

A compression band may be used across the chest. Employ suspended expiration.

Right-left markers

Place the R marker in the right superior border of the film.

Technical tips

To emphasize the inferior portion of the sternoclavicular articulations, place the forearms above the head.

Structures demonstrated

Anterior (P-A) view of the sternoclavicular joints.

Note:

For acromioclavicular separation, make unilateral anteroposterior erect views of each shoulder while the patient is holding a 5-pound sandbag in each hand. Center the horizontal central ray through each acromioclavicular joint.

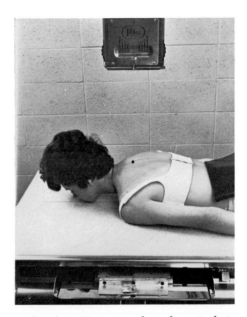

Fig. 12-49. Clavicle—anterior (P-A) position, sternoclavicular articulations.

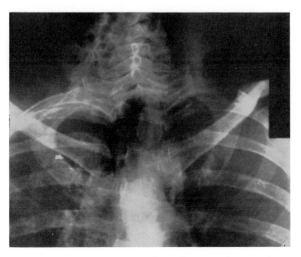

Fig. 12-50. Clavicle—anterior (P-A) view, sternoclavicular articulations. (Courtesy Dr. E. I. L. Cilley, Dr. T. W. Crowell, Dr. R. E. Waud, and Dr. G. H. Hoffman.)

Clavicle—anterior (P-A) oblique view, sternoclavicular articulation
(Figs. 12-51 and 12-52)

> *Film size—8″ × 10″*   *Bucky*
> *Cassette*   *Extension cone*
> *Lengthwise*   *(fully extended)*

Technique

Factors	*Screen film cassette (par)*
Ma	100
Time	0.6
Mas	60
Thickness in cm	21
Kvp	78
Distance	40

Patient preparation

Remove all garments down to the waist. Provide a gown for female patients.

Palpation points

Sternoclavicular articulations; shaft of the clavicle; manubrium.

Procedure

Place the patient in the prone or anterior (P-A) erect position. Elevate the side opposite the one being examined so that the midsagittal plane of the head and body forms a 45-degree angle with the tabletop. When the patient is prone, flex the knee and the elbow of the elevated side for support. Align the joint being examined over the center line of the table.

Central ray

Direct the central ray perpendicular through the sternoclavicular articulation to the center of the film holder.

Immobilization

Place a sponge or sandbag under the flexed knee. Employ suspended expiration.

Right-left markers

Burn the correct marker in the superior center border of the film holder above the cone field after the exposure is made.

Technical tips

The sternoclavicular articulation is on the same transverse plane as the spinous process of the 3rd thoracic vertebra.

Structures demonstrated

Anterior (P-A) oblique views of the sternoclavicular articulation and of the manubrium.

Note:

Both right and left views should be made for comparison.

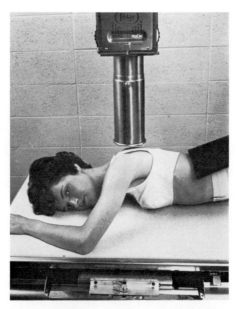

Fig. 12-51. Clavicle—anterior (A-P) oblique position, sternoclavicular articulation.

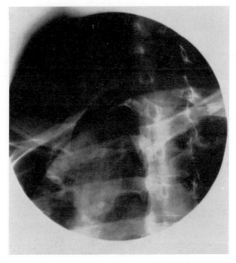

Fig. 12-52. Clavicle—anterior (P-A) oblique view, sternoclavicular articulation. (Courtesy Dr. E. I. L. Cilley, Dr. T. W. Crowell, Dr. R. E. Waud, and Dr. G. H. Hoffman.)

Sternum
Sternum—anterior (P-A) oblique view (Figs. 12-53 and 12-54)

Film size—10″ × 12″	*Bucky*
Cassette	*Cone to cover*
Lengthwise	*(rapid shallow breathing technique)*

Technique

Factors	Screen film cassette (par)
Ma	25
Time	1.0
Mas	25
Thickness in cm	25
Kvp	82
Distance	30

Patient preparation
Remove all garments down to the waist. Provide a gown for female patients.

Palpation points
Manubrium and xiphoid processes of the sternum.

Procedure
Place the patient in the prone position. Elevate the left side of the body approximately 30 degrees and flex the left knee and elbow for support. Align the long axis of the sternum over the center line of the table. Place a wedge sponge under the elevated thoracic cage. Instruct the patient to extend the left arm down the body and simultaneously relax the left shoulder and roll it anteriorly.

Central ray
Direct the central ray perpendicular through a point halfway between the manubrium and xiphoid process to the center of the film holder.

Immobilization
Place a wedge sponge or a sandbag under the flexed knee. A compression band may be used across the thoracic cage. Employ rapid shallow breathing during the radiographic exposure.

Right-left markers
Place the L marker on the left lateral center border of the film holder.

Technical tips
For left anterior oblique position, reduce the kvp 4 kilovolts.

Structures demonstrated
Anterior (P-A) oblique view of the sternum.

Note:
A short focal-film distance with the rapid shallow breathing technique will blur out surrounding structures.

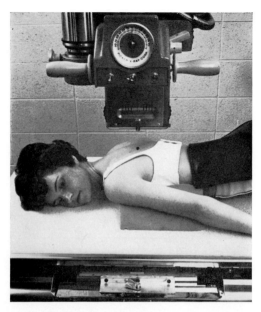

Fig. 12-53. Sternum—anterior (P-A) oblique position.

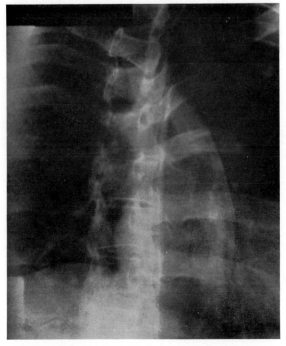

Fig. 12-54. Sternum—anterior (P-A) oblique view. (Courtesy Dr. E. I. L. Cilley, Dr. T. W. Crowell, Dr. R. E. Waud, and Dr. G. H. Hoffman.)

Sternum—lateral view (Figs. 12-55 and 12-56)

Film size—10″ × 12″   *Bucky (erect)*
Cassette   *Cone to cover*
Lengthwise

Technique

Factors	*Screen film cassette (par)*
Ma	100
Time	0.6
Mas	60
Thickness in cm	30
Kvp	80
Distance	40

Patient preparation

Remove all garments down to the waist. Provide a gown for female patients.

Palpation points

Manubrium and xiphoid processes of the sternum.

Procedure

Place the patient in a lateral erect position, either standing or sitting. Place the arms behind the back and clasp the hands together. Relax the shoulders and roll them posteriorly. Align the long axis of the sternum over the center line of the table.

Central ray

Direct the central ray perpendicular through a point halfway between the manubrium and the xiphoid process to the center of the film holder.

Immobilization

Place a compression band around the patient's body. Employ suspended inspiration.

Right-left markers

Place the correct marker on the anterior center border of the film holder.

Technical tips

Measurements for technique should be made transversely across the entire anterior chest wall.

Structures demonstrated

Lateral view of the sternum.

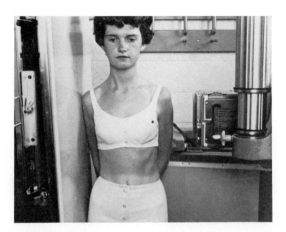

Fig. 12-55. Sternum—lateral position.

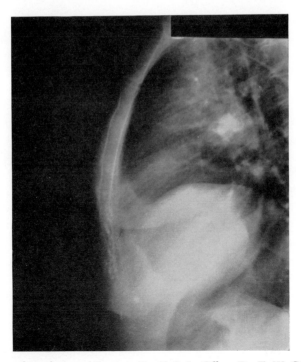

Fig. 12-56. Sternum—lateral view. (Courtesy Dr. E. I. L. Cilley, Dr. T. W. Crowell, Dr. R. E. Waud, and Dr. G. H. Hoffman.)

Scapula

Scapula—posterior (A-P) view (Figs. 12-57 and 12-58)

> *Film size—10″ × 12″*   *Bucky*
> *Cassette*   *Cone to cover*
> *Lengthwise*

Technique

Factors	Screen film cassette (*par*)
Ma	100
Time	0.3
Mas	30
Thickness in cm	16
Kvp	76
Distance	40

Patient preparation

Remove all garments down to the waist. Provide a gown for female patients.

Palpation points

Acromion process, spine, and apex of the scapula; spinous processes of the thoracic vertebrae.

Procedure

Place the patient in the supine position. Center a point halfway between the midline of the body and the lateral border of the shoulder over the center line of the table. Extend the arm at the side of the body with the palm up.

Central ray

Direct the central ray perpendicularly to enter a point halfway between the top of the shoulder and the apex of the scapula, to the center of the film holder.

Immobilization

Place one sandbag under and a second on top of the hand. Employ suspended inspiration.

Right-left markers

Place the correct marker on the lateral center border of the film holder.

Technical tips

To better demonstrate the axillary border of the scapula being radiographed, place that forearm over the head.

Structures demonstrated

Posterior (A-P) views of the scapula and lateral clavicle.

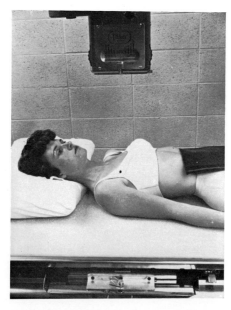

Fig. 12-57. Scapula—posterior (A-P) position.

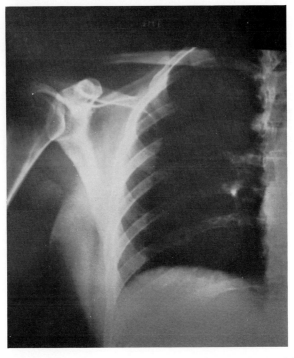

Fig. 12-58. Scapula—posterior (A-P) view. (Courtesy Dr. E. I. L. Cilley, Dr. T. W. Crowell, Dr. R. E. Waud, and Dr. G. H. Hoffman.)

Scapula—lateral view (Figs. 12-59 and 12-60)

> *Film size—10″ × 12″*   *Bucky (erect)*
> *Cassette*   *Cone to cover*
> *Lengthwise*

Technique

Factors	*Screen film cassette (par)*
Ma	100
Time	0.6
Mas	60
Thickness in cm	16
Kvp	78
Distance	40

Patient preparation

Remove all garments down to the waist. Provide a gown for female patients.

Palpation points

Acromion process, spine, and apex of the scapula; spinous processes of the thoracic vertebrae.

Procedure

Place the patient in an erect position, either sitting or standing, with the shoulder being examined against the erect Bucky. Flex the elbow nearer to the film and place the arm behind the patient with the back of hand against the posterior ribs. Instruct the patient to grasp the edge of the table with the opposite hand and to roll the opposite shoulder anteriorly. Rotate the body slightly to align the flat surface of the scapula so that it is perpendicular to and over the center line of the upright Bucky.

Central ray

Direct the central ray perpendicularly to enter a point halfway between the top of the shoulder and the apex of the scapula, to the center of the film holder.

Immobilization

A compression band may be placed around the patient's lower thoracic region. Employ suspended expiration.

Right-left markers

Place the correct marker on the anterior center border of the film holder.

Technical tips

For uniform radiographic density, use $\frac{1}{10}$ mm copper filter internally plus an increase of 10 kvp.

Structures demonstrated

Lateral view of the scapula projected away from the rib cage.

Note:

For supine patients, elevate the side being examined 25 degrees, placing that forearm over the head; align the central ray perpendicularly through the mid-scapula to the center of the film holder.

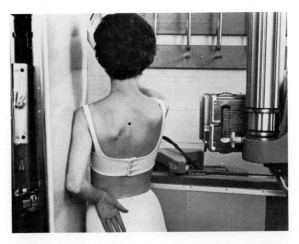

Fig. 12-59. Scapula—lateral position.

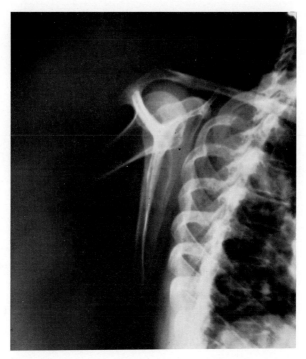

Fig. 12-60. Scapula—lateral view. (Courtesy Dr. E. I. L. Cilley, Dr. T. W. Crowell, Dr. R. E. Waud, and Dr. G. H. Hoffman.)

Ribs

Ribs—posterior (A-P) or anterior (P-A) view above the diaphragm
(Figs. 12-61 and 12-62)

> *Film size—14″ × 17″* *Bucky*
> *Cassette* *Cone to cover*
> *Crosswise*

Technique

Factors	Screen film cassette (*par*)
Ma	100
Time	0.4
Mas	40
Thickness in cm	20
Kvp	70
Distance	40

Patient preparation

Remove all garments down to the waist. Provide a gown for female patients.

Palpation points

Vertebra prominens; lateral ribs.

Procedure

Place the patient either in the prone or the supine position with the side being examined nearer the table. Center the midline of the body over the center line of the table. Extend both arms down the sides of the body. Align the top of the cassette 2 inches above the vertebra prominens (seventh cervical vertebra).

Central ray

Direct the central ray perpendicular to the center of the film holder.

Immobilization

Employ suspended expiration.

Right-left markers

Place the R marker on the right lateral center border of the film holder.

Technical tips

Complete expiration will produce lung-tissue concentration and provide for more uniform object density.

Structures demonstrated

Posterior (A-P) or anterior (P-A) view of the upper two thirds of the bilateral rib cage.

Note:

Make erect views if the patient has any difficulty in assuming the positions described above.

For patients measuring less than 19 cm, use chest positioning, microline grid, and optimum kvp chest technique.

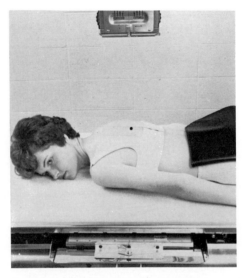

Fig. 12-61. Ribs—anterior (P-A) position, above the diaphragm.

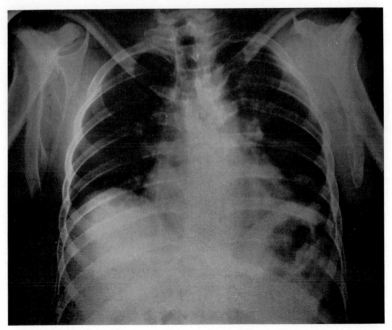

Fig. 12-62. Ribs—anterior (P-A) view, above the diaphragm. (Courtesy Dr. E. I. L. Cilley, Dr. T. W. Crowell, Dr. R. E. Waud, and Dr. G. H. Hoffman.)

Ribs—anterior (P-A) oblique (L.A.O.-R.A.O.) view (Figs. 12-63 and 12-64)

> *Film size—14″ × 17″*   *Bucky*
> *Cassette*   *Cone to cover*
> *Lengthwise*

Technique

Factors	Screen film cassette (par)
Ma	100
Time	0.4
Mas	40
Thickness in cm	23
Kvp	76
Distance	40

Patient preparation

Remove all garments down to the waist. Provide a gown for female patients.

Palpation points

Vertebra prominens; lateral ribs.

Procedure

Place the patient in the prone position. Elevate the side being examined 35 degrees, and flex the elbow and knee for support. Center a point midway between the spine and the lateral margin of the ribs of the side being examined over the center line of the table. Align the top of the film holder with the vertebra prominens (seventh cervical vertebra).

Central ray

Direct the central ray perpendicular to the center of the film holder.

Immobilization

Employ suspended expiration.

Right-left markers

Place the correct marker on the anterior center border of the film holder.

Technical tips

Complete expiration will produce lung-tissue concentration and provide for more uniform object density.

Structures demonstrated

Axillary view of the unilateral rib cage.

Note:

Make erect views if the patient has any difficulty in assuming the positions described above.

For patients measuring less than 19 cm, use chest positioning, microline grid, and optimum kvp chest technique.

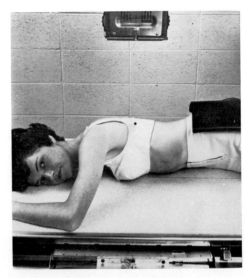

Fig. 12-63. Ribs—anterior (P-A) oblique (R.A.O.) position.

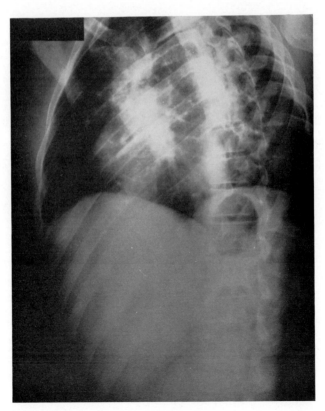

Fig. 12-64. Ribs—anterior (P-A) oblique (R.A.O.) view. (Courtesy Dr. E. I. L. Cilley, Dr. T. W. Crowell, Dr. R. E. Waud, and Dr. G. H. Hoffman.)

Ribs—posterior (A-P) or anterior (P-A) view below the diaphragm
(Figs. 12-65 and 12-66)

        Film size—14″ × 17″   *Bucky*
        Cassette   *Cone to cover*
        Crosswise

Technique

Factors	*Screen film cassette (par)*
Ma	100
Time	0.5
Mas	50
Thickness in cm	22
Kvp	78
Distance	40

Patient preparation

Remove all garments down to the waist. Provide a gown for female patients.

Palpation points

Iliac crest; lateral ribs.

Procedure

Place the patient in either the prone or the supine position with the side being examined nearer the table. Extend the arms down the sides of the body. Align the bottom of the cassette with the iliac crest.

Central ray

Direct the central ray perpendicular to the center of the film holder.

Immobilization

Employ suspended expiration.

Right-left markers

Place the R marker on the right lateral center border of the film holder.

Technical tips

Complete expiration will produce lung-tissue concentration and provide for more uniform object density.

Structures demonstrated

Posterior (A-P) or anterior (P-A) view of the lower two thirds of the bilateral rib cage.

Note:

Make erect views if the patient has any difficulty in assuming the positions described above.

For patients measuring less than 19 cm, use chest positioning, microline grid, and optimum kvp chest technique.

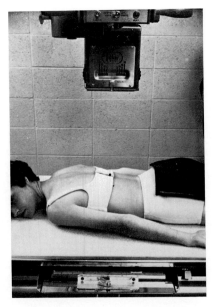

Fig. 12-65. Ribs—anterior (P-A) position, below the diaphragm.

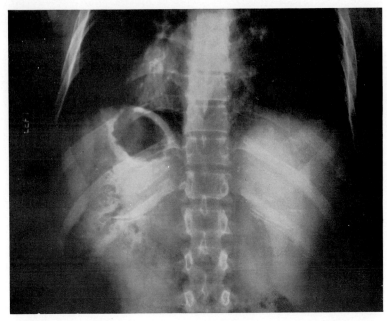

Fig. 12-66. Ribs—anterior (P-A) view, below the diaphragm. (Courtesy Dr. E. I. L. Cilley, Dr. T. W. Crowell, Dr. R. E. Waud, and Dr. G. H. Hoffman.)

Chest

Chest—anterior (P-A) view (Figs. 12-67 and 12-68)

Film size—14″ × 17″	*Erect film holder*
Cassette	*Cone to cover*
Lengthwise	

Technique

Factors	Screen film cassette (par)
Ma	200
Time	1/20
Mas	10
Thickness in cm	20
Kvp	60
Distance	72

Patient preparation

Remove all garments down to the waist. Provide a gown for female patients.

Palpation points

Acromion processes; lateral ribs; apex of the scapula.

Procedure

Place the patient in the erect position with the anterior surface of the chest against the cassette. Center the midline of the body over the center line of the film holder. Align the top of the cassette 3 inches above the acromion processes. Elevate the chin so that it rests on top of the film holder. Place the backs of the hands on the hips. Roll the shoulders anteriorly as far as possible.

Central ray

Direct the central ray horizontally, perpendicular to the center of the film holder.

Immobilization

A compression band may be used across the thoracic cage. Employ deep suspended inspiration.

Right-left markers

Place the *L* marker in the left superior corner of the film holder.

Technical tips

The spinous process of the seventh thoracic vertebra is on the same plane as the apex of the scapula and the midportion of the lung field.

Structures demonstrated

Anterior (P-A) views of the lungs, heart, and the rib structures above the diaphragm.

Note:

For heart series, make a routine chest series; include the patient's weight, height, and age on the protocol.

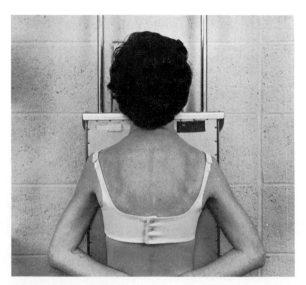

Fig. 12-67. Chest—anterior (P-A) position.

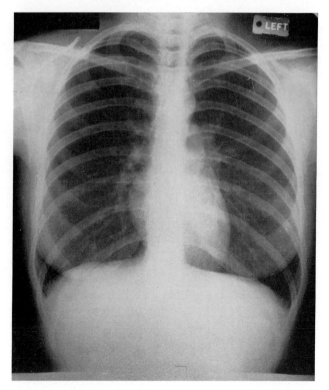

Fig. 12-68. Chest—anterior (P-A) view. (Courtesy Dr. E. I. L. Cilley, Dr. T. W. Crowell, Dr. R. E. Waud, and Dr. G. H. Hoffman.)

Chest—lateral view (Figs. 12-69 and 12-70)

Film size—14″ × 17″   *Erect film holder*
Cassette   *Cone to cover*
Lengthwise

Technique

Factors	Screen film cassette (par)
Ma	200
Time	0.1
Mas	20
Thickness in cm	30
Kvp	72
Distance	72

Patient preparation

Remove all garments down to the waist. Provide a gown for female patients.

Palpation points

Acromion processes; posterior ribs; sternum.

Procedure

Place the patient in the erect position with the lateral surface of the chest against the cassette. Center the midaxillary line of the body over the center line of the film holder. Align the top of the cassette 3 inches above the acromion process. Cross the arms over the head and rest the forearms on top of the head. Rotate the body into a true lateral position.

Central ray

Direct the central ray horizontally, perpendicular to the center of the film holder.

Immobilization

Brace the shoulder against the cassette. A compression band may be used across the thoracic cage. Employ deep suspended inspiration.

Right-left markers

Place the correct marker in the left superior corner of the film holder.

Technical tips

Holding the breath on the second inspiration will ensure a greater area of lung visualization.

Structures demonstrated

Lateral views of both lungs superimposed, heart and aorta, and the midthoracic spine.

Note:

Make a left lateral view unless otherwise directed.

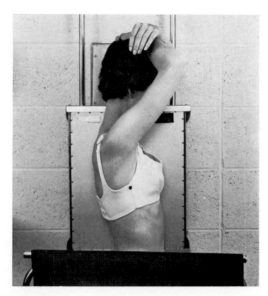

Fig. 12-69. Chest—lateral position.

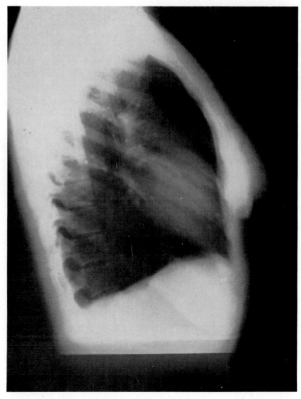

Fig. 12-70. Chest—lateral view. (Courtesy Dr. E. I. L. Cilley, Dr. T. W. Crowell, Dr. R. E. Waud, and Dr. G. H. Hoffman.)

Chest—anterior (P-A) oblique view (Figs. 12-71 and 12-72)

Film size—14″ × 17″	*Erect film holder*
Cassette	*Cone to cover*
Lengthwise	

Technique

Factors	Screen film cassette (par)
Ma	200
Time	1/20
Mas	10
Thickness in cm	26
Kvp	70
Distance	72

Patient preparation

Remove all garments down to the waist. Provide a gown for female patients.

Palpation points

Acromion processes; lateral ribs; spinous processes of the thoracic vertebrae.

Procedure

Place the patient in the erect position with the anterior surface of the chest against the cassette. Align the top of the cassette 3 inches above the acromion process. Rotate the side of the chest being examined away from the cassette 45 degrees; flex that elbow and place the hand on top of the film holder. Flex the opposite elbow and place the hand on the hip. Align a point midway between the spine and the lateral margin of the side of the chest being examined over the center line of the film holder.

Central ray

Direct the central ray horizontally, perpendicular to the center of the film holder.

Immobilization

A compression band may be used across the thoracic cage. Employ deep suspended inspiration.

Right-left markers

Place the *L* marker in the left superior corner of the film holder.

Technical tips

Holding the breath on the second inspiration will ensure a greater area of lung visualization.

Structures demonstrated

Right anterior oblique—maximum view of the left lung field, the trachea, and entire right bronchial tree; left atrium and both ventricles of the heart. When filled with barium sulfate, the esophagus is well demonstrated in this view.

Left anterior oblique—maximum view of the right lung field, the trachea, and left bronchial tree.

Note:

For supine patients, elevate the side opposite the one being radiographed 45 degrees. Use a 72-inch focal-film distance if possible.

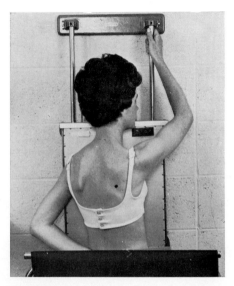

Fig. 12-71. Chest—left anterior oblique (L.A.O.) position.

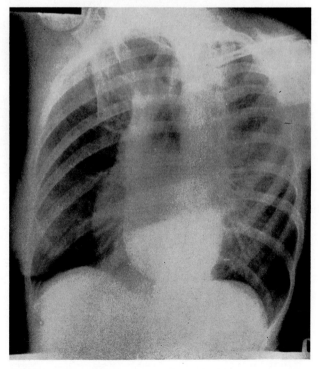

Fig. 12-72. Chest—left anterior oblique (L.A.O.) view. (Courtesy Dr. E. I. L. Cilley, Dr. T. W. Crowell, Dr. R. E. Waud, and Dr. G. H. Hoffman.)

Chest—apical lordotic view (Figs. 12-73 and 12-74)

Film size—14″ × 17″	*Erect film holder*
Cassette	*Cone to cover*
Lengthwise	

Technique

Factors	Screen film cassette (*par*)
Ma	200
Time	1/20
Mas	10
Thickness in cm	23
Kvp	68
Distance	72

Patient preparation

Remove all garments down to the waist. Provide a gown for female patients.

Palpation points

Acromion processes; lateral ribs; sternum.

Procedure

Place the patient in the erect posterior (A-P) position 1 foot in front of the erect film holder. Align the top of the cassette 2 inches above the acromion processes. Place the backs of the hands on the hips, and roll the shoulders anteriorly as far as possible. Instruct the patient to lean backward and rest the tops of his shoulders against the cassette. Center the median line of the body over the center line of the film holder.

Central ray

Direct the central ray horizontally, perpendicular to the center of the film holder.

Immobilization

Employ deep suspended inspiration.

Right-left markers

Place the R marker in the left superior border of the film holder.

Technical tips

If the patient is incapable of assuming complete extension for this position, angle the central ray 10 degrees cephalad.

Structures demonstrated

Semiaxial view of the lungs visualizing the apices.

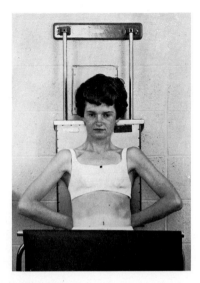

Fig. 12-73. Chest—apical lordotic position.

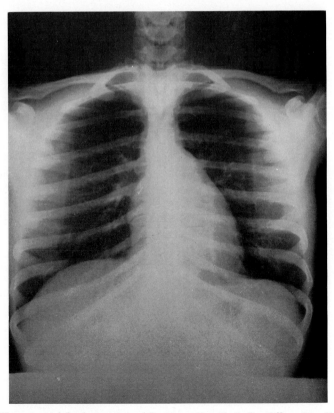

Fig. 12-74. Chest—apical lordotic view. (Courtesy Dr. E. I. L. Cilley, Dr. T. W. Crowell, Dr. R. E. Waud, and Dr. G. H. Hoffman.)

Chapter 13

Bones of the skull

Cranial bones

The superior surface of the skull is oval or circular in appearance. Frequently, variations of these types occur. The average skull is *mesocephalic*. A wide skull is *brachycephalic*. The transverse diameter of a brachycephalic skull is more than eight tenths of its anteroposterior diameter. An elongated skull is *dolichocephalic*. There are three sutures on the superior surface of the skull: *coronal*, at the junction of the frontal with the parietal bones; *sagittal*, between the parietal bones and at right angles to the coronal and lambdoidal sutures; and *lambdoidal*, at the junction of the occipital and the parietal bones and paralleling the coronal suture in direction.

The upper part of the skull, *calvarium** (skull cap) includes parts of four bones and all of two bones: the squama of the occipital, frontal, and temporal bones, and all of the two parietal bones. The cranial case includes eight bones: one frontal, two parietal, two temporal, one occipital, one sphenoid, and one ethmoid. The cranial floor includes parts of six bones: the sphenoid, ethmoid, both temporals, the occipital, and frontal.

Frontal bone

Two parts make up the frontal bone. The horizontal *(orbital)* part lies between the nasal cavity and the eye orbits. The *squama* curves toward its perimeter from the anterior portion of the orbital part. The *frontal eminences* are on the anterior surface of the squama, above the *supraorbital ridges* and bilateral to the midsagittal line. The *glabella* is raised and smooth and is located between the *superciliary arches*. The frontal bone articulates inferiorly with both nasal bones, forming a suture, the midpoint of which is called the *nasion*. The frontal processes of the maxillae and the nasal bones all lie above the nasal process, which terminates in the *nasal spine*. The supraorbital margin is the line of demarcation between the squama and the orbital portion. (See Figs. 13-1 and 13-2.) The *ethmoidal notch* is between the orbital plates and contains the *cribriform plate* of the ethmoid bone. The superior surfaces of the eye orbits are the orbital plates. The *frontal sinus* is directly behind the glabella and is usually separated into two parts by a septum. The frontal sinus and the squama are demonstrated radiographically by the use of the frontal-ethmoidal (modified Caldwell) and lateral sinus views. The frontal bone articulates with the ethmoid bone, sphenoid bone,

---

*The calvarium is that portion of the skull lying above a plane extending through the supraorbital ridges anteriorly and the superior nuchal lines (of the occipital bone) posteriorly.

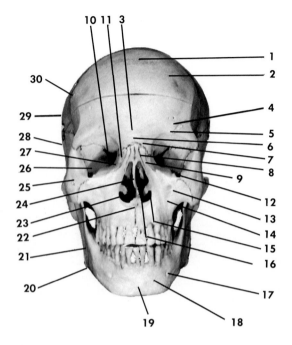

Fig. 13-1. Skull, anterior aspect.

1. Frontal bone
2. Frontal eminence
3. Glabella
4. Supercilliary arch
5. Supraorbital notch
6. Nasion
7. Nasofrontal suture
8. Nasal bone
9. Frontal process of maxilla
10. Superior orbital fissure
11. Lacrimal bone
12. Inferior oribital fissure
13. Infraorbital foramen
14. Maxilla
15. Nasal turbinate (inferior concha)
16. Middle concha
17. Mental foramen
18. Body of mandible
19. Symphysis mandibulus (menti)
20. Angle of mandible
21. Ramus of mandible
22. Inferior nasal spine
23. Vomer
24. Perpendicular plate of ethmoid
25. Zygoma
26. Great wing of sphenoid (orbital part)
27. Lamina papyraceae of ethmoid
28. Squama of temporal bone
29. Parietal bone
30. Coronal suture

both maxillae, both zygomatic bones, both parietal bones, both nasal bones, and both lacrimal bones.

Ethmoid bone

The ethmoid bone occupies the space surrounded by the frontal bone, the maxillae, and the sphenoid bone. The cribriform plate is horizontal between the orbital plates of the frontal bone. The *perpendicular plate* forms the major portion of the *nasal septum*. The *laminae papyraceae*, on the lateral surfaces of the two *lateral masses*, articulate in the eye orbit in the space surrounded by the maxillae, palatine bones, lacrimal bones, sphenoid bone, and frontal bone. The *crista galli* extends superiorly above the cribriform plate. The *ethmoid cells* are

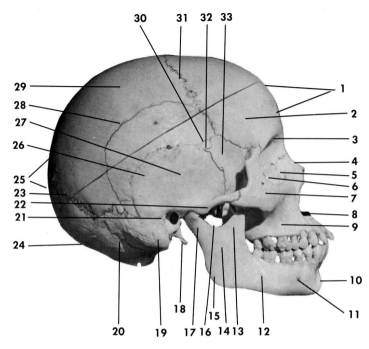

Fig. 13-2. Skull, lateral surface.

1. Sinciput
2. Frontal bone
3. Supraorbital foramen
4. Nasal bone
5. Lacrimal bone
6. Ethmoid
7. Zygoma (malar)
8. Anterior nasal spine
9. Maxilla
10. Symphysis mandibulus
11. Mental foramen
12. Mandibular body
13. Coronoid process
14. Ramus
15. Angle
16. Mandibular notch
17. Condylar process
18. Styloid process
19. Mastoid process
20. Occipitomastoid suture
21. E.A.M. (external auditory meatus)
22. Zygomatic arch
23. Lambdoidal suture
24. Occipital bone
25. Occiput
26. Squamosal suture
27. Squama of temporal bone
28. Inferior temporal line
29. Parietal bone
30. Epipteric bone
31. Coronal suture
32. Pterion
33. Sphenoid

in the middle concha. The cells and the ethmoid bone are demonstrated radiographically by the use of the frontal-ethmoidal (modified Caldwell) and lateral sinus views. The ethmoid bone articulates with the frontal bone, sphenoid bone, both sphenoidal conchae, both nasal bones, both maxillae, both palatine bones, both lacrimal bones, vomer, and both inferior nasal turbinate bones.

Sphenoid bone

The sphenoid bone occupies the space in the floor of the cranium anterior to the occipital and temporal bones and posterior to the frontal bone and ethmoid

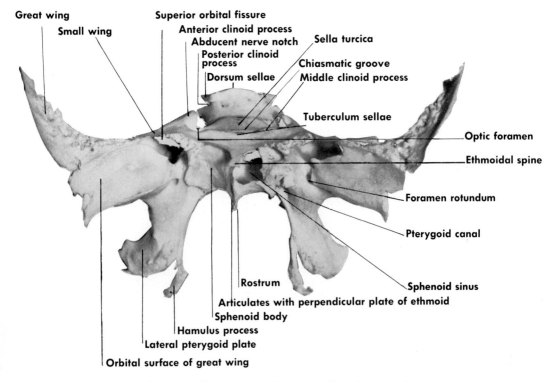

Great wing
Small wing
Superior orbital fissure
Anterior clinoid process
Abducent nerve notch
Sella turcica
Posterior clinoid process
Chiasmatic groove
Dorsum sellae
Middle clinoid process
Tuberculum sellae
Optic foramen
Ethmoidal spine
Foramen rotundum
Pterygoid canal
Sphenoid sinus
Rostrum
Articulates with perpendicular plate of ethmoid
Sphenoid body
Hamulus process
Lateral pterygoid plate
Orbital surface of great wing

Fig. 13-3. Sphenoid, supero-oblique aspect. (Courtesy Clay-Adams, Inc.)

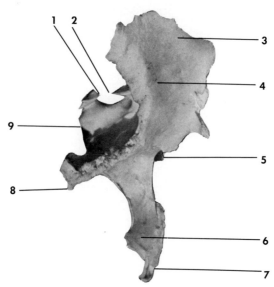

Fig. 13-4. Sphenoid, lateral surface.

1. Posterior clinoid process
2. Anterior clinoid process
3. Great wing
4. Temporal fossa
5. Articulates with vomer
6. Pterygoid process
7. Pterygoid hamulus
8. Spina angularis
9. Dorsum sellae

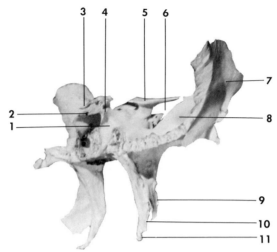

Fig. 13-5. Sphenoid, latero-oblique aspect.

1. Body
2. Dorsum sellae
3. Anterior clinoid process
4. Posterior clinoid process
5. Small wing
6. Superior orbital fissure
7. Great wing, lateral surface
8. Great wing, orbital part
9. Lateral pterygoid process
10. Medial pterygoid process
11. Hamulus process

bone. It is irregularly shaped. From its body project two *great wings,* two *small wings,* and two *pterygoid processes.* (See Figs. 13-3 to 13-5.) The body is hollow. A septum divides this space into the *sphenoidal sinuses,* which are inferior to the *sella turcica.* The sella turcica is the saddle-shaped part of the sphenoid bone which contains the pituitary gland. The cribriform plate of the ethmoid bone articulates with the *ethmoid spine,* which extends above the body. The chiasmatic groove is posterior to the ethmoid spine in a smooth, raised part and is anterior to the *tuberculum sellae.* The sella turcica* is directly behind and below the tuberculum sellae. It is bounded anteriorly by the *middle* and *anterior clinoid processes* and posteriorly by the dorsum sellae, which terminates superiorly in the *posterior clinoid process.* The *petrosal process* is inferior to the *dorsum sellae.* The apex of the *petrous portion* of the temporal bone articulates with the petrosal process. The *clivus* is posterior to the dorsum sellae and articulates posteriorly with the basilar part of the occipital bone. The perpendicular plate of the ethmoid bone articulates posteriorly with the sphenoidal crest, which joints the *rostrum* of the sphenoid bone. The lower lateral margins of the anterior surface form parts of the eye orbits. Between the alae of the vomer is the sphenoidal rostrum. On both sides a portion of the lateral wall of the skull is formed by a part of the greater wing of the sphenoid. This portion occupies the space between the temporal and frontal bones and between the parietal and zygomatic bones. The *spina angularis* is an inferior projection adajacent to both the squamosal and petrous portions of the temporal bone. The *pterion* is a point at the

---

*Other names for the sella turcica are the pituitary fossa and the hypophyseal fossa.

junction of the frontal, parietal, and temporal bones and great wing of the sphenoid bone, about 3 cm posterior to the external angular process of the orbit. Frequently, a point is formed by the junction of the parietal, temporal, and sphenoid bones; however, in many skulls this part of the sphenoid bone is broad and separates the frontal bone from the temporal bone. The smaller wings are superior to the body and extend bilaterally. They contain the *optic foramina* and form the anterior clinoid processes. The pterygoid processes are paired. They are inferior to the junction of the body and the greater wings. There are two sphenoidal conchae between the nasal cavity and the sphenoidal sinus, which permit the passage of air between the nasal cavity and the sinus. The sphenoid bone is demonstrated radiographically by the use of the open-mouth sphenoid and lateral sinus views. The anterior (P-A) view demonstrates the optic foramen. The sphenoid bone articulates with the parietal bones, zygomatic bones, palatine bones, temporal bones, vomer, ethmoid bone, frontal bone, and occipital bone. The maxillary tuberosities occasionally articulate with the sphenoid bone.

Occipital bone

The occipital bone forms parts of the posterior and inferior, or basal, portions of the cranium. It consists of three parts: the *basilar,* which articulates anteriorly with the basilar part of the sphenoid bone; the *lateral,* which are situated bilateral to the *foramen magnum;* and the *squamous,* which lies posterior, superior, and anterior to the foramen magnum and contributes to the formation of the lambdoidal suture. The *occipital condyles* are located on the inferior surfaces of the lateral parts and articulate with the superior articular facets of the atlas. The squama of the occipital bone, like the squama of the frontal bone, curves toward its perimeter. Its cranial surface faces the posterior part of the brain. The medulla spinalis passes through the foramen magnum to connect with the brain. The occiput is demonstrated radiographically by the use of the occipital view. The occipital bone articulates with both temporal bones, both parietal bones, the atlas, and the sphenoid bone.

Parietal bone

The paired parietal bones articulate with each other in the midsagittal plane, forming the sagittal suture. Each bone articulates inferiorly with the temporal bone, posteriorly with the occipital bone, and anteriorly with the frontal bone. Near the sagittal and lambdoidal sutures, each parietal bone contains a small foramen called the *parietal foramen.* These foramina are not always visualized. The junction of the sagittal and coronal sutures is named the *anterior fontanelle* (bregma), and the junction of the lambdoidal and sagittal sutures is named the *posterior fontanelle* (lambda). The parietal bone is demonstrated radiographically by the use of the lateral skull position. Each parietal bone articulates with the temporal bone, sphenoid bone, frontal bone, occipital bone, and opposite parietal bone.

Temporal bone

Obtaining radiographs that demonstrate well the numerous parts of the temporal bones requires both anatomic knowledge and radiographic skill. Careful study of the anatomy of the temporal bone is essential. Although not demon-

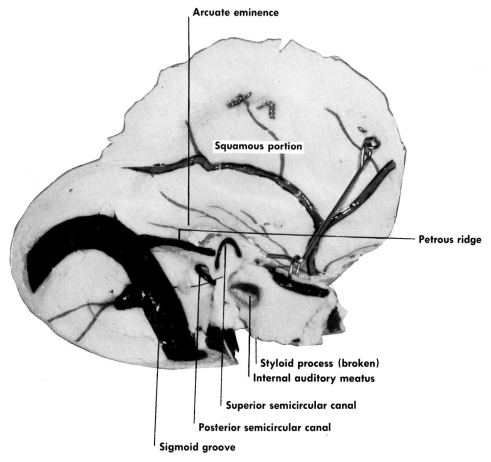

Arcuate eminence

Squamous portion

Petrous ridge

Styloid process (broken)
Internal auditory meatus

Superior semicircular canal

Posterior semicircular canal

Sigmoid groove

Fig. 13-6. Left temporal, internal surface. (Courtesy Clay-Adams, Inc.)

strable radiographically, the *auditory ossicles* are in the cavity of the tympanum. These bones are the *malleus, incus,* and *stapes.*

The temporal bones are inferior to the parietal bones between the occipital bone and great wing of the sphenoid bone. (See Figs. 13-6 and 13-7.) The *squama* of the temporal bone is surrounded by the sphenoid bone and parietal bone. The *zygomatic process* extends anteriorly from the inferior portion of the squama and articulates anteriorly with the zygomatic bone. The *mastoid portion* is posterior and inferior to the squama. The mastoid process contains the *mastoid cells* and extends posteriorly and inferiorly below the *external auditory meatus.* The *tympanic antrum* is medial to the cells and lateral and posterior to the *epitympanic recess.* Most of the important auditory organs, among which are the *semicircular canals* and *membranous labyrinth,* are in the petrous portion, which separates the occipital bone and sphenoid bone. The *styloid process* is directed inferiorly and anteriorly from beneath the tympanic part. The external auditory meatus is located in the petrous portion. The temporal bone is demonstrated radiographically by the use of the lateral skull view; the petrous ridges,

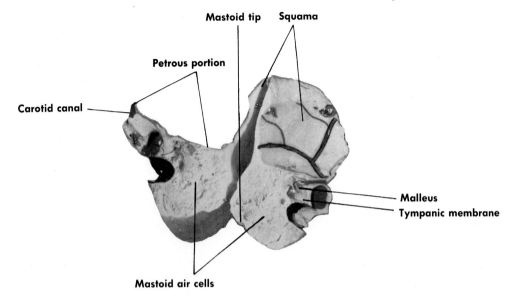

Mastoid tip   **Squama**

Petrous portion

Carotid canal

Malleus
Tympanic membrane

Mastoid air cells

Fig. 13-7. Left temporal, oblique section through mastoid and petrous portions. (Courtesy Clay-Adams, Inc.)

by the use of the posterior (A-P) axial view, anterior (P-A) axial view, and the occipital view; and the mastoids, by the use of the lateral view. The temporal bone articulates with the parietal bone, occipital bone, sphenoid bone, zygomatic bone, and mandible.

Points of importance

1. The floor of the cranium is formed by the ethmoid bone, sphenoid bone, both temporal bones, frontal bone, and occipital bone.
2. The flat bones of the skull cap are composed of three layers: *outer table, diploë,* and *inner table.* The diploë contains the major supply of the nerves and blood vessels of the skull cap. It is the nutrient layer for the entire outer table and for part of the inner table.
3. The foramen magnum in the occipital bone is surrounded by the lateral parts, basilar part, and squamous part.
4. The basilar part of the occipital bone articulates anteriorly with the basilar portion of the sphenoid bone.
5. The basilar portion of the sphenoid bone articulates anteriorly and inferiorly with the vomer.
6. The following bones and parts contribute to the formation of the nasal septum: nasal crests and frontal spine, perpendicular plate of the ethmoid, sphenoidal rostrum and vomer, and maxillary crests.
7. The sagittal suture is formed by the junction of the parietal bones.
8. The coronal suture is formed by the junction of the frontal bone with the parietal bones.
9. The anterior fontanelle (bregma) is at the junction of the sagittal and coronal sutures.

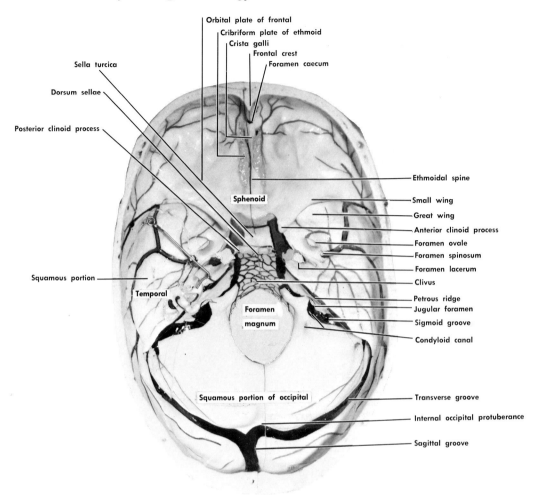

Fig. 13-8. Cranial floor, superior aspect. (Courtesy Clay-Adams, Inc.)

10. The posterior fontanelle (lambda) is at the junction of the sagittal and lamboidal sutures.
11. The lamboidal suture is situated between the occipital bone and the parietal bones.
12. The squamous sutures are between the temporal bones and parietal bones.
13. The pterion is located at the junction of the coronal and squamosal sutures.
14. The *asterion* is located at the junction of the lambdoidal and squamosal sutures.
15. The *obelion* is located at the junction of a line drawn between the parietal foramina with the sagittal suture.
16. The *inion* is the midpoint of the external occipital protuberance.

For a better understanding of the relation of the bones forming the base of the cranium, see Fig. 13-8. The verticosubmental view is frequently used to demonstrate the cranial floor.

Facial bones

Including the mandible, there are fourteen facial bones: two nasal, two zygomatic, two lacrimal, two maxillae, two palatine, two inferior nasal turbinate, mandible, and vomer. They are generally responsible for the shape and appearance of the face.

Nasal bones

The nasal bones are quite small and articulate with each other in the midsagittal plane. Each articulates with the corresponding frontal process of the maxilla. The lateral cartilage of the nose is inferior to each nasal bone. The vertical crest articulates with the frontal spine and the perpendicular plate of the ethmoid bone and extends below the sagittal border. The nasal bones are demonstrated radiographically by the use of the axial, anterior (P-A) (Waters) sinus views, and lateral nasal bone view. The nasal bone articulates with the frontal bone, ethmoid bone, maxilla, and opposite nasal bone.

Lacrimal bone

The smallest facial bone is the lacrimal bone. It occupies the space surrounded by the lamina papyracea of the ethmoid bone, two parts of the maxilla, frontal orbital plate, and inferior nasal turbinate and forms a part of the medial orbital wall. The lacrimal bones are not well demonstrated radiographically. The anterior (P-A) view is used.

Zygomatic (malar) bone

The zygomatic bone occupies the space bordering on the temporal bone, frontal bone, maxilla, and sphenoid bone and has processes that articulate with these bones. It is situated inferior and lateral to the outer canthus of the eye and is commonly called the cheek bone. It is concerned with the formation of the lateral border of the eye orbit in its articulation with the frontal bone and also with the formation of the zygomatic arch in its articulation with the zygomatic process of the temporal bone. The zygomatic bone is demonstrated radiographically by the use of the zygomatic arch, tangential view.

Maxillae

The second largest bones of the facial group are the maxillae, which form the upper jaw. The maxilla articulates with, and occupies the space bordering on, the nasal bone, lacrimal bone, zygomatic bone, inferior nasal turbinate bone, vomer, palatine bone, ethmoid bone, frontal bone, and opposite maxilla. It contains one of the *maxillary sinuses (nasal antra)* lateral to the median plane and superior to the bicuspid, when demonstrated in an anterior projection. It borders on the buccal, nasal, and orbital cavities. Each maxilla forms one half of the anterior nasal spine. The *frontal process* extends superiorly between the nasal and lacrimal bones and articulates with the frontal bone. The *zygomatic process* faces and articulates posteriorly with the zygomatic bone. The strong *palatine process* is horizontal. It articulates in the midsagittal plane with the palatine process of the opposite maxilla. Posteriorly each palatine process articulates with the horizontal portion of the palatine bone. The palatine processes of the maxillae with the horizontal parts of the palatine bones separate the nasal and buccal cavities and form the *hard palate.* The *alveolar process* is the ridge from which the teeth of the upper jaw erupt. The *alveolar arch* is composed of the two alveolar processes. The maxillary sinus will be described on pp. 270 and 271. The maxilla is demonstrated radiographically by the use of the oblique maxilla and anterior (P-A) (Waters) views. The antra are demonstrated by the use of the erect anterior (P-A) (Waters) view, whereas the maxillae, inferior (superoinferior) view demonstrates the hard palate and palatine processes.

Palatine bone

The palatine bone, above the roof of the mouth, occupies the space bordering on the palatine process of the maxilla, the opposite palatine bone, ethmoid bone, vomer, and inferior nasal turbinate bone and articulates with these bones. The palatine borders on the nasal and buccal cavities and the orbit of the eye. It is composed of five distinct parts: three processes (pyramidal, orbital, and sphenoidal) and a horizontal part and a vertical part. The *horizontal part* articulates with the corresponding part of the other palatine bone in the midsagittal plane. This articulation is described under the palatine processes of the maxillae. It is inferiorly placed on the palatine bone and extends medially from the main structure. The *vertical part* extends above the horizontal part and includes the orbital, sphenoidal, and pyramidal processes. The palatine bone is demonstrated radiographically by the use of the maxillae, inferior (superoinferior) view for the hard palate. The horizontal part of the palatine bones is always included in radiographs of the hard palate.

Inferior nasal turbinate bone (concha)

The inferior nasal turbinate bone resembles a conch shell and is truly osseous, while the middle and superior turbinate bones are chiefly cartilaginous. The middle and superior nasal turbinates are parts of the ethmoid. The inferior nasal turbinate bones are lateral and inferior in the nasal cavity, one turbinate bone being located on each lateral wall. This bone is best demonstrated radiographically in the anterior (P-A) skull view, although it may be visualized in the anterior (P-A) (Waters) sinus view. The inferior nasal turbinate bone articulates with the ethmoid bone, maxilla, lacrimal bone, and palatine bone.

Vomer

The vomer occupies the space surrounded by the ethmoid bone, sphenoid bone, both maxillae, and both palatine bones and articulates with these bones. It is near the center of the base of the skull. A lateral projection bears a fair resemblance to a blunt arrowhead, with the blunted end directed toward the *alveolar point.* The *choanae* (posterior nares) are separated by the posterior margin of the vomer. The vomer contributes to the formation of the nasal septum and is the most posterior part of the nasal septum. Although difficult to visualize, the vomer is demonstrated radiographically by the use of the lateral skull, submentovertex, and verticosubmental views.

Mandible

The largest bone of the facial section of the skull is the mandible. Ossification begins in two different centers in intrauterine life, and the mandibular body is in two parts at birth. In the first few months of extrauterine life, the two parts of the body are fused anteriorly in the midsagittal plane *(symphysis mandibulus)*. Superiorly on each side of the body is the *alveolar ridge (process)*, from which the teeth of the lower jaw erupt. From the posterior ends of the body the bone turns upward, forming the *ramus* on each side. This turn is called the *angle of the mandible*. The *condylar process* extends posteriorly and superiorly from the ramus to support the *head (condyle)*, which articulates in the mandibular fossa of the temporal bone, forming the *temporomandibular joint*. There is one head for each ramus. The *coronoid process* extends anteriorly and superiorly from the ramus. It has no articulation. There is one coronoid process for each ramus. The mandible is demonstrated radiographically by the use of the lateral and oblique mandible views, and the symphysis and rami are demonstrated by the use of the anterior (P-A) view. Frequently, it is inconvenient to obtain satisfactory views in the routine positioning. The use of dental films intraorally and extraorally is of extreme value in certain cases.

Hyoid bone

Although the hyoid bone is not one of the bones of the skull, it is usually discussed immediately following them. It is U shaped, has no osseous articulations, and is attached by ligaments to the styloid processes of the temporal

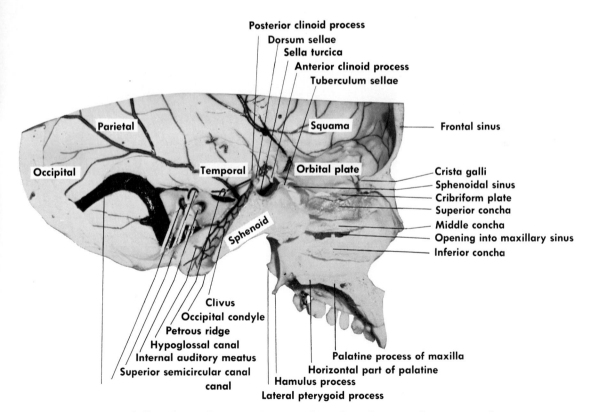

Fig. 13-9. Skull, midsagittal section, showing relationship of paranasal sinuses to other structures. (Courtesy Clay-Adams, Inc.)

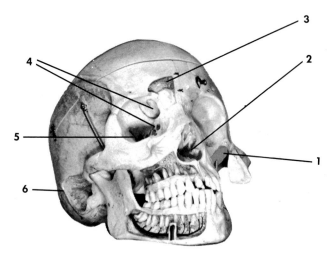

Fig. 13-10. Skull, antero-oblique aspect.

1. Maxillary sinus (anterior surface removed)
2. Nasal cavity
3. Frontal sinus (anterior surface removed)

4. Ethmoid air cells
5. Optic foramen
6. Mastoid air cells (lateral surface removed)

bones. It is superior to the thyroid cartilage and anterior to the base of the tongue. The hyoid bone is demonstrated radiographically by the use of the lateral cervical spine view.

Sinuses

The *paranasal sinuses (frontal, two ethmoid, sphenoid,* and *maxillary* or *nasal antra)* form a border of air spaces around the nasal cavity. Each sinus has openings into the nasal cavity. The sinuses are frequently examined radiographically. The major positions for examinations were mentioned briefly in conjunction with the description of their respective bones. In addition to these sinuses, a discussion of the *nasal cavity* is pertinent in this section. (See Figs. 13-9 and 13-10.)

Frontal sinus

The frontal sinus is located in the frontal bone posterior to the glabella and medially between the supraorbital ridges in the diploë.

Ethmoid sinuses

The two ethmoid sinuses are anterior and posterior to each other. They are located in the ethmoid bone superior and bilateral to the nasal septum and anterior and superior to the sphenoid sinus.

Sphenoid sinus

The sphenoid sinus is located in the sphenoid bone, anterior and inferior to the sella turcica.

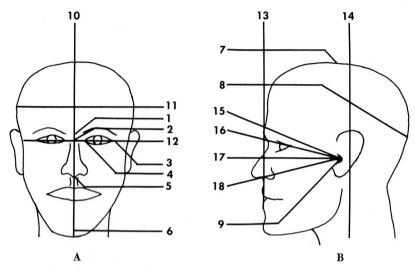

Fig. 13-11. Skull landmarks, **A**, and guidelines, **B**.

1. Glabella
2. Nasion
3. Outer canthus
4. Inner canthus
5. Acanthion (anterior nasal spine)
6. Mental (mandibular) symphysis
7. Vertex
8. External occipital protuberance (E.O.P.)
9. External acoustic meatus (E.A.M.)

10. Midsagittal (median) plane
11. Transverse plane
12. Interpupillary line
13. Glabelloalveolar line
14. Coronal plane
15. Glabellomeatal line
16. Orbitomeatal (canthomeatal) line
17. Infraorbitomeatal line
18. Acanthiomeatal line

Nasal antra

The nasal antra are located in the maxillae, bilateral to the nasal cavity and inferior to the orbital floors of the eye cavities.

Nasal cavity

The nasal septum divides the nasal cavity into two parts. It is situated between the buccal cavity and the cranial floor. The nasal bone, frontal spine, cribriform plate of the ethmoid bone, body of the sphenoid bone, sphenoidal conchae, alae of the vomer, and the palatine sphenoidal processes form the roof of the nasal cavity. The palatine processes of the maxillae and half of the horizontal parts of the palatine bones form the floor of the nasal cavity. The medial wall is the nasal septum and is described in item 6 under Points of Importance. The frontal process of the maxilla, lacrimal bone, ethmoid bone, body of the maxilla, inferior nasal turbinate bone, vertical plate of the palatine bone, and the medial pterygoid plate of the sphenoid bone form the lateral wall. The nasal cavity opens to the outside through the *anterior nares* (bony parts of the nose) and into the pharynx through the choanae (posterior nares). It is demonstrated radiographically by the use of the routine sinus views.

REFERENCES

Anthony, Catherine Parker: Textbook of anatomy and physiology, St. Louis, 1967, The C. V. Mosby Co.

Best, C. H., and Taylor, N. B.: The living body, New York, 1952, Henry Holt & Co., Inc.

Best, C. H., and Taylor, N. B.: The human body, New York, 1956, Henry Holt & Co., Inc.

De Coursey, Russell Myles: The human organism, New York, 1955, McGraw-Hill Book Co.

Goss, Charles M.: Gray's anatomy, ed. 28, Philadelphia, 1966, Lea & Febiger.

Greisheimer, Esther M.: Physiology and anatomy, Philadelphia, 1950, J. B. Lippincott Co.

Kimber, Diana Clifford, and Gray, Carolyn E.: Textbook of anatomy and physiology, New York, 1928, The Macmillan Co.

Meschan, Isadore: Normal radiographic anatomy, Philadelphia, 1951, W. B. Saunders Co.

Chapter 14

Positioning for the skull

Skull

Skull—anterior (P-A) view (Figs. 14-1 and 14-2)

> *Film size—10″ × 12″*   *Bucky*
> *Cassette*   *Cone to cover*
> *Lengthwise*

Technique

Factors	Screen film cassette (par)
Ma	100
Time	0.6
Mas	60
Thickness in cm	18
Kvp	78
Distance	40

Patient preparation

Remove all metallic and plastic articles from the head and neck region.

Palpation point

Vertex.

Procedure

Place the patient in the prone position with the median plane of the skull and body over the center line of the table. Place the hands in a comfortable position at the sides of the head. Place the forehead and nose on the table so that both the midsagittal plane and the canthomeatal line are perpendicular to the table-top. Align the top of the cassette 1½ inches above the vertex of the skull.

Central ray

Direct the central ray perpendicular through the nasion to the film holder.

Immobilization

Place large sponges on each side of the skull and hold them in place with sandbags or the patient's hands. Employ suspended expiration.

Right-left markers

Place the *R* marker on the right side, center border of the film holder.

Technical tips

For thin patients, place a pillow or positioning sponges under the anterior thorax.

Structures demonstrated

Anterior (P-A) view of the anterior wall of the cranium, the frontal sinuses, the ethmoid sinuses, and the crista galli. The petrous ridges should fill the lower two thirds of the eye orbits.

Note:

To demonstrate a larger area of the petrous portion, make an anteroposterior view, reversing the above procedure.

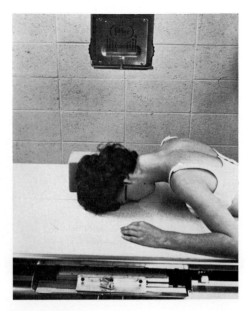

Fig. 14-1. Skull—anterior (P-A) position.

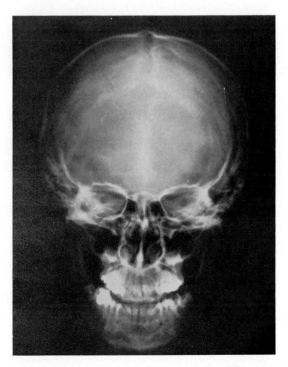

Fig. 14-2. Skull—anterior (P-A) view. (Courtesy Dr. E. I. L. Cilley, Dr. T. W. Crowell, Dr. R. E. Waud, and Dr. G. H. Hoffman.)

Skull—lateral view (Figs. 14-3 and 14-4)

> *Film size—10″ × 12″*   *Bucky*
> *Cassette*   *Cone to cover*
> *Crosswise*

Technique

Factors	Screen film cassette (par)
Ma	100
Time	0.5
Mas	50
Thickness in cm	15
Kvp	68
Distance	40

Patient preparation

Remove all metallic and plastic articles from the head and neck region.

Palpation point

Vertex.

Procedure

Place the patient in the prone position with the side of the skull being examined on the table. Elevate the opposite side of the body; flex this knee and elbow for support. The midsagittal plane of the skull is parallel with the tabletop. Flex the neck so that the canthomeatal line is perpendicular to the side of the table. Support the chin with a sponge or the patient's fist. On the canthomeatal line, center a point ¾ inch anterior and ¾ inch superior to the E.A.M. (external auditory meatus) over the center line of the table. Align the top of the cassette 1½ inches above the vertex of the skull.

Central ray

Direct the central ray perpendicular through the selected point to the film holder.

Immobilization

Place large sponges against the top and back of the skull; hold them in place with sandbags. Employ suspended expiration.

Right-left markers

Place the correct marker on the anterior center border of the film holder.

Technical tips

Make bilateral views on patients with traumatic injuries.

Structures demonstrated

Lateral view visualizing the anterior and posterior clinoid processes, sella turcica, dorsum sellae, and superimposed parietal bones.

Note:

For stereographic views, make two separate views, shifting the tube 2 inches inferior from the centering point and then 2 inches superior from the centering point. The patient *must retain the same position* for both radiographic exposures.

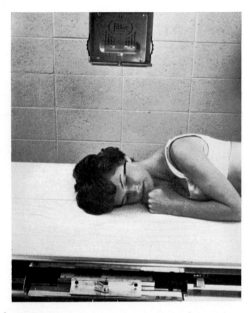

Fig. 14-3. Skull—lateral position.

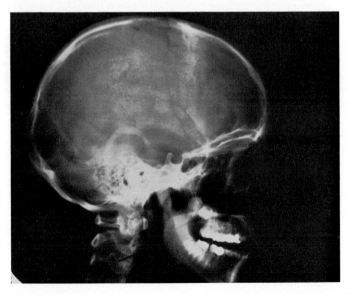

Fig. 14-4. Skull—lateral view. (Courtesy Dr. E. I. L. Cilley, Dr. T. W. Crowell, Dr. R. E. Waud, and Dr. G. H. Hoffman.)

Skull—occipital (Towne) view (Figs. 14-5 and 14-6)

      Film size—10″ × 12″   *Bucky*

      Cassette   *Cone to cover*

      Lengthwise

Technique

Factors	*Screen film cassette (par)*
Ma	100
Time	0.7
Mas	70
Thickness in cm	23
Kvp	80
Distance	40

Patient preparation

Remove all metallic and plastic articles from the head and neck region.

Palpation point

Vertex.

Procedure

Place the patient in the supine position with the median plane of the skull and body over the center line of the table. The midsagittal plane is perpendicular to the tabletop. Flex the chin so that the canthomeatal line is perpendicular to the tabletop. Align the top of the cassette with the vertex of the skull.

Central ray

Direct the central ray 35 degrees caudad through a point in line with the E.A.M. (external auditory meatus) to the film holder.

Immobilization

Place a sandbag on top of the chin and chest and instruct the patient to hold the sandbag in place. Employ suspended expiration.

Right-left markers

Place the *R* marker on the right lateral center border of the film holder.

Technical tips

The posterior clinoid processes will be demonstrated within the foramen magnum when the view is exact.

Structures demonstrated

Posterior (P-A) view of the occipital region visualizing the bilateral petrous pyramids, foramen magnum, dorsum sellae, occipital squama, and the posterior portions of both parietal bones.

Note:

For prone patients, place the forehead on the tabletop and reverse the central ray angulation described above.

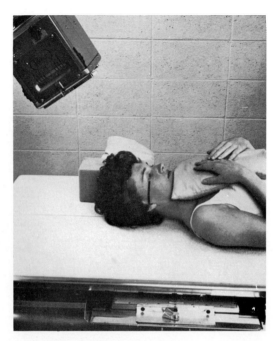

Fig. 14-5. Skull—occipital (Towne) position.

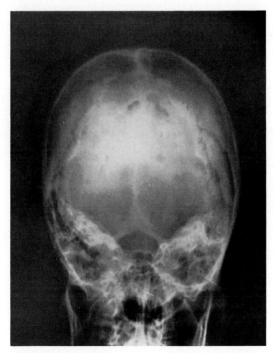

Fig. 14-6. Skull—occipital (Towne) view. (Courtesy Dr. E. I. L. Cilley, Dr. T. W. Crowell, Dr. R. E. Waud, and Dr. G. H. Hoffman.)

Skull—basilar (submentovertex) view (Figs. 14-7 and 14-8)

> *Film size—10″ × 12″*   *Bucky*
> *Cassette*   *Cone to cover*
> *Lengthwise*

Technique

Factors	Screen film cassette (*par*)
Ma	100
Time	0.8
Mas	80
Thickness in cm	23
Kvp	80
Distance	40

Patient preparation

Remove all metallic and plastic articles from the head and neck region.

Palpation points

Vertex; mandibular angles.

Procedure

Place the patient in the supine position on a large cushion or pillow with the median plane of the skull and body over the center line of the table. Extend the head backward so that the vertex of the skull rests on the tabletop. The midsagittal plane is perpendicular to the tabletop.

Central ray

Direct the central ray perpendicular to the infraorbitomeatal line, to enter a point midway between the angles of the mandible, and to the center of the film holder.

Immobilization

Place sponges supported by sandbags against the forehead. Flex both knees and place both feet on the table to relieve neck strain. Employ suspended expiration.

Right-left markers

Place the R marker on the right lateral center border of the film holder.

Technical tips

For a better demonstration of the jugular foramen, decrease the cervical extension 20 degrees.

Structures demonstrated

Axial view of the basilar region visualizing the bilateral petrous ridges, mastoid processes, atlas, sphenoidal sinuses, maxillary sinuses, mandible, and the bilateral zygomatic arches.

Note:

For elderly or wheelchair patients, use an erect table or a film holder with the patient seated.

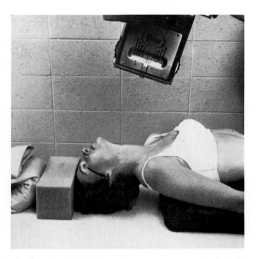

Fig. 14-7. Skull—basilar (submentovertex) position.

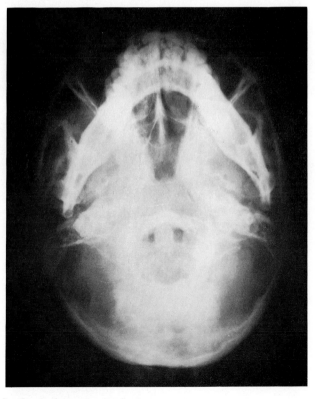

Fig. 14-8. Skull—basilar (submentovertex) view.

Skull—verticosubmental view (Figs. 14-9 and 14-10)

>   *Film size—10″ × 12″*   *Bucky*
>   *Cassette*   *Cone to cover*
>   *Lengthwise*

Technique

Factors	Screen film cassette (par)
Ma	100
Time	0.8
Mas	80
Thickness in cm	23
Kvp	80
Distance	40

Patient preparation

Remove all metallic and plastic articles from the head and neck region.

Palpation points

Vertex; mandibular condyles.

Procedure

Place the patient in the prone position with the median plane of the skull and body over the center line of the table. Place the hands on the table at the sides of the head. Extend the chin as far as possible and rest it on the center line of the table. The midsagittal plane of the skull is perpendicular to the tabletop.

Central ray

Direct the central ray perpendicular to the infraorbitomeatal line, through a point in line with the condyles of the mandible, and to the center of the film holder.

Immobilization

Place large sponges against the sides of the skull, and sandbags against the sponges; instruct the patient to hold the sandbags in place with his hands. Employ suspended expiration.

Right-left markers

Place the R marker on the right lateral center border of the film holder.

Technical tips

Use of a grid cassette or portable Bucky will reduce both magnification and distortion of the image.

Structures demonstrated

Axial view of the base of the skull visualizing the spenoidal sinuses and anterior cranial base.

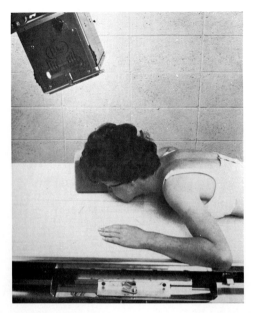

Fig. 14-9. Skull—verticosubmental position.

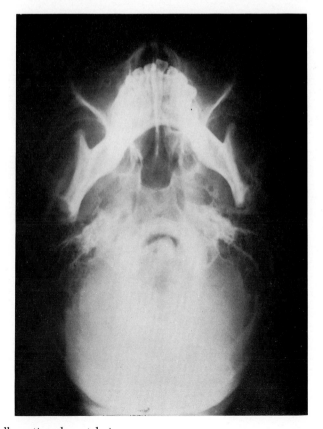

Fig. 14-10. Skull—verticosubmental view.

Sinuses

Sinuses—maxillary (Waters) view (Figs. 14-11 and 14-12)

Film size—8″ × 10″	*Erect Bucky*
Cassette	*Extension cone*
Lengthwise	

Technique

Factors	Screen film cassette (par) Bucky	Screen film cassette (par) tabletop
Ma	100	100
Time	0.5	0.25
Mas	50	25
Thickness in cm	21	21
Kvp	78	78
Distance	30	30

Patient preparation

Remove all metallic and plastic articles from the head and neck region.

Palpation point

Acanthion.

Procedure

Seat the patient facing the erect Bucky with the median plane of the skull over the center line of the erect Bucky. Extend the chin both upward and forward to rest against the center line of the erect Bucky. The canthomeatal line forms a 37-degree angle with the erect Bucky, and the midsagittal plane of the skull is perpendicular to it.

Central ray

Direct the central ray perpendicular through the anterior nasal spine to the center of the film holder.

Immobilization

Instruct the patient to grasp each side of the table with his hands. Place the extension cone against the back of the skull (shock-proof equipment only). Employ suspended expiration.

Right-left markers

Burn the erect and *L* markers in the upper left border of the film holder above the cone field after the exposure is made.

Technical tips

Increase the cervical extension to decrease the amount of petrous portion demonstrated.

Structures demonstrated

Anterior (P-A) views of the maxillary antra to demonstrate possible fluid levels, the nasal septum, and the posterior walls of the eye orbits.

Note:

Prone positioning will allow for better immobilization but will not demonstrate fluid level.

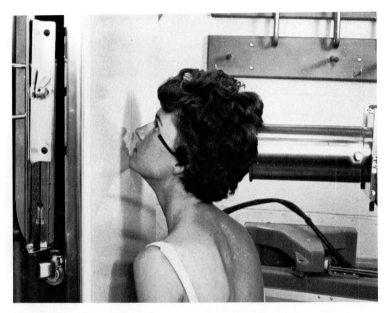

Fig. 14-11. Sinuses—maxillary (Waters) erect position.

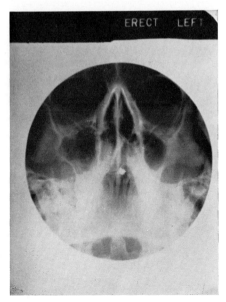

Fig. 14-12. Sinuses—maxillary (Waters) erect view. (Courtesy Dr. E. I. L. Cilley, Dr. T. W. Crowell, Dr. R. E. Waud, and Dr. G. H. Hoffman.)

Sinuses—frontal-ethmoidal (modified Caldwell) view (Figs. 14-13 and 14-14)

Film size—8″ × 10″	*Bucky*
Cassette	*Extension cone*
Lengthwise	

Technique

Factors	Screen film cassette (par) Bucky	Screen film cassette (par) tabletop
Ma	100	100
Time	0.5	0.25
Mas	50	25
Thickness in cm	19	19
Kvp	74	74
Distance	30	30

Patient preparation

Remove all metallic and plastic articles from the head and neck region.

Palpation points

Glabella; nasal bones.

Procedure

Place the patient in the prone position with the median plane of the skull and body over the center line of the table. Place the hands at the sides of the head. Place the forehead and nose on the center line of the table. Both the canthomeatal line and the midsagittal plane are perpendicular to the tabletop.

Central ray

Direct the central ray 15 degrees caudad through the nasion to the center of the film holder.

Immobilization

Place large sponges against the sides of the skull; instruct the patient to hold them in place with his hands, or hold them in place with sandbags. Employ suspended expiration.

Right-left markers

Burn the *L* marker in the upper left border of the film holder above the cone field after the exposure is made.

Technical tips

For thin patients, place a pillow or positioning sponges under the anterior thorax.

Structures demonstrated

Anterior (P-A) view of the frontal sinuses, anterior ethmoid cells, and the superior optic fissures.

Note:

For a true Caldwell view, angle the central ray 23 degrees caudad through the glabella to the center of the film holder.

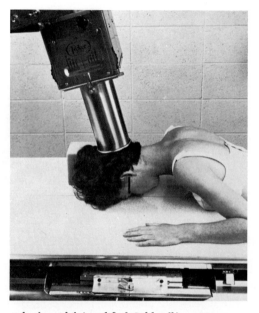

Fig. 14-13. Sinuses—frontal-ethmoidal (modified Caldwell) position.

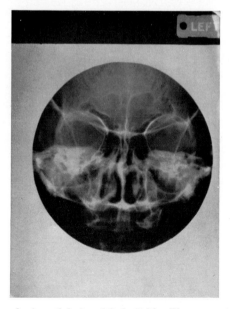

Fig. 14-14. Sinuses—frontal-ethmoidal (modified Caldwell) view. (Courtesy Dr. E. I. L. Cilley, Dr. T. W. Crowell, Dr. R. E. Waud, and Dr. G. H. Hoffman.)

Sinuses—lateral view (Figs. 14-15 and 14-16)

>   *Film size—8″ × 10″*   *Bucky*
>   *Cassette*   *Extension cone*
>   *Lengthwise*

Technique

Factors	*Screen film cassette (par)* *Bucky*	*Screen film cassette (par)* *tabletop*
Ma	100	100
Time	0.2	0.1
Mas	20	10
Thickness in cm	15	15
Kvp	62	62
Distance	30	30

Patient preparation

Remove all metallic and plastic articles from the head and neck region.

Palpation point

Lateral margin of bony orbit.

Procedure

Place the patient in the prone position with the side of the head being examined on the table. Elevate the opposite side of the body and flex this knee and elbow for support. The midsagittal plane of the head is parallel with the tabletop. Flex the neck so that the canthomeatal line is perpendicular to the side of the table. Support the chin with a sponge or the patient's fist. Center a point ½ inch posterior to the outer canthus of the eye over the center line of the table.

Central ray

Direct the central ray perpendicular through the selected point to the center of the film holder.

Immobilization

Place large sponges against the top and back of the head and hold them in place with sandbags. Employ suspended expiration.

Right-left markers

Burn the correct marker in the upper center border of the film holder above the cone field after the exposure is made.

Technical tips

The rim of the extension cone should just clear the anterior border of the E.A.M.

Structures demonstrated

Lateral view of the paranasal sinuses and sella turcica.

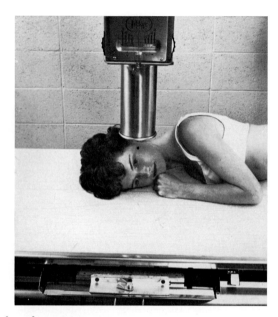

Fig. 14-15. Sinuses—lateral position.

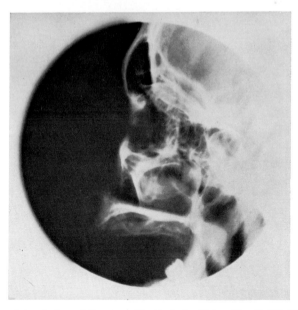

Fig. 14-16. Sinuses—lateral view. (Courtesy Dr. E. I. L. Cilley, Dr. T. W. Crowell, Dr. R. E. Waud, and Dr. G. H. Hoffman.)

Sinuses—open-mouth, sphenoid view (Figs. 14-17 and 14-18)

Film size—8″ × 10″	*Bucky*
Cassette	*Extension cone*
Lengthwise	

Technique

Factors	Screen film cassette (*par*) Bucky	Screen film cassette (*par*) tabletop
Ma	100	100
Time	0.5	0.25
Mas	50	25
Thickness in cm	21	21
Kvp	76	76
Distance	30	30

Patient preparation

Remove all metallic and plastic articles from the head and neck region.

Palpation point

Temporal bone.

Procedure

Place the patient in the prone position with the median plane of the head and body over the center line of the table. Place the hands at the sides of the head. Have the patient open the mouth as far as possible and place it on the center line of the table. The midsagittal plane is perpendicular to the tabletop.

Central ray

Direct the central ray 23 degrees caudad through the sella turcica and the center of the open mouth to the center of the film holder.

Immobilization

Place large sponges against the sides of the head, and instruct the patient to hold them in place with his hands, or use sandbags. Employ suspended expiration.

Right-left markers

Burn the *L* marker in the upper left border of the film holder above the cone field after the exposure is made.

Technical tips

Decreased central-ray angulation may be necessary to align the sella turcica with the center of the open mouth.

Structures demonstrated

Anterior (P-A) view of the sphenoidal sinuses projected through the open mouth.

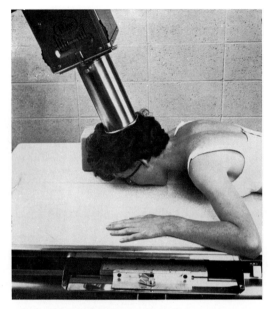

Fig. 14-17. Sinuses—sphenoid (open-mouth) position.

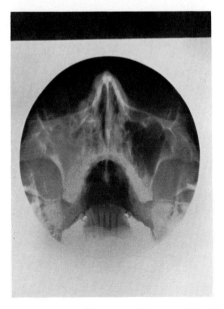

Fig. 14-18. Sinuses—sphenoid (open-mouth) view. (Courtesy Dr. E. I. L. Cilley, Dr. T. W. Crowell, Dr. R. E. Waud, and Dr. G. H. Hoffman.)

Mastoids

Mastoids—lateral (15°-15° Law's) view (Figs. 14-19 and 14-20)

> *Film size—8″ × 10″*   *Bucky*
> *Cassette*   *Extension cone*
> *Lengthwise*

Technique

Factors	Screen film cassette (par) Bucky	Screen film cassette (par) tabletop
Ma	100	100
Time	0.4	0.2
Mas	40	20
Thickness in cm	18	18
Kvp	70	64
Distance	30	30

Patient preparation

Remove all metallic and plastic articles from the head and neck region.

Palpation points

Mastoid processes.

Procedure

With a wax pencil make a mark 1 inch posterior to the E.A.M. (external auditory meatus) on each side of the head in line with the infraorbitomeatal line; tape the auricle of each ear forward. Place the patient in the prone position with the side of the head being examined on the table. Elevate the opposite side of the body, and flex this knee and elbow for support. The midsagittal plane is parallel with the tabletop. Rotate the face downward so that the midsagittal plane of the head forms a 15-degree angle with the tabletop. The infraorbitomeatal line is perpendicular to the side of the table. Center the lower pencil mark over the center line of the table.

Central ray

Direct the central ray 15 degrees caudad through the lower pencil mark to the center of the film holder.

Immobilization

Support the patient's chin with a sponge. Employ suspended expiration.

Right-left markers

Burn the correct marker in the upper center border of the film holder above the cone field after the exposure is made.

Technical tips

To improve centering accuracy, precenter the central ray to a point on the table and down to the film center. Position the selected mark on the patient over the point on the table.

Structures demonstrated

Lateral view of the mastoid air cells, and of the superimposed internal and external auditory meatuses.

Note:

Make bilateral views for comparison.

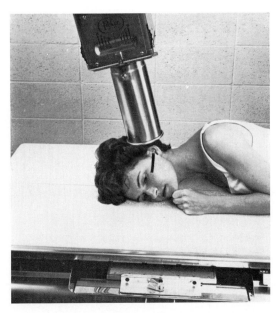

Fig. 14-19. Mastoids—lateral (15°-15° Law's) position.

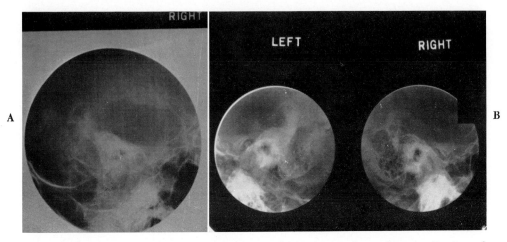

Fig. 14-20. Mastoids. **A,** Lateral (15°-15° Law's) view—Bucky technique. **B,** Lateral (15°-15° Law's) view—angle-board technique. (Courtesy Dr. E. I. L. Cilley, Dr. T. W. Crowell, Dr. R. E. Waud, and Dr. G. H. Hoffman.)

Pars petrosa, petrous portion—posterior (A-P) oblique (Arcelin's) view (Figs. 14-21 and 14-22)

> *Film size—8″ × 10″*   *Bucky*
> *Cassette*   *Extension cone*
> *Lengthwise*

Technique

Factors	Screen film cassette (par) Bucky	Screen film cassette (par) tabletop
Ma	100	100
Time	0.4	0.3
Mas	40	30
Thickness in cm	16	16
Kvp	70	56
Distance	30	30

Patient preparation

Remove all metallic and plastic articles from the head and neck region.

Palpation points

Mastoid processes.

Procedure

With a wax pencil make a mark 1 inch anterior to the E.A.M. (external auditory meatus) on the canthomeatal line on each side of the head. Place the patient in the supine position. Rotate the head 45 degrees away from the side being examined. The infraorbitomeatal line is perpendicular to the side of the table. Center the pencil mark on the upper side of the skull over the center line of the table.

Central ray

Direct the central ray 15 degrees caudad through the upper pencil mark to the center of the film holder.

Immobilization

Place a wedge sponge under the face; hold the sponge in place with a sandbag. A compression band may be placed across the head. Employ suspended expiration.

Right-left markers

Burn the correct marker in the upper center border of the film holder above the cone field after the exposure is made.

Technical tips

To improve centering accuracy, precenter the central ray to a point on the table and down to the film center. Position the selected mark on the patient over the point on the table.

Structures demonstrated

Posterior (A-P) view of the petrous pyramid, apex, internal acoustic canal, antral and labyrinthal areas, and mastoid air cells.

Note:

Make bilateral views for comparison.

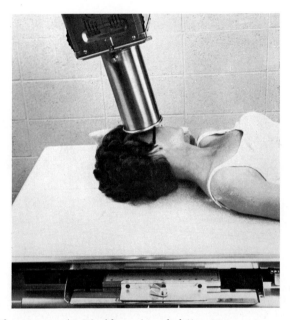

Fig. 14-21. Mastoids—posterior (A-P) oblique (Arcelin's) position.

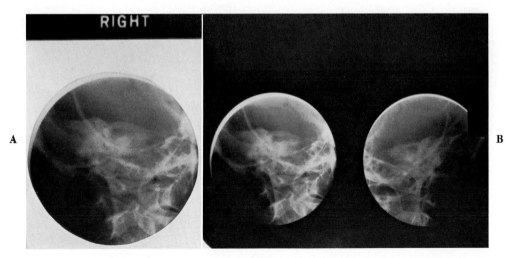

Fig. 14-22. Mastoids. **A,** Posterior (A-P) oblique (Arcelin's) view—Bucky technique. **B,** Posterior (A-P) oblique (Arcelin's) view—angle-board technique. (Courtesy Dr. E. I. L. Cilley, Dr. T. W. Crowell, Dr. R. E. Waud, and Dr. G. H. Hoffman.)

Petrous portion—anterior (P-A) oblique (Stenver's) view (Figs. 14-23 and 14-24)

> *Film size—8″ × 10″*   *Bucky*
> *Cassette*   *Extension cone*
> *Lengthwise*

Technique

Factors	Screen film cassette (par) Bucky	Screen film cassette (par) tabletop
Ma	100	100
Time	0.4	0.3
Mas	40	30
Thickness in cm	16	16
Kvp	70	56
Distance	30	30

Patient preparation

Remove all metallic and plastic articles from the head and neck region.

Palpation points

Mastoid processes.

Procedure

With a wax pencil make a mark 1 inch anterior to the E.A.M. (external auditory meatus) on the infraorbitomeatal line on each side of the head. Place the patient in the prone position with the forehead and nose on the tabletop. Place the hands at the sides of the head. Turn the side of the head being examined downward so that the midsagittal plane forms a 45-degree angle with the tabletop. The infraorbitomeatal line is perpendicular to the side of the table. Center the lower pencil mark over the center line of the table.

Central ray

Direct the central ray 12 degrees cephalad through the lower pencil mark to the center of the film holder.

Immobilization

Place a wedge sponge under the posterior portion of the head and instruct the patient to hold the sponge in place with his hand, or use a sandbag. Employ suspended expiration.

Right-left markers

Burn the correct marker in the upper center border of the film holder above the cone field after the exposure is made.

Technical tips

The superior and horizontal semicircular canals should be clearly defined when positioning accuracy is achieved.

Structures demonstrated

Anterior (P-A) view of the petrous pyramid, apex, internal acoustic canal, antral and labyrinthal areas, and mastoid air cells.

Note:

Make bilateral views for comparison.

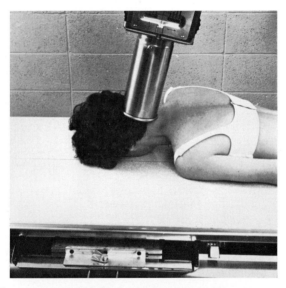

Fig. 14-23. Mastoids—anterior (P-A) oblique (Stenver's) position.

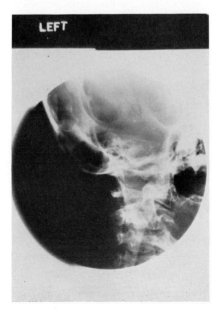

Fig. 14-24. Mastoids—anterior (P-A) oblique (Stenver's) view. (Courtesy Dr. E. I. L. Cilley, Dr. T. W. Crowell, Dr. R. E. Waud, and Dr. G. H. Hoffman.)

Petrous portion—axial (Mayer's) view (Figs. 14-25 and 14-26)

> *Film size—8″ × 10″*   *Bucky*
> *Cassette*   *Extension cone*
> *Lengthwise*

Technique

Factors	Screen film cassette (par) Bucky	Screen film cassette (par) tabletop
Ma	100	100
Time	0.6	0.3
Mas	60	30
Thickness in cm	22	22
Kvp	78	60
Distance	30	30

Patient preparation

Remove all metallic and plastic articles from the head and neck region.

Palpation points

Mastoid processes.

Procedure

With a wax pencil make a mark behind each ear on the posterior border of the E.A.M. (external auditory meatus). Tape the auricle of each ear forward. Place the patient in the supine position with the median plane of the body over the center line of the table. Rotate the head 45 degrees toward the side being examined. The infraorbitomeatal line is perpendicular to the tabletop. Place the lower pencil mark over the center line of the table.

Central ray

Direct the central ray 45 degrees caudad through the lower pencil mark to the center of the film holder.

Immobilization

Place a wedge sponge under the face and hold the sponge in place with sandbags. Employ suspended expiration.

Right-left markers

Burn the correct marker in the upper center border of the film holder above the cone field after the exposure is made.

Technical tips

For stocky patients with short necks, use an angle board on the tabletop to minimize distortion.

Structures demonstrated

Axial views of the internal and external auditory canals, the labyrinthal area, the mastoid cells, and the carotid canal.

Note:

Make bilateral views for comparison.

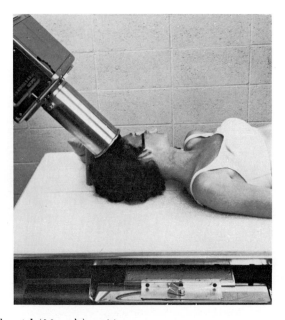

Fig. 14-25. Mastoid—axial (Mayer's) position.

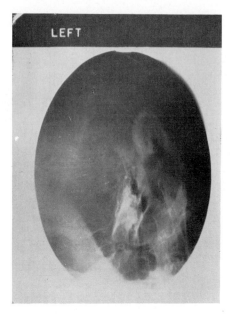

Fig. 14-26. Mastoid—axial (Mayer's) view. (Courtesy Dr. E. I. L. Cilley, Dr. T. W. Crowell, Dr. R. E. Waud, and Dr. G. H. Hoffman.)

Temporomandibular joints

Temporomandibular joints—lateral (T.M.J.) view (mouth open and mouth closed) (Figs. 14-27 and 14-28)

> *Film size—8″ × 10″*   *Bucky*
> *Cassette*   *Extension cone*
> *Lengthwise*

Technique

Factors	Screen film cassette (par) Bucky	Screen film cassette (par) tabletop
Ma	100	100
Time	0.5	3/20
Mas	50	15
Thickness in cm	18	18
Kvp	68	66
Distance	30	30

Patient preparation

Remove all metallic and plastic articles from the head and neck region.

Palpation points

Lateral mandibular condyles.

Procedure

Closed—With a wax pencil make a mark ¾ inch anterior to the E.A.M. (external auditory meatus) on each side of the head. Place the patient in the prone position. Place the side of the head being examined on the table. Elevate the opposite side of the body and flex this knee and elbow for support. Place the lower pencil mark over the center line of the table. The midsagittal plane is parallel with the tabletop. The acanthiomeatal line is perpendicular to the side of the table. The jaw must be closed.

Open—Open the mouth and insert a sterile cork. Recheck the acanthiomeatal line for position.

Central ray

Direct the central ray 15 degrees caudad through the lower pencil mark to the center of the film holder.

Immobilization

Place a fist or sponge under the chin. Employ suspended expiration.

Right-left markers

Burn the correct marker in the upper center border of the film holder above the cone field.

Technical tips

To improve centering accuracy, precenter the central ray to a point on the table and down to the film center. Position the selected mark on the patient over the point on the table.

Structures demonstrated

Lateral views of the condyle in relationship to the mandibular fossa.

Note:

Make bilateral views for comparison.

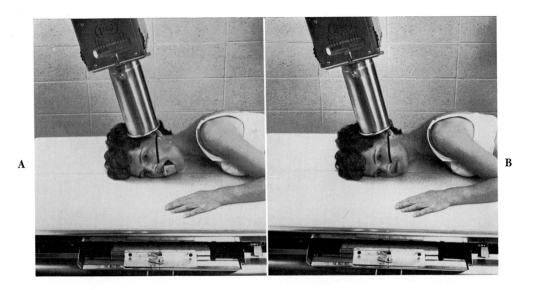

A

B

Fig. 14-27. Temporomandibular joint positions. **A,** Lateral (T.M.J.) position, mouth open. **B,** Lateral (T.M.J.) position, mouth closed.

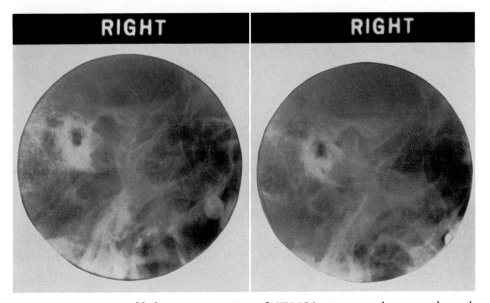

Fig. 14-28. Temporomandibular joint views. Lateral (T.M.J.) views, mouth open and mouth closed. (Courtesy Dr. E. I. L. Cilley, Dr. T. W. Crowell, Dr. R. E. Waud, and Dr. G. H. Hoffman.)

Facial bones
Facial bones—zygomatic arch, tangential view (Figs. 14-29 and 14-30)

> *Film size—8″ × 10″*   *Tabletop*
> *Cassette*   *Extension cone*
> *Lengthwise*

Technique

Factors	Screen film cassette (par)
Ma	100
Time	0.2
Mas	20
Thickness in cm	20
Kvp	54
Distance	30

Patient preparation

Remove all metallic and plastic articles from the head and neck region.

Palpation points

Lateral wall of the cranial vault; zygomatic arch; angle and body of the mandible.

Procedure

Place the patient in the prone position with the chest supported by a folded pillow. Extend the chin as far as possible and place it on the cassette face. The center of the zygomatic arch being examined is over the center line of the cassette. Shift the mandible to the opposite side; instruct the patient to bite down to hold the mandible in place. Tilt the head toward the opposite side so that a tangent from the side of the skull to the side of the mandible is perpendicular to the face of the cassette.

Central ray

Direct the central ray perpendicular to the infraorbitomeatal line, through the zygomatic arch, and to the center of the film holder.

Immobilization

Place the patient's thumbs on the anterior corners of the cassette to hold it in place. Extend the cone to contact the head. Employ suspended expiration.

Right-left markers

Burn the correct marker in the upper center border of the film holder above the cone field after the exposure is made.

Technical tips

For better demonstration of the zygomatic bone, angle the central ray 20 degrees toward the anterior (face).

Structures demonstrated

Tangential view of the zygomatic arch.

Note:

Make bilateral views for comparison.

For supine patients, make a submentovertex skull view on 10″ × 12″ film with a tabletop technique.

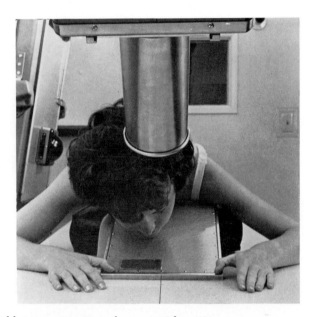

Fig. 14-29. Facial bones: zygomatic arch—tangential position.

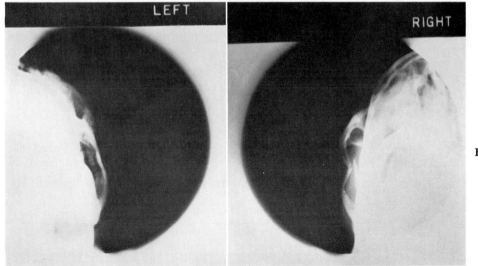

Fig. 14-30. Facial bones: zygomatic arch—tangential view. **A,** Normal. **B,** With fracture. (Courtesy Dr. E. I. L. Cilley, Dr. T. W. Crowell, Dr. R. E. Waud, and Dr. G. H. Hoffman.)

Facial bones—orbital ridges, anterior (P-A) view (Figs. 14-31 and 14-32)

> *Film size—8″ × 10″*   *Bucky*
> *Cassette*   *Cone to cover*
> *Lengthwise*

Technique

Factors	Screen film cassette (par)
Ma	100
Time	0.5
Mas	50
Thickness in cm	20
Kvp	76
Distance	30

Patient preparation

Remove all metallic and plastic articles from the head and neck region.

Palpation point

Acanthion.

Procedure

Place the patient in a prone position with the median plane of the head and body over the center line of the table. Extend the chin both upward and forward to rest on the center line of the table. The canthomeatal line forms a 37-degree angle with the tabletop, and the midsagittal plane of the head is perpendicular to it.

Central ray

Direct the central ray perpendicular through the anterior nasal spine to the center of the film holder.

Immobilization

Place sponges on each side of the head. Instruct the patient to hold them in place with his hands, or use sandbags. Employ suspended expiration.

Right-left markers

Place the R marker on the right lateral center border of the film holder.

Technical tips

For a variation of this view, angle the central ray 10 degrees caudad.

Structures demonstrated

Anterior (P-A) view of the orbits, nasal bones, nasal septum, zygomas, and maxillary antra.

Note:

This view may be used as a survey film for a foreign body in the eye.

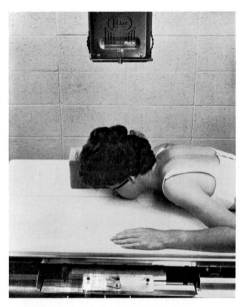

Fig. 14-31. Facial bones: orbital ridges—anterior (P-A) position.

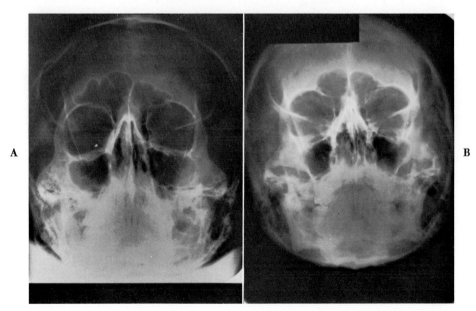

Fig. 14-32. Facial bones: orbital ridges—anterior (P-A) view. **A,** With 90-degree (perpendicular) angle. **B,** With 10-degree caudad angle. (Courtesy Dr. E. I. L. Cilley, Dr. T. W. Crowell, Dr. R. E. Waud, and Dr. G. H. Hoffman.)

Facial bones—lateral view (Figs. 14-33 and 14-34)

> *Film size—8″ × 10″*   *Bucky*
> *Cassette*   *Cone to cover*
> *Lengthwise*

Technique

Factors	*Screen film cassette (par)*
Ma	100
Time	0.2
Mas	20
Thickness in cm	15
Kvp	62
Distance	30

Patient preparation

Remove all metallic and plastic articles from the head and neck region.

Palpation point

Lateral ridge of the eye orbit.

Procedure

Place the patient in the prone position with the side of the head being examined on the table. Elevate the opposite side of the body and flex this knee and elbow for support. The midsagittal plane of the head is parallel with the tabletop. The canthomeatal line is perpendicular to the side of the table. Center a point ½ inch posterior to the outer canthus over the center line of the table.

Central ray

Direct the central ray perpendicular through the selected point to the center of the film holder.

Immobilization

Instruct the patient to brace the tip of the chin with his fist, or use a sponge. Place large sponges on the top of and behind the skull, and hold them in place with sandbags. Employ suspended expiration.

Right-left markers

Place the correct marker on the anterior center border of the film holder.

Technical tips

For better visualization of soft tissue structures, use a cardboard film holder on the tabletop.

Structures demonstrated

Lateral view of the bones of the face with the right and left sides superimposed.

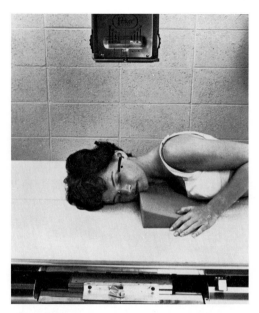

Fig. 14-33. Facial bones—lateral position.

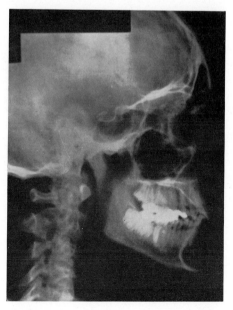

Fig. 14-34. Facial bones—lateral view. (Courtesy Dr. E. I. L. Cilley, Dr. T. W. Crowell, Dr. R. E. Waud, and Dr. G. H. Hoffman.)

Facial bones—nasal bones, axial view (Figs. 14-35 and 14-36)

> *Film size—occlusal*   *Intraoral*
> *Dental type*   *Extension cone*
> *Lengthwise*

Technique

Factors	No-screen film occlusal (fast)
Ma	100
Time	0.2
Mas	20
Thickness in cm	—
Kvp	64
Distance	30

Patient preparation

Remove all metallic and plastic articles from the face region.

Palpation points

Glabella; nasion; acanthion.

Procedure

Seat the patient at the end of the table. Place both elbows on the table with the forearms in the vertical plane and the fists together. Place the lower part of the chin on the fists, and insert half of the length of the occlusal film between the teeth.

Central ray

Direct the central ray perpendicular along the glabelloalveolar line to the film holder.

Immobilization

Place the extension cone in contact with the forehead. Employ suspended expiration.

Right-left markers

Place a *small letter r* in the right anterior corner of the film holder.

Technical tips

For a film substitute, use a regular dental film, or the corner of a cardboard film holder and the finger technique.

Structures demonstrated

Axial view of the nasal bones that extend beyond the glabelloalveolar line.

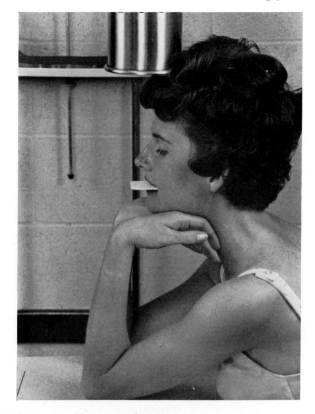

Fig. 14-35. Facial bones: nasal bones—axial position.

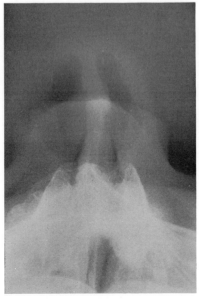

Fig. 14-36. Facial bones: nasal bones—axial view. (Courtesy Dr. E. I. L. Cilley, Dr. T. W. Crowell, Dr. R. E. Waud, and Dr. G. H. Hoffman.)

Facial bones—nasal bones, lateral view (Figs. 14-37 and 14-38)

> *Film size—8″ × 10″*   *Tabletop*
> *Cardboard*   *Extension cone*
> *Lengthwise*   *(half extended)*

Technique

Factors	Screen film cardboard	No-screen film occlusal (fast)
Ma	100	100
Time	0.7	0.2
Mas	70	20
Thickness in cm	3	3
Kvp	56	60
Distance	30	30

Patient preparation

Remove all metallic and plastic articles from the face region.

Palpation point

Nasion.

Procedure

Place the patient in the prone position with the side of the face being examined on the table. Elevate the opposite side of the body and flex this knee and elbow for support. The midsagittal plane of the head is parallel with the tabletop. The canthomeatal line is perpendicular to the side of the table. Center the nasion over the center of the cardboard film holder.

Central ray

Direct the central ray percendicular through the nasion to the center of the film holder.

Immobilization

Brace the tip of the chin with the patient's fist, or use a sponge. Employ suspended expiration.

Right-left markers

Burn the correct marker in the upper center border of the film holder above the cone field after the exposure is made.

Technical tips

For a film substitute, use a dental or occlusal film, inserting the corner of the film gently into the inner canthus of the eye.

Structures demonstrated

Lateral view of the nasal bones and of the soft tissue structures of the nose.

Note:

Some routines call for bilateral views on one radiograph.

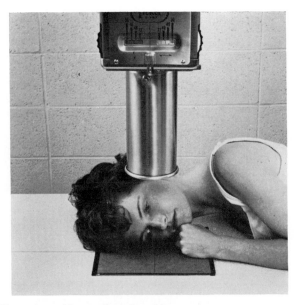

Fig. 14-37. Facial bones: nasal bones—lateral position.

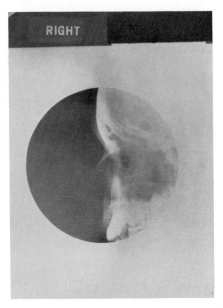

Fig. 14-38. Facial bones: nasal bones—lateral view. (Courtesy Dr. E. I. L. Cilley, Dr. T. W. Crowell, Dr. R. E. Waud, and Dr. G. H. Hoffman.)

Facial bones—optic foramen, anterior (P-A) view (Figs. 14-39 and 14-40)

    Film size—8″ × 10″   *Bucky*
    Cassette   *Extension cone*
    Lengthwise

Technique

Factors	Screen film cassette (par) Bucky	Screen film cassette (par) tabletop
Ma	100	100
Time	0.4	0.2
Mas	40	20
Thickness in cm	18	18
Kvp	70	64
Distance	30	30

Patient preparation

Remove all metallic and plastic articles from the head region.

Palpation point

Lateral ridge of the eye orbit.

Procedure

Place the patient in the prone position with the median plane of the head and body over the center line of the table. Place the hands at the sides of the head. Rotate the head 40 degrees toward the side being examined. The acanthiomeatal line is perpendicular to the side of the table. Center a point ¼ inch medial to the outer canthus of the eye being examined over the center line of the table.

Central ray

Direct the central ray perpendicular through the selected point to the center of the film holder.

Immobilization

Place a wedge sponge under the lower side of the head, and instruct the patient to hold this in place with his hand, or use sandbags. Place the extension cone in contact with the head. Employ suspended expiration.

Right-left markers

Burn the correct marker in the upper center border of the film holder above the cone field after the exposure is made.

Technical tips

To project the optic foramen lower in the orbit, increase the cervical extension; to project the optic foramen lateral in the orbit, increase the head rotation.

Structures demonstrated

Anterior (P-A) view of the optic foramen projected in the lower lateral area of the orbit.

Note:

Make bilateral views for comparison.

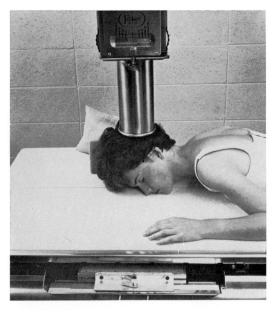

Fig. 14-39. Facial bones: optic foramen—anterior (P-A) position.

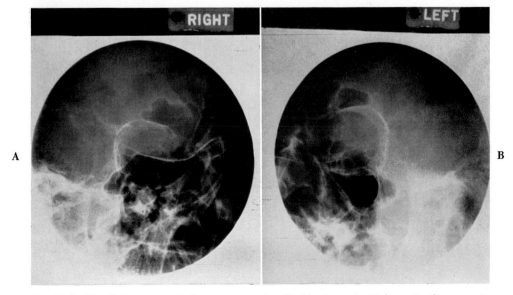

Fig. 14-40. Facial bones: optic foramen—anterior (P-A) view. **A,** Right optic foramen. **B,** Left optic foramen. (Courtesy Dr. E. I. L. Cilley, Dr. T. W. Crowell, Dr. R. E. Waud, and Dr. G. H. Hoffman.)

Facial bones—maxilla, oblique view (Figs. 14-41 and 14-42)

Film size—occlusal　　　　　　　*Intraoral*
Dental type　　　　　　　　　　*Extension cone*
Lengthwise

Technique

Factors	No-screen film occlusal (fast)
Ma	100
Time	0.2
Mas	20
Thickness in cm	—
Kvp	70
Distance	30

Patient preparation

Remove all metallic and plastic articles from the face region.

Palpation point

Maxillary bone.

Procedure

Seat the patient at the end of the table. Place both elbows on the table with the forearms in a vertical plane and the fists together. Place the lower part of the chin on fists, and insert the occlusal film between the teeth of the side being examined.

Central ray

Direct the central ray 45 degrees from vertical toward the face and 45 degrees from anterior toward the median plane through the maxilla being examined to the film holder.

Immobilization

Employ suspended expiration.

Right-left markers

Place the correct marker in the anterior lateral corner of the film holder.

Technical tips

To better demonstrate the posterior portion of the maxilla, direct the central ray 60 degrees from the anterior toward the median plane.

Structures demonstrated

Oblique views of the alveolar process and hard palate, and of the bicuspids and molars of the side of the maxilla being examined.

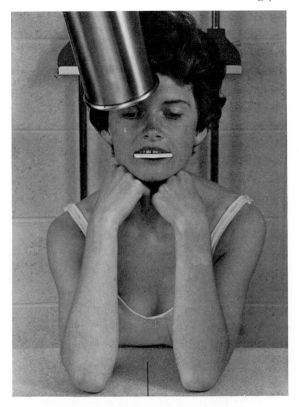

Fig. 14-41. Facial bones: maxilla—oblique position.

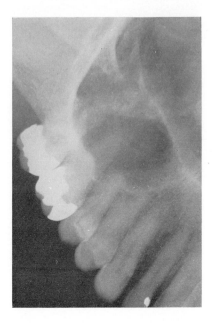

Fig. 14-42. Facial bones: maxilla—oblique view. (Courtesy Dr. E. I. L. Cilley, Dr. T. W. Crowell, Dr. R. E. Waud, and Dr. G. H. Hoffman.)

Facial bones—maxillae, inferior (superoinferior) view (Figs. 14-43 and 14-44)

Film size—occlusal   *Intraoral*
Dental type   *Extension cone*
Lengthwise

Technique

Factors	No-screen film occlusal (fast)
Ma	100
Time	0.2
Mas	20
Thickness in cm	—
Kvp	70
Distance	30

Patient preparation

Remove all plastic and metallic articles from the face region.

Palpation point

Maxillary bone.

Procedure

Seat the patient at the end of the table. Place both elbows on the table with the forearms in a vertical plane and the fists together. Place the lower part of the chin on the fists, and insert the occlusal film as far as possible between the teeth.

Central ray

Direct the central ray 45 degrees from vertical toward the face through the anterior nasal spine to the film holder.

Immobilization

Employ suspended expiration.

Right-left markers

Place a *small letter r* in the right anterior corner of the film holder.

Technical tips

For a film substitute, use a regular dental film or the corner of a cardboard film holder.

Structures demonstrated

Inferior (superoinferior) view of the upper incisors, the alveolar processes, and the hard palate.

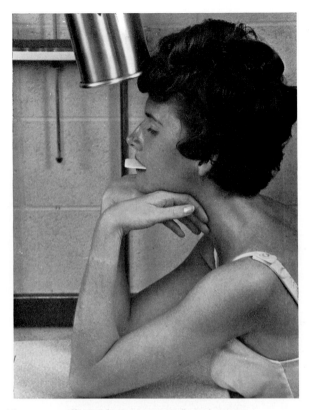

Fig. 14-43. Facial bones: maxillae—inferior (superoinferior) position.

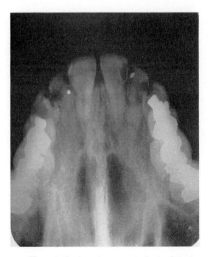

Fig. 14-44. Facial bones: maxillae—inferior (superoinferior) view. (Courtesy Dr. E. I. L. Cilley, Dr. T. W. Crowell, Dr. R. E. Waud, and Dr. G. H. Hoffman.)

Facial bones—mandible (rami), anterior (P-A) view (Figs. 14-45 and 14-46)

> *Film size—8″ × 10″*   *Bucky*
> *Cassette*   *Cone to cover*
> *Lengthwise*

Technique

Factors	Screen film cassette (par) Bucky	Screen film cassette (par) tabletop
Ma	100	100
Time	0.5	0.4
Mas	50	40
Thickness in cm	16	16
Kvp	66	56
Distance	40	40

Patient preparation

Remove all metallic and plastic articles from the head and neck region.

Palpation points

Mandibular rami and angles; spinous processes of the cervical vertebrae.

Procedure

Place the patient in the prone position with the median plane of the head and body over the center line of the table. Place the hands at the sides of the head. Place the forehead and nose on the center line of the table. The cantho-meatal line is perpendicular to the tabletop, and the midsagittal plane is perpendicular to the tabletop.

Central ray

Direct the central ray perpendicularly in line with the angles of the mandible, to the center of the film holder.

Immobilization

Place large sponges on each side of the head, and instruct the patient to hold them in place with his hands, or use sandbags. Employ suspended expiration.

Right-left markers

Place the R marker on the right lower lateral side of the film holder.

Technical tips

For thin patients, elevate the thorax with a pillow or sponges.

Structures demonstrated

Anterior (P-A) view of the mandibular body and rami. The mental area is demonstrated superimposed on the cervical vertebrae.

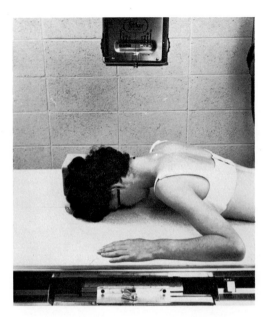

Fig. 14-45. Facial bones: mandible (rami)—anterior (P-A) position.

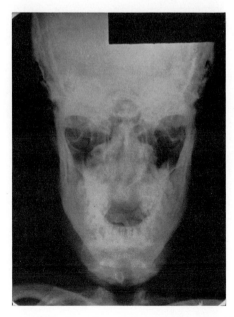

Fig. 14-46. Facial bones: mandible (rami)—anterior (P-A) view. (Courtesy Dr. E. I. L. Cilley, Dr. T. W. Crowell, Dr. R. E. Waud, and Dr. G. H. Hoffman.)

Facial bones—mandible (condyles), anterior (P-A) view (Figs. 14-47 and 14-48)

       Film size—8″ × 10″   *Bucky*
       Cassette   *Cone to cover*
       Lengthwise

Technique

Factors	Screen film cassette (par) Bucky	Screen film cassette (par) tabletop
Ma	100	100
Time	0.5	0.4
Mas	50	40
Thickness in cm	16	16
Kvp	66	56
Distance	40	40

Patient preparation

Remove all metallic and plastic articles from the head and neck region.

Palpation points

Mandibular rami and angles; spinous processes of the cervical vertebrae.

Procedure

Place the patient in the prone position with the median plane of the head and body over the center line of the table. Place the hands at the sides of the head. Place the forehead and nose on the center line of the table. The cantho-meatal line is perpendicular to the tabletop, and the midsagittal plane is perpendicular to the tabletop. Open the patient's mouth as far as possible and insert a sterile cork between the teeth.

Central ray

Direct the central ray 12 degrees cephalad through the nasion to the center of the film holder.

Immobilization

Place large sponges on each side of the head and instruct the patient to hold them in place with his hands, or use sandbags. Employ suspended expiration.

Right-left markers

Place the *R* marker on the right lower lateral side of the film holder.

Technical tips

If the base of the occiput is superimposed over the condyles, increase cervical flexion 5 degrees.

Structures demonstrated

Anterior (P-A) view of the mandibular body, rami, and condyles.

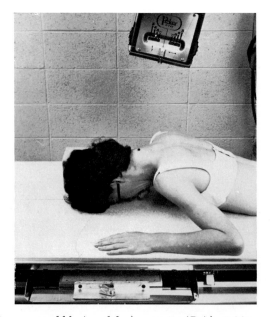

Fig. 14-47. Facial bones: mandible (condyles)—anterior (P-A) position.

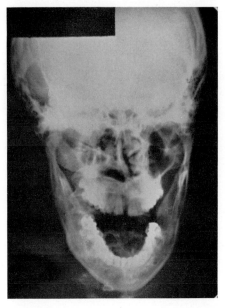

Fig. 14-48. Facial bones: mandible (condyles)—anterior (P-A) view. (Courtesy Dr. E. I. L. Cilley, Dr. T. W. Crowell, Dr. R. E. Waud, and Dr. G. H. Hoffman.)

Facial bones—mandible, lateral view (Figs. 14-49 and 14-50)

Film size—8″ × 10″	*Erect film holder*
Cassette	*Cone to cover*
Lengthwise	

Technique

Factors	Screen film cassette (par)
Ma	100
Time	0.3
Mas	30
Thickness in cm	8
Kvp	64
Distance	72

Patient preparation

Remove all metallic and plastic articles from the head and neck region.

Palpation points

Mandibular rami, angles, and bodies.

Procedure

Place the patient in the erect position, either sitting or standing, with the side of the face being examined against the center of the erect film holder. Place a sandbag in each hand of the patient and instruct him to extend each arm down the side of the body. Extend the chin upward and inward so that the long axis of the mandibular body being examined is parallel with both the erect film holder and the floor. Tilt the head 25 degrees, and rest the parietal region against the erect film holder.

Central ray

Direct a horizontal central ray perpendicular through the center of the mandibular body to the center of the film holder.

Immobilization

A compression band may be used across the patient's head. Employ suspended expiration.

Right-left markers

Place the correct marker on the anterior center border of the film holder.

Technical tips

To eliminate superimposition of mandibular bodies, increase the tilt of the head.

Structures demonstrated

Mediolateral (lateral) view of the mandibular body. The symphysis and ramus may be demonstrated with a variation in head rotation.

Note:

Make bilateral views for comparison.

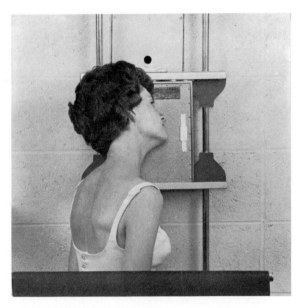

Fig. 14-49. Facial bones: mandible—lateral position.

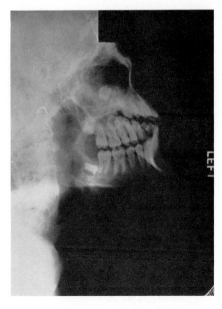

Fig. 14-50. Facial bones: mandible—lateral view. (Courtesy Dr. E. I. L. Cilley, Dr. T. W. Crowell, Dr. R. E. Waud, and Dr. G. H. Hoffman.)

Facial bones—mandible (symphysis), submentovertical view (Figs. 14-51 and 14-52)

Film size—occlusal   *Intraoral*
Dental type   *Extension cone*
Lengthwise

Technique

Factors	No-screen film occlusal (fast)
Ma	100
Time	0.2
Mas	20
Thickness in cm	5
Kvp	66
Distance	30

Patient preparation

Remove all metallic and plastic articles from the face and neck region.

Palpation point

Mandibular symphysis.

Procedure

Place the patient in a supine position on a large cushion or folded pillows, with the vertex of the head against the table. Insert half the length of the occlusal film between the teeth.

Central ray

Direct the central ray perpendicular through the mandibular symphysis to the film holder.

Immobilization

Place a sandbag against the forehead. Employ suspended expiration.

Right-left markers

Place a *small letter r* on the right anterior corner of the film holder.

Technical tips

For a film substitute, use a regular dental film, or the corner of a cardboard film holder and the finger technique.

Structures demonstrated

Submentovertical view of the mandibular symphysis.

Note:

For a variation of this view, place an occlusal film beneath the chin and direct the central ray superoinferior, 45 degrees from perpendicular, through the symphysis to the center of the film holder.

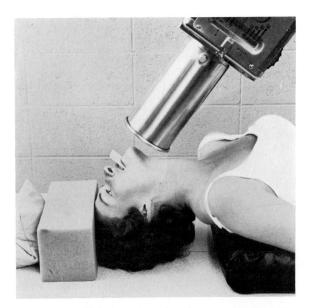

Fig. 14-51. Facial bones: mandible (symphysis)—submentovertical position.

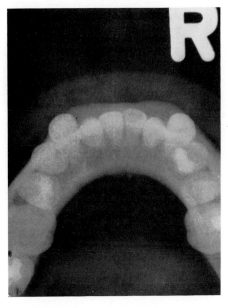

Fig. 14-52. Facial bones: mandible (symphysis)—submentovertical view. (Courtesy Dr. E. I. L. Cilley, Dr. T. W. Crowell, Dr. R. E. Waud, and Dr. G. H. Hoffman.)

Chapter 15

Anatomic physiology

Digestive system

The major parts of the digestive system form a canal that is open at both ends. The tract passes through the thoracic and abdominal cavities. Beginning with the mouth and terminating with the anus, this canal, commonly known as the *gastrointestinal tract*, is 840 to 1,020 cm* (28 to 34 feet) in length. The chief organs of digestion are the mouth, pharynx, esophagus, stomach, and small and large intestines. (See Fig. 15-1.) The accessory organs, which are contained within, or open into, the gastrointestinal tract, include the teeth, tongue, salivary glands, pancreas, liver, gallbladder, and appendix. The digestive system receives and prepares food for absorption and use by all of the body cells. In the mouth the food is masticated and mixed with saliva into a *bolus*, which, through the act of *deglutition*, passes into the stomach. *Peristaltic motion* then conducts the *bolus* through the stomach into the duodenum, jejunum, ileum, and finally the large intestine, from which it is eliminated as waste. After the bolus has undergone gastric digestion, it is called *chyme*. After undergoing intestinal digestion, the *chyle*, a milky fluid taken from the food during digestion, is absorbed by the lacteals.

Buccal cavity

The buccal cavity (mouth) is bounded laterally by the cheeks, anteriorly by the lips, superiorly by the hard and soft palates, inferiorly by the tongue and associated muscles, and posteriorly by the pharynx and uvula. It contains the teeth, which masticate the food; the tongue, which aids in mastication and deglutition; and the salivary glands, which manufacture and excrete saliva through their openings into this cavity. The salivary excretion contains *salivary amylase*, an enzyme that attacks starch and hydrolyzes it into maltose, and *mucin*, a very sticky substance that mixes with the food to form the bolus. There are three pairs of salivary glands: the *parotids*, which are inferior and anterior to the ears and are emptied by the *parotid (Stensen's) ducts*, which drain into the buccal cavity through small orifices in the cheeks (the orifices are near the upper second molars); the *submandibulars* (submaxillaries), which are on the posterior portions of the floor of the mouth near the angles of the mandibles and are emptied by the *submandibular (Wharton's) ducts*, which drain into the anterior part of the buccal cavity inferior to the tongue; and the *sublinguals*,

---

*Use 1 foot as being equal to 30 cm.

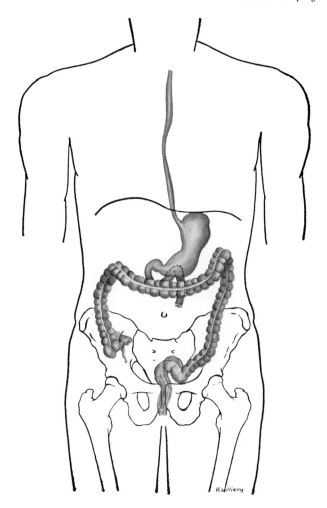

Fig. 15-1. Normal position of some of the digestive organs. (From Francis, Carl C: Introduction to human anatomy, St. Louis, 1968, The C. V. Mosby Co.)

which are in the floor of the mouth inferior to the free end of the tongue and empty into this cavity through several small ducts and direct openings. Special radiographic studies of the salivary glands are discussed in Chapter 16.

Teeth

The normal adult mouth contains thirty-two teeth, sixteen in each jaw. These teeth are called the *permanent teeth,* while those of the child, which are shed at various ages, are called *deciduous teeth.* The name of each tooth and the number per jaw are given in Table 15-1.

The teeth are contained in the alveolar processes of the mandible and maxilla. The plane of closing the teeth is called the *occlusal plane.* In dental radiography, emphasis is placed on the periodontal membrane, roots, and neck. There is less radiographic interest in the crown. It is extremely important to prevent elongation

Table 15-1. Dentition*

Name of tooth	Number per jaw deciduous set	Number per jaw permanent set
Central incisors	2	2
Lateral incisors	2	2
Cuspids (canines)	2	2
Premolars (bicuspids)	0	4
Molars (tricuspids)	4	6
Total per jaw	10	16
Total per set	20	32

*From Anthony, C. P.: Textbook of anatomy and physiology, St. Louis, 1967, The C. V. Mosby Co.

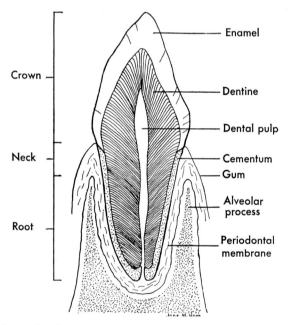

Fig. 15-2. Incisor, longitudinal section. (From Francis, Carl C: Introduction to human anatomy, St. Louis, 1968, The C. V. Mosby Co.)

or foreshortening of the roots. The construction and placement of a tooth in its alveolar socket is shown in Fig. 15-2.

Pharynx

The pharynx is a muscular structure common to both the digestive and respiratory systems and aids in the act of deglutition. It is about 12.5 cm long and lies between the cranial floor and the esophagus anterior to the cervical spine. Each eustachian tube opens into the sides of the *nasopharynx;* the choanae open into the anterior part of the nasopharynx; the buccal cavity opens into the anterior part of the *oropharynx;* and the pharynx opens posteroinferiorly into the

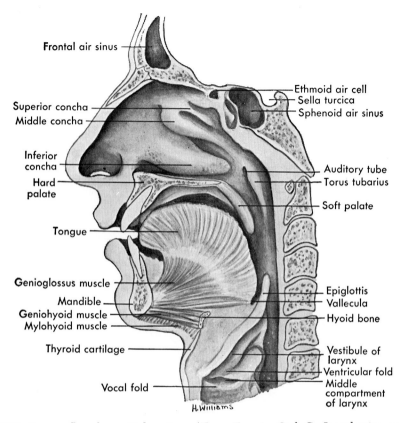

Fig. 15-3. Face and neck, sagittal section. (From Francis, Carl C: Introduction to human anatomy, St. Louis, 1968, The C. V. Mosby Co.)

larynx *(laryngopharynx)* and anteroinferiorly into the esophagus. The opening from the mouth is called the *fauces*. (See Fig. 15-3.) The pharynx is demonstrated radiographically by use of the lateral projection for the esophagus.

Esophagus

The esophagus is a muscular tube located chiefly in the thoracic cavity and partially in the abdominal cavity. It serves as the connection between the pharynx and the stomach and is approximately 22.5 to 27.5 cm in length. It passes through the *diaphragm* in the *esophageal hiatus* and is located posterior to the trachea and heart. True peristalsis does not begin in the esophagus, although a peristaltic-like action ·begins in the upper third of the esophagus and conveys the bolus into the stomach. Lateral and oblique positions (sometimes erect) are used to demonstrate the esophagus radiographically.

Stomach

The stomach is inferior to the diaphragm on the left side of the median line in the abdominal cavity. Its capacity varies from 500 to 1,000 ml. It is located chiefly in the epigastrium, but small parts are in the left hypochondrium and umbilical regions. The superior opening, called the *cardiac orifice,* is the junction of the esophagus with the stomach and is near the level of the eleventh thoracic vertebra. The inferior opening (outlet), the *pylorus,* opens into the first part of the duodenum. The stomach has three divisions: the *cardiac third (fundus),* which is that part superior to a horizontal plane passing through the cardiac orifice; the *pyloric third,* which is the distal portion; and the *body,* which is the portion between the cardiac and pyloric thirds. The shorter margin of the stomach between the cardiac and pyloric orifices is called the *lesser curvature,* while the opposite, longer margin is called the *greater curvature.* Throughout the stomach are heavy folds of mucosa called *rugae,* the majority of which extend the length of the stomach. The circular muscle in the cardiac orifice is called the cardiac sphincter. A similar muscle in the pylorus is called the pyloric sphincter. Numerous glands located throughout the entire gastric mucosa excrete the gastric juices. The principal excretions of the stomach are *hydrochloric acid,* which acidifies the gastric juice and aids in proteolytic hydrolysis; pepsinogen, a precursor to *pepsin,* which hydrolyzes proteins to proteoses and peptones; *lipase,* which hydrolyzes some of the emulsified fats to fatty acids and glycerol; and *rennin* in infants, which acts upon caseinogen to form paracasein. (See Fig. 15-4.)

Small intestine

Duodenum. The duodenum is the first part of the small intestine and is approximately 22.5 cm long. The major percentage of true digestion, or absorption, occurs in the *villi* of its walls. It is divided into four parts: *bulb (cap), descending, transverse,* and *ascending.* The bulb is attached to the pylorus, and the ascending portion attaches to the jejunum. The duodenum is located primarily in the epigastrium to the right of the stomach and is the only part of the small intestine not completely attached to the mesentery. Approximately 7.5 cm inferior

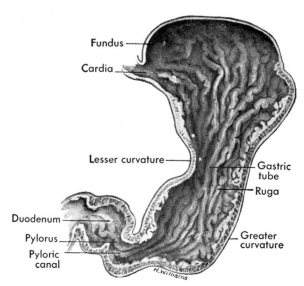

Fig. 15-4. Stomach, frontal section. (From Francis, Carl C: Introduction to human anatomy, St. Louis, 1968, The C. V. Mosby Co.)

to the pylorus and on the posteromedial surface is the *ampulla of Vater,* through which the bile and pancreatic juice enter the duodenum. The principal intestinal juices are *peptidase,* which hydrolyzes peptones and peptides to amino acids; *lactase,* which hydrolyzes lactose to glucose and galactose; *maltase,* which hydrolyzes maltose to glucose; and *sucrase,* which hydrolyzes sucrose to glucose and fructose. The head of the pancreas is enveloped by the loop of the duodenum. The duodenum joins the jejunum in the *duodenojejunal flexure* approximately on the level of the second lumbar vertebra and slightly left of the aorta. Radiographic examination of the esophagus, stomach, and duodenum comprises an upper gastrointestinal tract study, often called an E.S.D. or U.G.I.

Jejunum. The jejunum is about 270 cm long and lies in the umbilical, left lumbar, and left iliac regions. It joins distally with the ileum. The villi become progressively smaller at this junction. Some digestion occurs in the ileum and jejunum. (See Fig. 15-5.)

Ileum. The ileum is the distal part of the small intestine. It is approximately 390 cm long and begins with the jejunum and terminates in its junction with the cecum. It is located primarily in the pelvic cavity. The junction with the cecum contains the *ileocecal valve,* which prevents regurgitation of the feces into the ileum. When this valve is *patent,* it has lost its function, and feces may enter the ileum. *Meckel's diverticulum* extends from the ileum in a very small

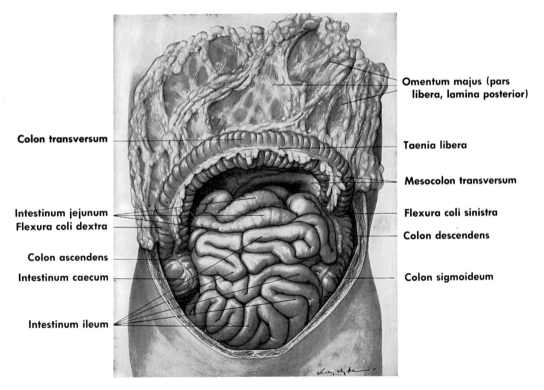

Fig. 15-5. Abdominal viscera. (From Anson, B. J., and Maddock, W. G.: Callander's surgical anatomy, Philadelphia, 1958, W. B. Saunders Co.)

percentage of persons. It is located about 90 cm above the ileocecal valve. The jejunum and ileum are examined radiographically following the procedures for E.S.D. studies.

Bile ducts and gallbladder

This system of ducts and glands plays an important part in radiography. The gallbladder is located beneath the right lobe of the liver. It has three divisions: the *fundus,* which is inferior, and the *body* and *neck,* which extend above the fundus. The gallbladder is drained by the *cystic duct,* which is very short. It stores and concentrates the bile and is stimulated to contract and excrete the bile by a hormone *(cholecystokinin)* secreted in the intestinal mucosa. The *hepatic duct* from the liver originates from two branches, one each from the right and left lobes. The short hepatic duct joins the cystic duct to form the *common bile duct.* The latter is about as long as the combined lengths of the cystic and hepatic ducts. The common bile duct joins with the pancreatic duct *(duct of Wirsung)* to form the hepatopancreatic ampulla (of Vater), which is extremely short. The choledochal *sphincter (of Oddi)* is in the terminus of the common bile duct. The hepatopancreatic ampulla opens into the duodenum through the major *duodenal papilla.* The accessory pancreatic duct *(duct of Santorini)* opens into the duodenum slightly above the ampulla. (See Fig. 15-6.) The bile ducts and gallbladder are demonstrated radiographically by cholecystography and cholangiography.

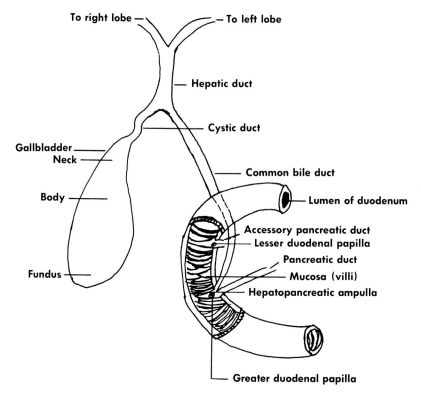

Fig. 15-6. Diagram of biliary tract.

Pancreas

The pancreas excretes juices into the duodenum via the duct of Wirsung. Included with these juices are the enzymes *trypsin, amylase,* and *lipase.* In addition, the pancreas contains several groups of specialized cells, called the *islands of Langerhans,* which secrete a hormone, *insulin.* The pancreas lies posteriorly in the epigastric and left hypochondriac regions in a transverse position. (See Fig. 15-7.) Its head lies within the curve of the duodenum, with the tail extending to the left.

Large intestine

The large intestine, which begins with the cecum and terminates in the anus, is between 150 and 180 cm in length. It consists of the *cecum, colon (ascending, transverse, descending, iliac,* and *sigmoid* portions), *rectum,* and *anal canal.*

The cecum is located in the right iliac region and has about the same capacity as the stomach. The ileum enters the large intestine at the junction of the cecum with the colon. The fundus of the cecum is directed inferiorly. The appendix projects distally from the cecum and is infrequently demonstrated radio-

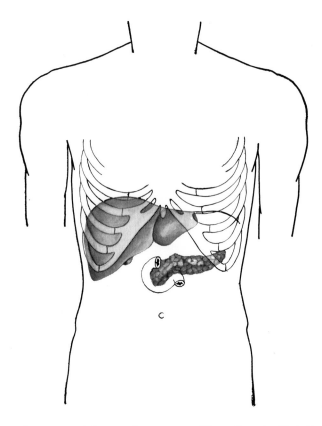

Fig. 15-7. Normal position of liver and pancreas. (From Francis, Carl C: Introduction to human anatomy, St. Louis, 1968, The C. V. Mosby Co.)

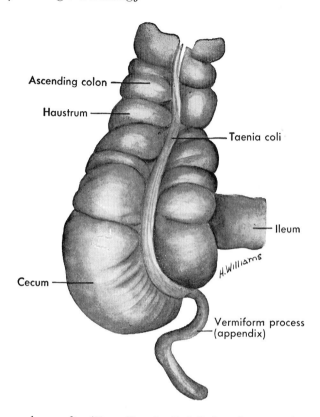

Ascending colon

Haustrum

Taenia coli

Ileum

H. Williams

Cecum

Vermiform process (appendix)

Fig. 15-8. Cecum and appendix. (From Francis, Carl C: Introduction to human anatomy, St. Louis, 1968, The C. V. Mosby Co.)

graphically during the course of examination with barium enemas. (See Fig. 15-8.) The ascending colon extends from the cecum to the right lobe of the liver. At this point the colon bends, forming the *hepatic flexure*. Then it passes across the abdomen (transverse portion), approximately in line with the division between the epigastric and umbilical regions, making another bend in the left hypochondrium (the *splenic flexure*). The splenic flexure is usually higher than the hepatic flexure and is attached to the diaphragm on a level between the tenth and eleventh ribs. From the splenic flexure, the colon extends down through the left hypochondrium and left lumbar regions as the descending colon. Below the left kidney the descending colon extends medially toward the crest of the left ilium. At this point it becomes the iliac colon (frequently included as a part of the descending colon by various authors). The short iliac colon becomes the sigmoid colon as it enters into the lesser pelvis. The sigmoid colon is usually entirely in the pelvis. It is S shaped and terminates in the rectum. The rectum projects down and back to terminate in the anal canal. The anal canal is very short and terminates with the anus. The large intestine is demonstrated radiographically by the use of radiopaque and contrast media. The media of choice are barium sulfate and air.

For descriptive purposes the abdominal cavity may be divided in two ways:

Table 15-2. Major viscera of the nine regions of the abdomen

Right hypochondrium	*Epigastrium*	*Left hypochondrium*

Most of right lobe of liver
Hepatic flexure of colon
Part of right renal body
	Most of left lobe and remainder
	  of right lobe of liver
	Gallbladder
	Most of stomach, duodenum, and
	  pancreas
	Part of spleen
	Suprarenals
	Parts of renals
		Greater curvature of stomach
		Remainder of spleen
		Tail of pancreas
		Splenic flexure of colon
		Part of left renal body

Right lumbar	*Umbilical*	*Left lumbar*
Ascending colon Most of right renal body	Most of transverse colon Parts of duodenum, jejunum, and ileum Parts of renal bodies Most of ureters	Descending colon Part of jejunum Most of left renal body
Right iliac	*Hypogastrium*	*Left iliac*
Cecum Appendix Terminal end of ileum Ileocecal valve	Ileum Flexure of sigmoid colon	Sigmoid colon Jejunum Ileum Iliac colon

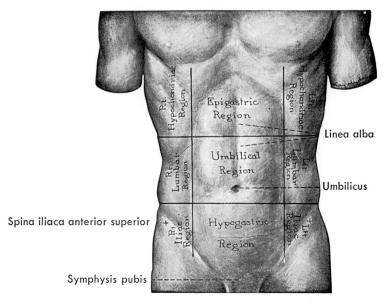

Fig. 15-9. The nine regions of the abdomen. (From Anson, B. J., and Maddock, W. G.: Callander's surgical anatomy, Philadelphia, 1958, W. B. Saunders Co.)

four quadrants or *nine regions*. Both divisions include all or most of the pelvic cavity. Sagittal and transverse lines at right angles to each other and through the *umbilicus* (navel) outline the four quadrants. The nine regions are as follows: right hypochondrium, epigastrium, left hypochondrium, right lumbar, umbilical, left lumbar, right iliac, hypogastrium, and left iliac. In Table 15-2 are listed the more important parts of the viscera according to the regions shown in Fig. 15-9. There are many other portions of the abdominal viscera that are not mentioned in relation to each of these regions since they are of little importance to x-ray technologists.

Genitourinary system

The genital and urinary systems are considered together since both systems share a common outlet in both sexes. Also, the procedure of radiographic examination is similar in both sexes and in both systems.

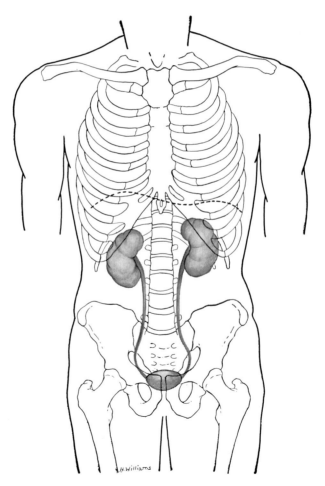

Fig. 15-10. Normal position of urinary organs. (From Francis, Carl C: Introduction to human anatomy, St. Louis, 1968, The C. V. Mosby Co.)

Urinary system

The urinary system is a rather complex excretory system and has two distinct functions: filtration of the urine from the blood and elimination of the urine from the body. It is vitally concerned with the maintenance of *homeostasis* and includes two kidneys, two ureters, the urinary bladder, and the urethra. (See Fig. 15-10.)

Kidneys. The paired kidneys are located bilateral to the midsagittal plane behind the parietal peritoneum of the abdomen in the area of the twelfth thoracic to the third lumbar vertebra. The right kidney is slightly lower and smaller than the left. The kidney is a bean-shaped organ approximately 10 cm in total length. Its concave surface faces the midsagittal plane. In the center of this concavity is located the *hilar space,* through which the nerves, blood vessels, and ureters pass. The waste products of the kidneys may either be liquid or be suspended in liquid. The functional unit of the kidneys is called the *nephron.*

Frequently, requests are made for erect films of the kidneys and ureters for the demonstration of any possible ptosis of either of the kidneys or ureters. The kidneys are sometimes demonstrated radiographically without opacification but are always opacified for study. Opacification is obtained by either of two methods: by intravenous injection of a radiopaque medium and utilization of the normal function of blood filtration, called *intravenous pyelography,* or by the injection of a radiopaque substance into the kidneys directly through catheters placed in the kidneys, called *retrograde pyelography.* After opacification the *calyces* and the *renal pelves* are visualized radiographically. The renal pelvis narrows inferiorly to form the *ureter,* which drains the kidney. (See Fig. 15-11.)

Ureters. The ureters are about 27.5 cm in length and are quite small in diameter. Their walls are muscular. They are located bilateral to the midsagittal

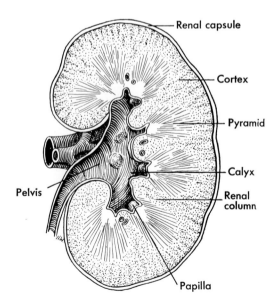

Fig. 15-11. Kidney, coronal section. (From Anthony, Catherine Parker: Textbook of anatomy and physiology, St. Louis, 1963, The C. V. Mosby Co.)

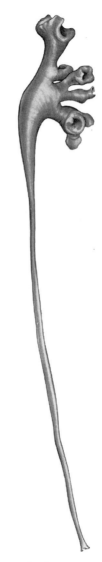

Fig. 15-12. Left ureter, renal pelvis, and calyces, anterior view. (From Francis, Carl C: Introduction to human anatomy, St. Louis, 1968, The C. V. Mosby Co.)

plane, are extraperitoneal, and connect the hilar spaces of the kidneys to the posterior surface of the bladder. (See Fig. 15-12.) The urine is moved through the ureters into the bladder by peristalsis. The ureteral orifices are located laterally and posteriorly in the bladder. These, together with the urethral orifice (anteriorly), form the *trigone*.

Bladder. The urinary bladder receives urine from the ureters. Its capacity has been stated to be from 400 to 600 ml. The total quantity of urine eliminated in a 24-hour period has been stated to be from 1 to 2 liters. The urinary bladder has a *vertex*, which is ventral and slightly superior, and a *fundus*, which is dorsal and slightly inferior. In the male the bladder is superior to the prostate. In the female it is inferior to the uterus and anterior to the vagina. (See Figs.

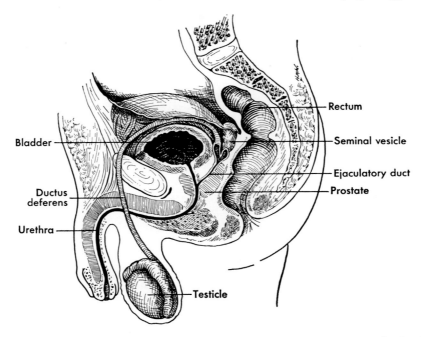

Fig. 15-13. Male pelvis, sagittal section. (From Anthony, Catherine Parker: Textbook of anatomy and physiology, St. Louis, 1963, The C. V. Mosby Co.)

15-13 and 15-14.) Radiographic examinations of the bladder are called *cystograms,* and the visual examination is called *cystoscopy.* The procedure of radiographic examination may be either intravenous or retrograde.

Urethra. In both sexes the bladder is drained by the urethra, which extends between the urinary bladder and the external urethral orifice. In the male the external orifice *(meatus)* is in the distal end of the penis, while in the female, it is between the labia minora and posterior to the glans clitoris. (See Figs. 15-13 and 15-14.) In the male the urethra is approximately 18 cm long, whereas in the female it is approximately 4 cm long. The urethra is the excretory canal of the bladder for the urine. In the male it also serves as the excretory duct for the semen. The male urethra passes directly from the urinary bladder through the prostate gland, where it receives the excretions from the ejaculatory ducts, vas deferens, and testes. Radiographic examination, *urethrography,* of the urethra in the female is seldom requested; however, this procedure is not infrequent in the male. Urethrography is also a method of examination of the *prostate* in certain cases.

Reproductive system

Male. The male reproductive system consists of the testes, ductus deferens, seminal vesicles, ejaculatory ducts, and penis and includes the accessory prostate and bulbourethral (Cowper's) glands. (See Fig. 15-13.) There are no radiographic procedures (other than urethrography) that are peculiar to the male reproductive system.

Female. The female reproductive system consists of the ovaries, salpinges

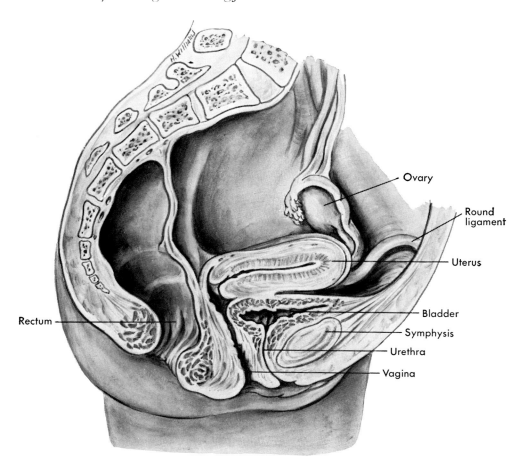

Fig. 15-14. Female pelvis, sagittal section. (From Anthony, Catherine Parker: Textbook of anatomy and physiology, St. Louis, 1963, The C. V. Mosby Co.)

(fallopian tubes), uterus, vagina, clitoris, and vulva, along with the associated accessory glands. (See Fig. 15-14.) From the radiographic viewpoint, interest lies in the technique of *uterosalpingography*, which is radiography of the uterus and salpinges following opacification with an iodized oil. The uterine walls are thick and muscular. The *uterus* separates the rectum and urinary bladder and opens into the vagina through the *cervix*. The fundus is anterior and superior to the body of the uterus. The *salpinges* join the uterus superiorly and bilaterally in the cornu. They are not directly attached to the ovaries but have a funnel-like terminus called the *fimbria*, which catches the ova from the ovaries. The salpinges (less than 13 cm long) extend bilaterally from the uterus in the broad ligament.

Circulatory system

In recent years the circulatory system has presented many interesting radiographic studies, among which are angiograms, venograms, arteriograms, and angiocardiograms. In addition to the lymphatic system, which willl be discussed in the following section, the circulatory system consists of three distinct, closely interrelated systems: the *pulmonary circulation,* which is the flow of blood from the heart to the lungs and back to the heart for the purpose of gaseous exchange; the *portal circulation,* which is the flow of blood from the digestive viscera to the liver, and from the liver to the inferior vena cava, allowing the blood to absorb the nutrients that feed the body cells; and the *systemic circulation,* which is the flow of blood to the remainder of the body cells to deliver nutrition and oxygen and to return waste materials and carbon dioxide. The organs of the circulatory system include the heart, arteries, veins, capillaries, and lymphatic vessels.

Pulmonary circulation

The right atrium receives blood from the superior and inferior vena cavas during the same period that the left atrium is receiving blood from the pulmonary veins. These chambers are in *diastole* during the filling period. The atria begin to contract, or begin the *systole,* and force the blood into the corresponding ventricles, which are now in diastole. When the atria are completely contracted, they begin to relax, and the ventricles begin the systole, which forces the blood from the right ventricle into the pulmonary artery and from the left ventricle into the aorta. The blood in the pulmonary artery is forced into the lungs, where the carbon dioxide is exchanged for oxygen. From the lungs the blood flows via the pulmonary veins into the left atrium. The blood in the aorta flows into the systemic and portal systems to all of the body cells.

Portal circulation

The blood from the systemic circulation enters the spleen, pancreas, stomach, small bowel, and greater part of the large bowel but does not directly return to the right atrium. It flows via the portal vein to the liver and into the liver sinusoids and from the liver via the hepatic vein to the inferior vena cava. This portal system is a vital part of the digestive and nutritive processes.

Systemic circulation

The systemic circulation is that which leaves the left ventricle, circulates through the body, and returns to the right atrium. It is this system that receives the various radiopaque media injected for radiographic studies.

Heart

The heart is a very muscular organ located in the thoracic cavity in the mediastinum and enveloped by the pericardium. It resembles an inverted cone and lies posterior to the sternum, with about twice as much to the left of the midsagittal plane as to the right. The *apex* is inferior to and slightly to the right of the left nipple. The heart is divided into four chambers: right and left *atria* (or auricles) and right and left *ventricles.* Blood from the vena cavas enters the right atrium, passes to the right ventricle through the *tricuspid valve,* and then passes from the right ventricle to the lungs via the pulmonary arteries. From the lungs via the pulmonary veins it enters the left atrium, passes into the left ventricle through the *bicuspid valve,* and then passes from the left

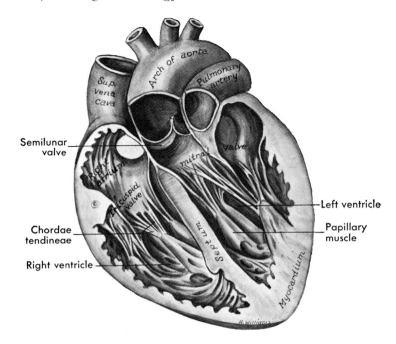

Fig. 15-15. Heart, frontal section. (From Anthony, Catherine Parker: Textbook of anatomy and physiology, St. Louis, 1963, The C. V. Mosby Co.)

ventricle via the aorta. Semilunar valves are located in the inferior vena cava, pulmonary vein, pulmonary artery, and aortic orifices. (See Fig. 15-15.) The heart is demonstrated radiographically without opacification in the routine chest exposures. However, it is always opacified by the injection of suitable radiopaque media for certain studies. These studies usually precede surgery.

Major arteries

The aorta arises from the left ventricle and makes an arch to the left of the median line. From this arch the aorta begins its descent. The coronary arteries for the heart muscles rise from the ascending portion. There are three major arteries arising from the arch: innominate (brachiocephalic), which branches into the right common carotid and right subclavian arteries; left common carotid; and left subclavian. The carotid arteries supply the head and neck along with the vertebral arteries, and the subclavian arteries supply the upper extremities. After the aorta begins its descent, it is called the descending or thoracic aorta in the thorax and the abdominal aorta in the abdomen. A little below the umbilicus the aorta branches into the two common iliac arteries, which are the major arteries supplying the lower extremities. The subclavian arteries, abdominal artery, and iliac arteries all branch into many smaller arteries, which supply various organs and parts. (See Fig. 15-16.)

The femur, tibia, and other long bones contain small nutrient foramina, located usually near the center of the shaft. One of the arterial branches, the

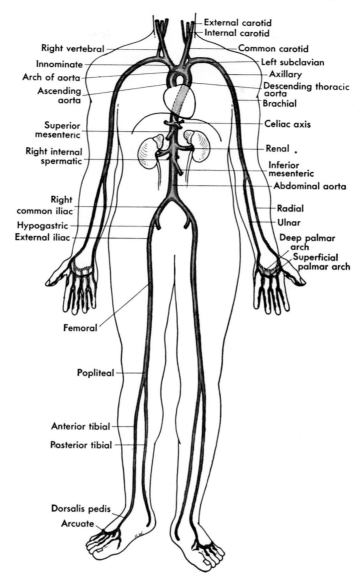

Fig. 15-16. Chief arteries. (From Anthony, Catherine Parker: Textbook of anatomy and physiology, St. Louis, 1963, The C. V. Mosby Co.)

nutrient artery, enters a foramen to supply the marrow of the bone. The tibial nutrient artery is one of the larger of these.

Major veins

The arteries all terminate in minute vessels known as capillaries, which join with the venules that join with each other to form veins. The veins receive other veins and become progressively larger as they approach the heart. The

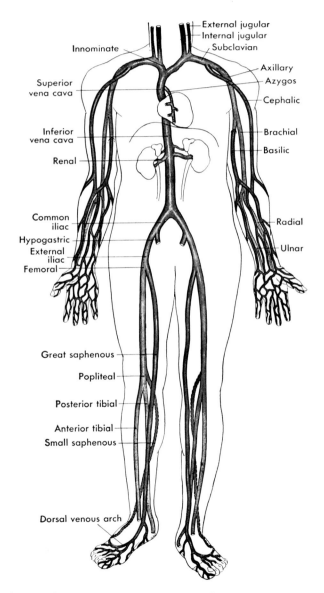

Fig. 15-17. Chief veins. (From Anthony, Catherine Parker: Textbook of anatomy and physiology, St. Louis, 1963, The C. V. Mosby Co.)

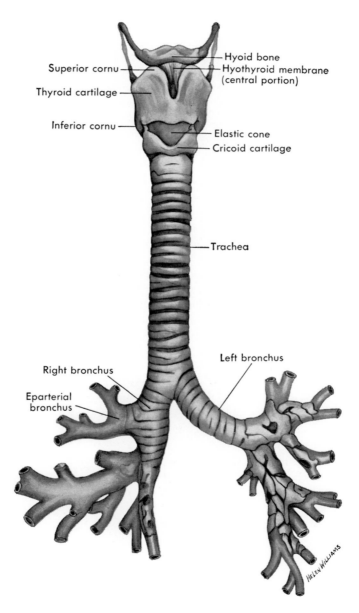

Superior cornu

Hyoid bone

Hyothyroid membrane
(central portion)

Thyroid cartilage

Inferior cornu

Elastic cone

Cricoid cartilage

Trachea

Right bronchus

Left bronchus

Eparterial
bronchus

HELEN WILLIAMS

Fig. 15-18. Larynx and bronchial tree, anterior view. (From Francis, Carl C: Introduction to human anatomy, St. Louis, 1968, The C. V. Mosby Co.)

veins of major importance in radiography are those into which the contrast media are injected. In the lower extremity the anterior and posterior tibial veins join to form the popliteal vein, which receives the lesser saphenous vein superior to the knee on the posterior surface. The popliteal vein receives the greater saphenous vein just inferior to the inguinal region and becomes the femoral vein, which later becomes the external iliac vein. The external iliac vein receives the hypogastric vein and becomes the common iliac vein; the two common iliac veins join to form the inferior vena cava. The inferior vena cava receives numerous other veins as it approaches the right atrium. In the upper extremities the radial and ulnar veins join just superior to the elbow to form the brachial vein. The brachial vein receives the basilic vein to form the axillary vein. Just above the portion called the axillary vein, the subclavian vein receives the cephalic vein. The subclavian vein receives the jugular vein from the head and neck to form the innominate (brachiocephalic) vein; the two brachiocephalic veins join to form the superior vena cava. (See Fig. 15-17.) As the veins pass through the anterior surface of the elbow, they are easily palpated. It is in this area, called the *antecubital space,* that intravenous injections are usually administered. The veins and arteries are usually named after the particular region of the body in which they are located or after a bone or organ in that particular region.

Lymphatic system

The lymphatic system is actually a part of the circulatory system, but the lymph flows only toward the heart: from the extremities and head to the subcalvian veins. The thoracic duct drains all of the left side of the head, neck, thorax, the left upper extremity, and all of the remainder of the body into the left subclavian vein. The lymphatic duct drains the right side of the head, neck, thorax, and the upper right extremity into the right subclavian vein. There are major concentrations of lymph nodes in the inguinal, mediastinal, axillary, subclavicular, supraclavicular, and cervical regions.

Respiratory system

The respiratory system includes the nose, pharynx, larynx, trachea, bronchi, and lungs. (See Fig. 15-18.) All of the organs of respiration are contained in the thorax, head, and neck, with the external openings (anterior nares) in the nose.

Nose

The nose opens into the nasal cavity, which opens directly into the pharynx through the choanae. The nasal septum was discussed elsewhere (p. 265). Air passes between the nasal cavities and the frontal, maxillary, ethmoid, and sphenoid sinuses. The formation of the nasal cavity was discussed on p. 271, and radiography of this cavity was discussed on p. 284.

Pharynx

The pharynx was described on pp. 328 and 329.

Larynx

The larynx enables us to speak. It is located between the trachea and the tongue in the neck in the area between the fourth and sixth cervical vertebrae.

The larynx connects the pharynx with the trachea. Its walls are composed of nine pieces of cartilage that contain the vocal cords within the cavity so formed. Among these cartilaginous parts are the *thyroid cartilage* (Adam's apple), *epiglottis* (lid) of the larynx, and the *cricoid cartilage*. The thyroid cartilage is very prominent in many males because of its more acute angle. The epiglottis prevents food from entering the trachea during deglutition. The cricoid cartilage forms the inferior surface of the larynx. The *glottis* is a space separating the true vocal cords. The vocal cords are fibers that expand and contract to control the frequency (pitch) of the voice. (See Fig. 15-3.)

Trachea

The *tracheal* walls contain incomplete circular cartilaginous rings that lend support to the walls and tend to keep the lumen of the trachea open at all times. The trachea is usually less than 12.5 cm long and occupies the area between the sixth cervical and fifth thoracic vertebrae. It bifurcates inferiorly, usually near the fifth thoracic vertebra, and the two major bronchi are formed at this bifurcation. The bronchi are of the same general construction as the trachea.

Bronchi

The *bronchi* enter the lungs through the *hila*. The right hilum is approximately opposite the fifth thoracic vertebra, and the left hilum is approximately opposite the sixth. The right bronchus extends almost directly into the right hilum, while the superior border of the left bronchus makes a more acute angle with the lateral margin of the trachea. In the lungs the bronchi branch into progressively smaller subdivisions, which are finally called *alveolar ducts*. The ducts are composed of *alveolar sacs*, which consist of many very small structures known as *alveoli*. The *gaseous exchange* takes place between the capillaries and the alveoli.

Lungs

The major respiratory organs, the *lungs*, are separated by the mediastinal viscera. The right lung is somewhat larger than the left and is divided into three lobes, whereas the left lung is divided into two lobes. Both lungs resemble cones. The *apex* of the lung is directed superiorly and is demonstrated radiographically by the use of the *apical lordotic position*. The base of each lung rests on the diaphragm. The medial surfaces of the lungs are concave and contain the hila. It is through the hila that all of the nerves and blood vessels as well as the bronchi enter the lungs. (See Fig. 15-19.) The major portion of the respiratory system is located in the thoracic cavity.

Thoracic cavity

The ribs and thoracic vertebrae form the posterior wall of the thoracic cavity, the ribs and related muscles form the lateral walls, and the ribs and sternum form the anterior wall. The superior border is narrowed and is bounded by the manubrium, the first ribs, and the first thoracic vertebra. The diaphragm forms the inferior border and separates the thoracic cavity from the abdominal cavity. The diaphragm is very important in respiration. It has three major openings

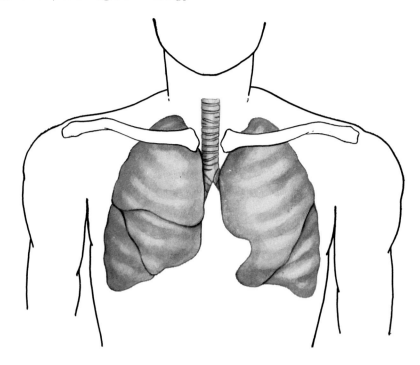

Fig. 15-19. Normal position of lungs and trachea. (From Francis, Carl C: Introduction to human anatomy, St. Louis, 1968, The C. V. Mosby Co.)

through it and several lesser openings that actually are posterior to it. The *aortic hiatus* is slightly to the left of the center and near the spine. The *esophageal hiatus* is slightly to the left of the midsagittal plane and nearly in the center. The *vena cavic foramen* is slightly anterior to the esophageal hiatus and to the right of the midsagittal plane. (See Fig. 15-20.) The diaphragm is a frequent object for radiographic study when *a diaphragmatic hernia* is suspected. Such herniations are demonstrable during gastrointestinal studies employing contrast media.

The thoracic cavity consists of three divisions: *pleural,* which contains the lungs; *mediastinal,* which contains the ascending aorta, descending aorta, aortic arch, inferior vena cava, thoracic duct, lymphatic duct, esophagus, bronchi, and azygos veins; and the *pericardial,* which contains the heart. These divisions are separated from each other by pleural partitions.

Nervous system and brain

The nervous system contains the *central* and *peripheral* divisions. The central nervous system includes the brain and spinal cord, while the peripheral system includes all the nerves of the body tissues and their connections to the central nervous system. Since nerves are radiolucent, they are difficult to radiograph. Opacification of surrounding tissues and insufflation of air surrounding the nerve tissue under consideration are the methods used in such radiographic techniques

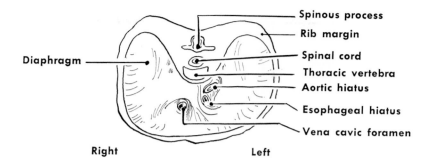

Fig. 15-20. Major openings of diaphragm.

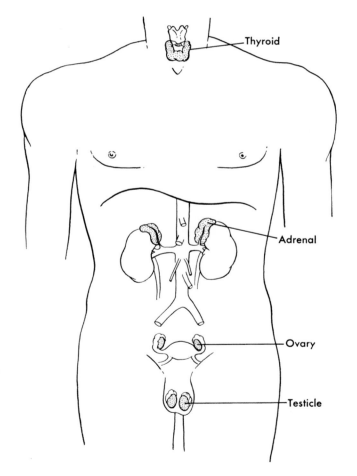

Fig. 15-21. Location of some of the endocrine glands. (From Anthony, Catherine Parker: Text-book of anatomy and physiology, St. Louis, 1963, The C. V. Mosby Co.)

Table 15-3. Endocrine glands

Gland	Location
Pituitary	Sella turcica in sphenoid
Thyroid	Anteriorly in neck, inferior to larynx
Parathyroids	Posterior surfaces of lobes of thyroid
Adrenals	Proximal poles of each kidney
Ovaries	Female pelvic cavity
Testes	Scrotum in male
Islands of Langerhans	Throughout pancreas
Indefinite glands	*Location*
Thymus	Posteriorly in neck from about C-6 to T-4
Pineal	Midbrain, superior and posterior to pituitary

as *myelography, encephalography,* and *ventriculography.* The spinal cord passes through the neural arches of the vertebral column, the formation of which is discussed in Chapter 11.

The medulla spinalis tapers in the conus medullaris and terminates near the level of the first lumbar vertebra to the second lumbar vertebra. The filum terminale interna continues below this level to terminate with the dura mater at the level of the first sacral vertebra. The filum terminale externa continues below the first sacral vertebra to terminate usually in the first coccygeal segment.

Endocrine system

The endocrine system is the system of the ductless glands, or the glands of hormone secretion. The names and anatomic locations of these glands are given in Table 15-3. (See also Fig. 15-21.)

REFERENCES

Anthony, Catherine Parker: Textbook of anatomy and physiology, St. Louis, 1967, The C. V. Mosby Co.
Best, C. H., and Taylor, N. B.: The living body, New York, 1952, Henry Holt & Co., Inc.
Best, C. H., and Taylor, N. B.: The human body, New York, 1956, Henry Holt & Co., Inc.
De Coursey, Russell Myles: The human organism, New York, 1955, McGraw-Hill Book Co.
Goss, Charles M.: Gray's anatomy, ed. 28, Philadelphia, 1966, Lea & Febiger.
Greisheimer, Esther M.: Physiology and anatomy, Philadelphia, 1950, J. B. Lippincott Co.
Kimber, Diana Clifford, and Gray, Carolyn E.: Textbook of anatomy and physiology, New York, 1928, The Macmillan Co.
Meschan, Isadore: Normal radiographic anatomy, Philadelphia, 1951, W. B. Saunders Co.

Chapter 16

Positioning for contrast studies

Contrast media

A contrast medium is a substance or material that makes it possible to examine by means of radiography specific organ systems and areas of the body that would otherwise have to be examined by actual observation or by relying on interpretation of the patient's symptoms.

There are many advantages to the use of contrast media:

1. They make the examination easier and faster in many cases and the diagnosis faster, more exact, and more complete.
2. In many cases the use of contrast media eliminates the necessity of resorting to surgery to study an organ or an area.
3. It can eliminate searching and probing on the part of the doctor; he can go directly to the area he wants to study and carry out his examination quickly and easily.
4. Completing a study using a contrast medium will in many cases give the patient peace of mind by reassuring him that there is no injury or disease to "worry about."

Normally, bone radiography presents no problem since the bone structures are sufficiently dense to present a good diagnostic demonstration on the x-ray film or the fluoroscopic screen. Since most internal organs and structures are composed of soft tissue, the demonstration of the organ or area is difficult unless it is filled with a medium that is either radiolucent or opaque to x-rays. For example, all the organs in the abdominal cavity are of about the same density, and it is difficult to distinguish one from the other on a routine radiograph. However, by filling the gallbladder with a radiopaque contrast medium, the gallbladder stands out in sharp contrast to the other organs in the abdominal cavity. This concentration of radiopaque chemicals in a certain area makes that area opaque to x-rays and so demonstrates the area on x-ray film.

Air or gas can be used as a contrast medium in certain areas, such as the brain ventricles, sinuses, and lungs. Air or gas makes the area of interest less opaque to x-rays than the surrounding areas; the presence of air causes the area to offer less resistance to the passage of x-rays than would be offered if the area were filled with fluid or with folds of tissue. On the film, the area is seen as having increased radiographic density (darker).

There are different forms of contrast media specific to examination of various areas and organs. Most forms—liquid, powder, pill forms—are opaque; air or gas, however, is used as a radiolucent (nonradiopaque) contrast medium. The

Table 16-1. Contrast media*

Viscera or structures	Examination name	Media
Cranial blood vessels	Cerebral angiography	Diodrast solution, Hypaque sodium, Urokon sodium
Paranasal sinuses	None	Iodochlorol, Lipiodol, Sinografin
Salivary ducts	Sialography	Diodrast solution, Lipiodol, Iodochlorol, Mulsopaque, Neo-Iopax, Sinografin
Esophagus, laryngopharynx	ESD, UGI, esophagus	Barium sulfate, Baropaque A, B, or C, Microtrast, Rugar, Baridol, Basolac, Barosperse, Esophatrast, Gastrografin
Articulations	Arthrograms	Diodrast solution, Lipiodol, Iodochlorol, Hypaque sodium
	Pneumoarthrograms	Oxygen or air
Heart and great vessels	Angiocardiography	Diodrast concentrate, Urokon sodium, Conray 400, Renografin 60
Arteries and veins	Arteriography, aortography, venography	Diodrast 70%, Diodrast solution, Hypaque sodium, Urokon sodium
Lymph vessels	Lymphangiography	Ethiodol
Lungs	Routine chest	Air
Bronchioles	Bronchography	Dionosil, Lipiodol, Iodochlorol
Breasts	Mammography	Diodrast solution, Lipiodol, Iodochlorol, Mulsopaque, Neo-Iopax
Stomach and small intestine	Gastrointestinal (GI) study	Barium sulfate, Baropaque A, B, or C, Micropaque, Baridol, Baroloid, Barotrast, Basolac, Gelobarin, Barosperse, Gastrografin
Stomach mucosa	GI study	Micropaque, Rugar, Umbrathor, Gastrografin
Spleen	Splenography	Air and Ethiodol
Gallbladder	Cholecystography	Telepaque, Cholografin sodium, Cholografin methylglucamine, GBD tablets, Oragrafin

*Note: Not all the media are listed in this Table, nor are all the media listed used routinely. The table simply presents ready reference material. The physician always orders a specific medium. Several preparations have been developed to aid the completion of certain studies. Among these preparations are Pitressin and Stamyl to aid in gas elimination and Cholex, Neo-Cholex, and Bilevac to substitute for the fatty meal following *filled* gallbladder radiographs.

Table 16-1. Contrast media—cont'd

Viscera or structures	Examination name	Media
Bile ducts	Cholangiography	Cholografin sodium, Cholografin methylglucamine, Diodrast solution, Iodochlorol, Lipiodol, Medopaque H, Mulsopaque, Neo-Iopax, Hypaque sodium
Intestinal mucosa	ESD, UGI, GI study, colon, barium enema (BE)	Micropaque, Rugar, barium sulfate, Umbrathor, Barosperse, Gastrografin
Colon	Barium enema (BE), colon	Barium sulfate, barium sulfate compound, Baropaque A and B, Barotrast, Micropaque, Baridol, Baroloid, Gastriloid, Umbrathor
Spinal canal	Myelography	Lipiodol, Pantopaque
Intervertebral discs	Discography	Pantopaque, Hypaque
Kidneys, ureters	IVP, retrograde pyelogram	Diodrast solution, Hypaque sodium solution, Renografin, Diodrast compound, Miokon sodium, Neo-Iopax, Conray 400, Urokon sodium
Urinary bladder, urethra	Cystogram, urethrogram	Diodrast solution, Hypaque sodium, Renografin, Diodrast compound, Miokon sodium, Neo-Iopax
Bladder mucosa	Bladder mucosa	Umbrathor, Urokon sodium
Seminal vesicles	Seminal vesicles	Diodrast solution, Lipiodol, Iodochlorol, Sinografin
Uterus and salpinges	Hysterosalpinography, uterosalpinography, uterography, salpinography	Diodrast solution, Ethiodol, Lipiodol, Salpix, Iodochlorol, Medopaque H
Draining sinuses, fistulae	None	Diodrast solution, Ethiodol, Lipiodol, Iodochlorol, Mulsopaque, Neo-Iopax, Sinografin

methods of introducing contrast media include intravenous injections, drinking in the form of liquids, ingesting orally in pill or granular form, injecting rectally in the form of an enema, and injecting the contrast medium directly into the space or area to be examined.

Characteristics of diagnostic opaques

Regardless of chemical composition, the contrast media (except, of course, air and gas) all contain some material or chemical that is opaque to x-rays. The type of diagnostic opaque to be used is selected with the foreknowledge that its radiopaque chemicals will concentrate in the area under consideration.

The radiopaque chemical in many contrast media is a form of iodine, usually in organic chemical combination. One disadvantage of this is that a small percentage of persons is overly sensitive to the iodine, so the contrast media should only be given following specific sensitivity tests.

Barium sulfate is a radiopaque mineral powder that is mixed with water and administered into the digestive system: it may be swallowed as a liquid, swallowed as a paste, or given in enema form to fill the colon.

Examples of contrast media and their uses are set out in Table 16-1.

Contrast studies

Contrast studies are increasing both in number and in the percentage of total studies performed as knowledge of assimilation and excretion of newer contrast media increases. One of the most common contrast studies, air contrast for lung detail, presents more practical application to Chapter 12 than to this chapter. Many contrast studies fall into the classification of special techniques. This chapter includes the more common contrast studies of the digestive, urinary, reproductive, respiratory, and nervous systems. The digestive system begins with the mouth, and the first contrast study is of the salivary glands and ducts.

Sialography

ROUTINE RADIOGRAPHIC POSITIONS

Salivary glands—submaxillary (submandibular) and sublingual, submentovertical view

Film size—occlusal	*Intraoral*
Dental type	*Extension cone*
Lengthwise	

Technique

Factors	*No-screen film occlusal (fast)*
Ma	100
Time	0.2
Mas	20
Thickness in cm	5
Kvp	64
Distance	30

Patient preparation

Remove all metallic and plastic articles from the head and neck region.

Contrast medium

Fill a sterile syringe with 1 ml of warmed iodized oil (Lipiodol).

Palpation points

Mandibular angles.

Procedure

Place the patient in the supine position, with shoulders elevated on a folded pillow. Extend the chin so that the vertex of the head rests on the table. Place the film lengthwise as far into the mouth as possible. The rough surface of the film packet must face the tube. (See Figs. 14-51 and 14-52).

Central ray

Direct the central ray cephalad and perpendicular through a point just anterior to the mandibular angles to the center of the film holder.

Immobilization

Place a sandbag against the patient's forehead. Employ suspended respiration.

Right-left markers

Tape an L or R on the corresponding corner of the film holder.

Examination

The doctor introduces a fine gold, chrome, or silver cannula into the duct orifice and injects the contrast medium until the patient experiences some discomfort. The radiographs must be made as quickly as possible in order to visualize the ducts before the oil diffuses into the alveoli.

Structures demonstrated

Submentovertical projection of the sublingual area to demonstrate pathology of the salivary ducts and alveoli. (See Fig. 16-1.)

Note:

This view is used in many routine series as a survey film for demonstrating calculi without the use of contrast media.

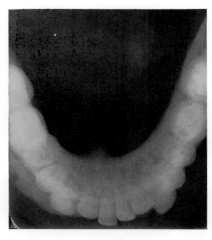

Fig. 16-1. Sialogram (salivary glands): submaxillary (submandibular) and sublingual glands —submentovertical view. (Courtesy Dr. James M. Hilton.)

Salivary glands—parotid gland, anterior (P-A) view

> *Film size—8″ × 10″*   *Erect film holder*
> *Cassette*   *Cone to cover*
> *Lenthwise*

Technique

Factors	*Screen film cassette (par)*
Ma	100
Time	0.3
Mas	30
Thickness in cm	10
Kvp	62
Distance	72

Patient preparation

Remove all metallic and plastic articles from the head and neck region.

Contrast medium

Fill a sterile syringe with 1 ml of warmed iodized oil (Lipiodol).

Palpation points

Mandibular angles.

Procedure

Place the patient in the prone or erect anterior (P-A) position. Rotate the head so that the long axis of the mandibular body of the side being examined is perpendicular to the film surface. Center that mandibular angle to the center of the film holder; the forehead and nose are in contact with the film holder. (See Fig. 16-2.)

Central ray

Direct the central ray perpendicular to the center of the film holder.

Immobilization

Place a positioning sponge against the opposite side of the face in contact with the film holder. Have the patient hold the sponge in place. Employ suspended respiration.

Examination

The doctor introduces a fine gold, chrome, or silver cannula into the duct orifice and injects the contrast medium until the patient experiences some discomfort. The radiographs must be made as quickly as possible in order to visualize the ducts before the oil diffuses into the alveoli.

Structures demonstrated

Anterior (P-A) projection of the parotid area to demonstrate pathology of the salivary ducts and alveoli. (See Fig. 16-3.)

Note:

This view is used in many routine series as a survey film for demonstrating calculi without the use of contrast media.

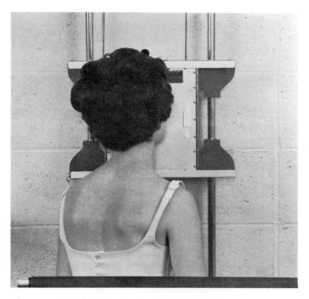

Fig. 16-2. Sialography: parotid gland—anterior (P-A) position.

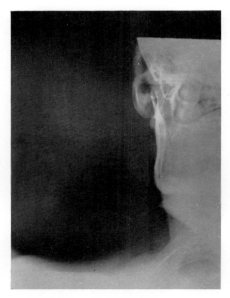

Fig. 16-3. Sialogram: parotid gland—anterior (P-A) view. (Courtesy Dr. E. I. L. Cilley, Dr. T. W. Crowell, Dr. R. E. Waud, and Dr. G. H. Hoffman.)

Salivary glands—parotid gland, posterior (A-P) view

Film size—8″ × 10″   *Tabletop*
Cassette   *Extension cone*
Lengthwise

Technique

Factors	Screen film cassette (par)
Ma	100
Time	0.2
Mas	20
Thickness in cm	10
Kvp	58
Distance	30

Patient preparation

Remove all metallic and plastic articles from the head and neck region.

Contrast medium

Fill a syringe with 1 ml of warmed iodized oil (Lipiodol).

Palpation points

Mandibular bodies and angles.

Procedure

Place the patient in the supine or erect posterior (A-P) position. Rotate the head so that the long axis of the mandibular body of the side being examined is perpendicular to the film holder. Center that mandibular angle to the center of the film holder; the canthomeatal line is perpendicular to the film holder. (See Fig. 16-4.)

Central ray

Direct the central ray perpendicular to the film holder.

Immobilization

Place a positioning sponge against the opposite side of the head. Have the patient hold the sponge in place. Employ suspended respiration.

Examination

The doctor introduces a fine gold, chrome, or silver cannula into the duct orifice and injects the contrast medium until the patient experiences some discomfort. The radiographs must be made as quickly as possible in order to visualize the ducts before the oil diffuses into the alveoli.

Structures demonstrated

Posterior (A-P) projection of the parotid area to demonstrate pathology of the parotid ducts and alveoli. (See Fig. 16-5.)

Note:

This view is used in many routine series as a survey film for demonstrating calculi without the use of contrast media.

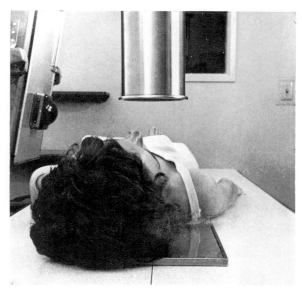

Fig. 16-4. Sialography: parotid gland—posterior (A-P) position.

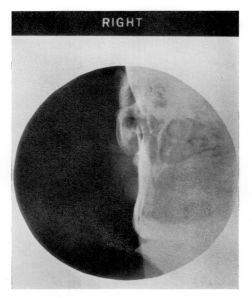

Fig. 16-5. Sialogram: parotid gland—posterior (A-P) view. (Courtesy Dr. E. I. L. Cilley, Dr. T. W. Crowell, Dr. R. E. Waud, and Dr. G. H. Hoffman.)

Salivary glands—parotid and submaxillary glands, lateral view

> *Film size—8″ × 10″*   *Erect film holder*
> *Cassette*   *Cone to cover*
> *Lengthwise*

Technique

Factors	Screen film cassette (par)
Ma	200
Time	0.1
Mas	20
Thickness in cm	11
Kvp	66
Distance	72

Patient preparation

Remove all metallic and plastic articles from the head and neck region.

Contrast medium

Fill a syringe with 1 ml of warmed iodized oil (Lipiodol).

Palpation points

Mandibular rami and bodies.

Procedure

Place the patient in the lateral erect position with the shoulder of the side being examined against the film holder. Extend the arms down the sides. The midsagittal plane of the head and body is parallel with the film holder. Elevate the chin so that the long axis of the mandibular body is parallel with the floor. Center a point 1 inch anterior to the E.A.M. (external auditory meatus) over the center of the film holder. (See Fig. 16-6.)

Central ray

Direct the central ray perpendicular through the selected point to the center of the film holder.

Immobilization

Place a rectangular sponge between the patient's head and the erect film holder. A compression band may be used around the head. Employ suspended respiration.

Examination

The doctor introduces a fine gold, chrome, or silver cannula into the duct orifice and injects the contrast medium until the patient experiences some discomfort. The radiographs must be made as quickly as possible in order to visualize the duct before the oil diffuses into the alveoli.

Structures demonstrated

Lateral projection of the salivary glands to demonstrate pathology of the parotid and submandibular glands, ducts, and alveoli. (See Fig. 16-7.)

Note:

This view is used in many routine series as a survey film for demonstrating calculi without the use of contrast media.

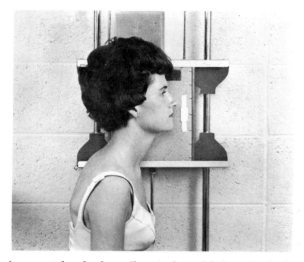

Fig. 16-6. Sialography: parotid and submaxillary (submandibular) glands—lateral position.

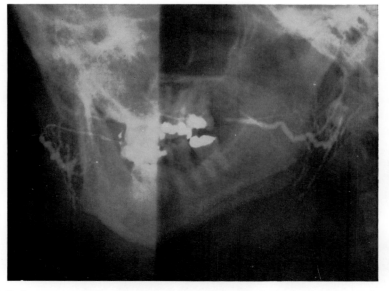

Fig. 16-7. Sialogram: parotid and submaxillary (submandibular) glands—tangential and lateral views. (Courtesy Dr. Earl L. Lawson.)

Gastrointestinal studies
Department routine

The first part of the morning is usually reserved for gallbladder, stomach, and colon studies. Each of these examinations requires previous appointments. After opening the department for the day, note the number of gallbladder and gastrointestinal studies scheduled and then prepare the barium for the day's examinations. Valuable time can be saved and department routine can be smoother when the barium mixtures are prepared correctly. The opacity of a given suspension of barium sulfate in water is in direct relation to the quantity of barium used. Use of a hydrometer especially designed to measure the specific gravity of barium sulfate suspensions assures consistent results from day to day.

Next, check the temperatures of the darkroom solutions, adjust if necessary, add replenishers, and completely mix and stir the solutions. Following this, prepare the previous day's unread films for interpretation. By this time one of the patients scheduled for gallbladder study should have arrived for radiography. If there is an interval of time between the completion of his radiographic examination and the arrival of the next patient, who is probably scheduled for gastrointestinal examination, file the previous day's films. To avoid confusion, accomplish filing between other duties and as often as possible. We do not intend to recommend departmental operation but to emphasize the need for a routine and to demonstrate or suggest how a routine enable one person to accomplish a large volume of work easily and thus aid his employer in maintaining a smooth, efficiently operating department.

Radiography of the viscera, or soft tissue radiography, requires considerably different combinations of factors than does bone radiography. Usually, higher peak kilovoltage and proportionally lower milliampere-seconds are required; however, the milliamperage is often quite high near the maximum capacity of the tube on the large focal spot. If the maximum milliamperage of the tube is 200, then 100 milliampere-seconds are usually used.

Various conditions limit or control the specific starting factors for visceral radiography: first, the radiologist must determine what combination of factors on any given machine will deliver the maximum tissue differentiation; second, the tube capacity and output of the transformer place limitations on the selected factors; third, the physiologic variability of the patients modifies many parts of the routine and selected factors.

Esophagus—fluoroscopic examination
Patient preparation

No special preparation of the patient is necessary. Remove all garments down to the waist. Provide a gown for female patients.

Contrast medium

Prepare approximately 4 ounces of regular barium sulfate mixture (two parts barium to one part water) with added flavoring if desired, or use flavored commercial preparations per instructions.

Equipment preparation

1. Lock a footstand on the fluoroscopy table.
2. Stand the fluoroscopy table erect and lock the Bucky diaphragm at the lower end of the table.
3. Unlock and position the fluoroscopy tower.
4. Insert a cassette into the spot-film device on the fluoroscopy tower and set the selector switch.
5. Place the foot switch to the left or right of the erect table, and position the radiologist's fluoroscopy stool in front of the table.
6. Close the line switch on the control panel and select the fluoroscopy technique (usually 3 to 5 ma).
7. Provide the mixed contrast medium, a tablespoon, an emesis basin, towels, a marking pencil, etc.
8. Darken the fluoroscopy room and energize the safelights.
9. Notify the radiologist that you are prepared and assist him with lead gloves and lead apron.

Note: If an *image intensifier* is used, attach the *intensifier* to the fluoroscopy tower according to instructions.

Examination

1. Introduce the radiologist to the patient.
2. Instruct the patient to stand on the footstand with his back against the table.
3. A cursory screening of the area under consideration may be performed by the doctor.
4. The technologist places a spoonful of the thick contrast medium mixture in the patient's mouth and cautions the patient to turn his face to the left and follow the doctor's instructions.
5. In most cases the doctor will make various *spot films* and require additional loaded cassettes.
6. Fluoroscopy may be conducted with the patient in the horizontal or Trendelenburg° positions with additional contrast medium mixture.
7. The doctor will instruct the technologist as to the number and kind of radiographic views desired.

°The head is lower than the feet.

ROUTINE RADIOGRAPHIC POSITION

Esophagus—right anterior oblique (R.A.O.) view

> *Film size— 14″ × 17″* *Bucky*
> *Cassette* *Cone to cover*
> *Lengthwise*

Technique

Factors	Screen film cassette (par)
Ma	300
Time	0.1
Mas	30
Thickness in cm	30
Kvp	80
Distance	40

Palpation points

Spinous processes of the thoracic vertebrae.

Procedure

Place the patient in the prone position. Flex the left elbow and knee, rotating the patient into a 35-degree right anterior oblique (R.A.O.) position. Center a point midway between the spinous processes and the vertebral border of the scapula on the elevated side over the midline of the table. Place the top of the film holder in line with the E.A.M.

Central ray

Direct the central ray perpendicular to the center of the film holder. (See Fig. 16-8.)

Immobilization

Employ suspended inspiration.

Right-left markers

Place an R.A.O. marker on the right lateral center border of the film holder.

Examination

1. Have the patient swallow one tablespoonful of thick contrast medium mixture.
2. Place a second tablespoonful of this mixture in the patient's mouth and caution him to swallow when instructed to by the doctor.
3. Energize the cathode and instruct the patient to suspend breathing on deep inspiration; then to swallow.
4. After the patient swallows, count one, two, and then make the exposure.
5. Inform the patient that a 1-ounce saline purgative and a copious amount of water may be necessary to eliminate the contrast medium.

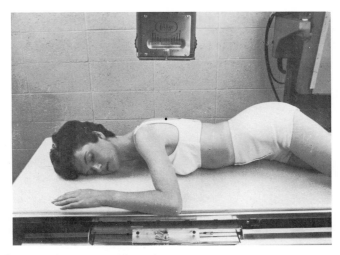

Fig. 16-8. Esophagus—right anterior oblique (R.A.O.) position.

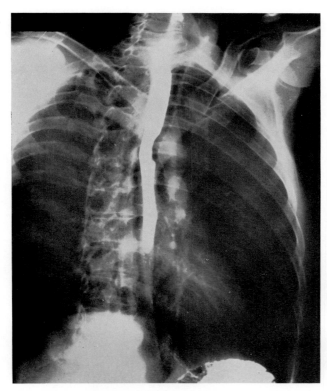

Fig. 16-9. Esophagus—right anterior oblique (R.A.O.) view. (Courtesy Dr. E. I. L. Cilley, Dr. T. W. Crowell, Dr. R. E. Waud, and Dr. G. H. Hoffman.)

Structures demonstrated

R.A.O. view of the entire esophagus and cardiac orifice filled with contrast medium. (See Fig. 16-9.)

Note:

For examination of the upper lateral esophagus, position the patient for a lateral cervical spine view (p. 188), using rapid exposure and thick contrast medium mixture.

Stomach and duodenum—fluoroscopic examination, upper G.I., barium meal, E.S.D.
Patient preparation

The patient is to have nothing by mouth after 10 P.M. the night prior to the examination. On the morning of the examination, remove all garments except shoes and socks. Provide a gown and instruct the patient to tie the open ends together in the back.

Make a 14″ × 17″ posterior (A-P) abdominal scout (survey) radiograph of the patient, centering at the iliac crest. (See p. 397.)

Contrast medium

Prepare approximately 8 ounces of regular barium sulfate mixture (one part barium to one part water) with added flavoring as desired, or use flavored commercial preparations per instructions.

Equipment preparation

1. Lock a footstand on the fluoroscopy table.
2. Stand the fluoroscopy table erect and lock the Bucky diaphragm at the lower end of the table.
3. Unlock and position the fluoroscopy tower.
4. Insert a loaded cassette into the spot-film device on fluoroscopy tower and set the selector switch.
5. Place the foot switch to the left or right of the erect table and position the radiologist's fluoroscopy stool in front of the table.
6. Close the line switch on the control panel and select the fluoroscopy technique (usually 3 to 5 ma).
7. Provide the mixed contrast medium, a drinking tube, an emesis basin, towels, a marking pencil, etc.
8. Darken the fluoroscopy room and energize the safelights.
9. Notify the radiologist that you are prepared and assist him with lead gloves and lead apron.

Note: If an *image intensifier* is used, leave the table horizontal and attach the *intensifier* to the fluoroscopy tower.

Examination

1. Introduce the radiologist to the patient.
2. Instruct the patient to stand on the footstand with his back against the table.
3. Instruct the patient to hold the glass of barium sulfate mixture in his left

hand and to rest the hand against his left shoulder, turn his face to the left, and follow the doctor's instructions.

4. A cursory screening of the area under consideration may be performed by the doctor.

5. In most cases the doctor will make various *spot films* and will require additional loaded cassettes.

6. Fluoroscopy may be conducted with the patient in the horizontal or Trendelenburg positions with the use of additional contrast medium and drinking tube.

7. The doctor will mark the region of interest and instruct the technologist as to the number and kind of radiographic views desired.

ROUTINE RADIOGRAHIC POSITIONS

Stomach—anterior (P-A) view

> Film size—10″ × 12″   Bucky
> Cassette   Cone to cover
> Crosswise

Technique

Factors	Screen film, cassette (par) Regular kvp—12:1 grid	Screen film, cassette (par) High kvp—16:1 grid
Ma	300	200
Time	0.2	1/20
Mas	60	10
Thickness in cm	20	20
Kvp	78	120
Distance	40	40

Palpation points

Spinous processes of the thoracic vertebrae.

Procedure

Place the patient in the prone position with the arms relaxed at the sides. Center a point 2½ inches to the left of the eleventh thoracic spinous process or xiphoid process over the center line of the table.

Central ray

Direct the central ray perpendicular through the selected point to the center of the film holder. (See Fig. 16-10.)

Immobilization

Employ suspended expiration.

Right-left markers

Markers are not necessary on this view.

Technical tips

For the hypersthenic (large, obese) patient, position the film holder crosswise and 2 or more inches higher than normal. For the asthenic (thin, slender) patient, position the film holder lengthwise and 2 or more inches lower than normal.

Structures demonstrated

Anterior (P-A) view of the entire stomach, including the terminal end of the esophagus and the duodenal cap (bulb) with the proximal duodenum. (See Fig. 16-11.)

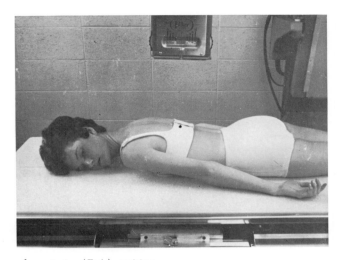

Fig. 16-10. Stomach—anterior (P-A) position.

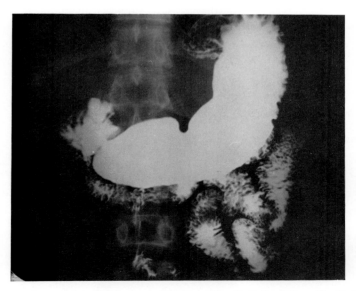

Fig. 16-11. Stomach—anterior (P-A) view. (Courtesy Dr. E. I. L. Cilley, Dr. T. W. Crowell, Dr. R. E. Waud, and Dr. G. H. Hoffman.)

Stomach—right anterior oblique (R.A.O.) view

Film size—10″ × 12″   *Bucky*
Cassette   *Cone to cover*
Lengthwise

Technique

Factors	Screen film cassette (par) Regular kvp—12:1 grid	Screen film cassette (par) High kvp—16:1 grid
Ma	300	200
Time	0.3	0.1
Mas	90	20
Thickness in cm	25	25
Kvp	85	120
Distance	40	40

Palpation points

Spinous processes of lumbar vertebrae; lateral ribs.

Procedure

Place the patient in the prone position. Flex the left elbow and knee, rotating the patient into a 45-degree right anterior oblique (R.A.O.) position. Center the area marked by the radiologist (during fluoroscopy) over the center line of the table. If no marks are present, center a point in line with the first lumbar vertebra and midway between the spinous processes and the lateral ribs on the elevated side over the center line of the table.

Central ray

Direct the central ray perpendicular to the center of the film holder. (See Fig. 16-12.)

Immobilization

Employ suspended expiration.

Right-left markers

Markers are not necessary on this view.

Technical tips

For the hypersthenic (large, obese) patient, position the film holder crosswise and 2 or more inches higher than normal. For the asthenic (thin, slender) patient, position the film holder lengthwise and 2 or more inches lower than normal.

Structures demonstrated

R.A.O. view of the entire stomach, including the terminal end of the esophagus and the duodenal cap (bulb) with the proximal duodenum. (See Fig. 16-13.)

Note:

Some routine series call for more than one radiograph in this position, at 2- or 3-minute time intervals and on inspiration as well as expiration. Also, many

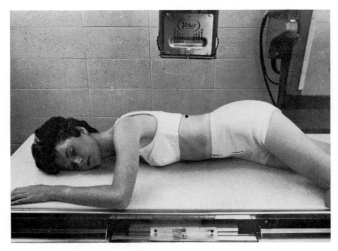

Fig. 16-12. Stomach—right anterior oblique (R.A.O.) position.

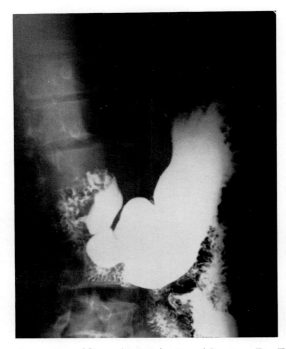

Fig. 16-13. Stomach—right anterior oblique (R.A.O.) view. (Courtesy Dr. E. I. L. Cilley, Dr. T. W. Crowell, Dr. R. E. Waud, and Dr. G. H. Hoffman.)

radiologists request that the patient return for a 2- or 3-hour *stasis* film; the patient is usually requested to abstain from anything to eat or drink during this period.

Upon completion of the entire radiographic procedure, inform the patient that a 1-ounce saline purgative and copious amounts of water may be necessary to eliminate the contrast medium.

Small intestine beyond duodenum—stasis, fluoroscopic examination

Patient preparation

The patient is to have nothing by mouth after 10 P.M. the night prior to the examination. On the morning of the examination, remove all garments except shoes and socks. Provide a gown and instruct the patient to tie the open ends together in the back. Make a 14″ × 17″ posterior (A-P) abdominal scout (survey) radiograph of the patient, centering at the iliac crest. (See p. 397.)

Contrast media

Prepare approximately 4 ounces of regular barium sulfate mixture (one part barium sulfate to one part water) with added flavoring as desired, or use flavored commercial preparations per instructions.

Equipment preparation

1. Lock a footstand on the fluoroscopy table.
2. Stand the fluoroscopy table erect and lock the Bucky diaphragm at the lower end of the table.
3. Unlock and position the fluoroscopy tower.
4. Insert a loaded cassette into the spot-film device on the fluoroscopy tower and set the selector switch.
5. Place the foot switch to the left or right of the erect table and position the radiologist's fluoroscopy stool in front of the table.
6. Close the line switch on the panel and select the fluoroscopy technique (usually 3 to 5 ma).
7. Provide the mixed contrast medium, an emesis basin, towels, a marking pencil, etc.
8. Darken the fluoroscopy room and energize the safelights.
9. Notify the radiologist that you are prepared and assist him with lead gloves and lead apron.

Note: If an *image intensifier* is used, leave the table horizontal and attach the *intensifier* to the fluoroscopy tower.

Examination

1. Introduce the radiologist to the patient.
2. Instruct the patient to stand on the footstand with his back against the table.
3. Instruct the patient to hold the glass of barium sulfate mixture in his left hand and to rest the hand against his left shoulder, turn his face to the left, and follow the doctor's instructions.
4. A cursory screening of the area under consideration may be performed by the doctor.

5. In most cases the doctor will instruct the patient to drink all of the contrast medium. (The technologist should note the approximate time required for Step 5).
6. In most cases the doctor will make various *spot films* and require additional loaded cassettes.
7. Fluoroscopy may be conducted with the patient in the horizontal or Trendelenburg positions.
8. The doctor will instruct the technologist as to the number and kind of radiographs desired.

Note: Many routines specify that the patient be given 8 ounces of cold isotonic saline solution or carbonated water after the initial fluoroscopic examination to accelerate the travel of the contrast medium through the small intestine.

ROUTINE RADIOGRAPHIC POSITION

Small intestine—posterior (A-P) view

> *Film size—14″ × 17″*   *Bucky*
> *Cassette*   *Cone to cover*
> *Lengthwise*

Technique

Factors	Screen film cassette (par) Regular kvp—12:1 grid	Screen film cassette (par) High kvp— 16:1 grid
Ma	300	200
Time	0.2	1/15
Mas	60	13.3
Thickness in cm	21	21
Kvp	80	120
Distance	40	40

Palpation points

Iliac crests.

Procedure

Place the patient in the supine position with the median line of the body over the center line of the table. Elevate the knees with sponges or sandbags to aid in patient comfort. Center the film holder to the crest of the ilium.

Central ray

Direct the central ray perpendicular to the center of the film holder (See Fig. 16-14.)

Immobilization

Employ suspended expiration.

Right-left markers

Place a right marker on the right lateral center border of the film holder.

Examination

The radiologist may request a progress film of this type every 30 to 60 minutes after the contrast medium has been ingested and until it reaches the cecum. Also, it may be routine for the radiologist to check the patient fluoroscopically prior to each progress film.

Structures demonstrated

Posterior (A-P) view of the abdomen demonstrating contrast medium at various stages of progression from the stomach through the small intestine. (See Fig. 16-15.)

Note:

Each progress film must have the time interval identified on it during exposure.

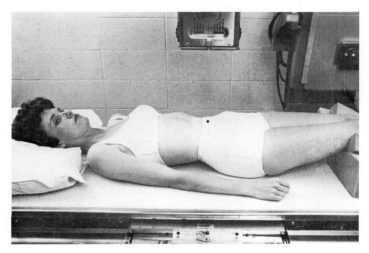

Fig. 16-14. Small intestine—posterior (A-P) position.

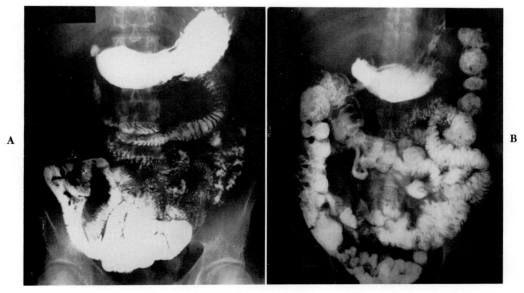

A

B

Fig. 16-15. Small intestine—posterior (A-P) view. **A,** One hour following barium meal. **B,** Two hours following barium meal. (Courtesy Dr. E. I. L. Cilley, Dr. T. W. Crowell, Dr. R. E. Waud, and Dr. G. H. Hoffman.)

Upon completion of the entire radiographic procedure, inform the patient that a 1-ounce saline purgative and copious amounts of water may be necessary to eliminate the contrast medium.

Large intestine—barium enema, fluoroscopic examination
Patient preparation

1. On the day prior to the examination, the patient should avoid eating roughage and dairy products. A liquid diet is desirable.
2. Between 3 and 5 P.M. on the day prior to the examination, the patient must take 2 ounces of castor oil. *This may be disguised with root beer or orange juice.*
3. He must take an enema consisting of 1½ to 2 pints of warm soapsuds at bedtime of the day prior to the examination.
4. On the morning of the examination he must take an enema consisting of one pint of warm water, repeated until a clear return is obtained.
5. He must omit breakfast except for a cup of black coffee or clear tea. (Omit this if a complete gastrointestinal study is to be made.)
6. When the patient is admitted, remove all garments except shoes and socks. Provide a gown and instruct the patient to tie the open ends together in the back.
7. Make a 14″ × 17″ posterior (A-P) abdominal scout (survey) radiograph of the patient, centering at the iliac crest. (See p. 397.)

Note: Ascertain from the patient whether he is able to retain an enema.

Contrast medium

Prepare approximately 1 quart of regular barium sulfate mixture (one part barium sulfate to two parts water), or use commercial preparations per instructions. Solution must be *tepid* (100° F) and mixed thoroughly.

Attach the enema tip to the tube. Pour the mixture into the enema container and allow it to run through the tube and tip before clamping off the tube. For commercial disposable containers, follow directions as indicated. (A hemostat makes an excellent clamp.)

Equipment preparation

1. Position and lock the Bucky diaphragm at the foot end of the horizontal table.
2. Unlock and position the fluoroscopy tower.
3. Insert loaded cassette into the spot-film device on the fluoroscopy tower and set the selector switch.
4. Place the foot switch to the center of the working side of the table.
5. Close the line switch on the control panel and select the fluoroscopy technique (usually 3 to 5 ma).
6. Provide the following:
   a. Enema container with tepid contrast medium
   b. Ceiling hook or I.V. stand for enema container
   c. Lubricant for enema tip (water-soluble preferred)
   d. Bedpan
   e. Paper towels

     f. A Bardex catheter with two hemostats in place of the regular enema tip if patient has difficulty in retaining an enema

7. Darken the fluoroscopy room and energize the safelights.
8. Notify the radiologist that you are prepared and assist him with lead gloves and lead apron.

Note: If an *image intensifier* is used, attach the *intensifier* to the fluoroscopy tower.

Examination

1. Introduce the radiologist to the patient.
2. Place the patient on the table on his left side with knees flexed.
3. Separate the gluteal folds and insert the well-lubricated enema tip (or Bardex catheter) into the rectum.
4. Instruct the patient to lie in the supine position. Recheck the enema tube to eliminate any twisting or kinking.
5. Explain the procedure to the patient and inform him that he may experience some cramping.
6. The technologist will stand to the right of the doctor and manipulate the barium sulfate mixture flow as directed.
7. A cursory screening of the area under consideration may be performed by the doctor.
8. In most cases the doctor will make various *spot films* during the barium sulfate mixture injection and will require additional loaded cassettes.
9. The fluoroscopy procedure is usually concluded when the contrast medium reaches the ileocecal valve.
10. The doctor will instruct the technologist as to the number and kind of radiographs desired.
11. After preevacuation radiographs have been made, the technologist will escort the patient to the lavatory to eliminate the enema mixture.

Note: If a disposable enema container is used, the contrast medium is returned to the container, thus eliminating Step 11 in some examinations.

ROUTINE RADIOGRAPHIC POSITION
Large intestine (colon)—anterior (P-A) views, preevacuation and postevacuation

     Film size—14″ × 17″   *Bucky*
     Casette   *Cone to cover*
     Lengthwise

Technique

Factors	Screen film cassette (par) Regular kvp—12:1 grid	Screen film cassette (par) High kvp—16:1 grid
Ma	300	200
Time	0.2	1/15
Mas	60	13.3
Thickness in cm	21	21
Kvp	80	115
Distance	40	40

Palpation points

Iliac crests.

Procedure

Place the patient in the prone position with the median line of the body over the center line of the table. Center the film holder to the crest of the ilium.

Central ray

Direct the central ray perpendicular to the center of the film holder. (See Fig. 16-16.)

Immobilization

Employ suspended expiration.

Right-left markers

Place a right marker on the right lateral center border of the film holder.

Technical tips

When the patient must eliminate the contrast medium in the lavatory, speed as well as accuracy is essential in radiographic procedures. Allow a sufficient amount of time for the elimination of the contrast medium before making the postevacuation exposures.

Structures demonstrated

Anterior (P-A) view of the large intestine demonstrating contrast medium between the rectum and the ileocecal junction. (See Figs. 16-17 and 16-18.)

Note:

For anterior (P-A) erect views, lower the film holder position 2 inches and increase the technique factors approximately 10 kvp or the equivalent. Upon completion of the entire radiographic procedure, inform the patient that a 1-ounce saline purgative and copious amounts of water may be necessary to eliminate the contrast medium.

Large intestine—double contrast (D.C. colon), fluoroscopic examination
Patient preparation

The patient is given the barium enema with the same procedure described in the preceding section (p. 376), except that after the scout (survey) film has been completed, instruct patient to ingest approximately 16 ounces of water in order to retard *flaking* (caused by dehydration) of the contrast medium in the colon.

Contrast medium

The contrast medium is the same as that used for the barium enema (p. 376).

Equipment preparation

The equipment needed is the same as that required for the barium enema (p. 376), except for the addition of a Bardex catheter with air insufflator.

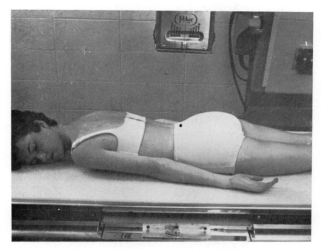

Fig. 16-16. Large intestine (colon)—anterior (P-A) position.

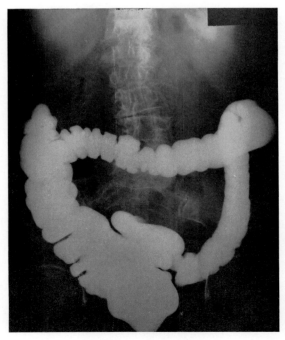

Fig. 16-17. Large intestine (colon)—anterior (P-A) view, preevacuation. (Courtesy Dr. E. I. L. Cilley, Dr. T. W. Crowell, Dr. R. E. Waud, and Dr. G. H. Hoffman.)

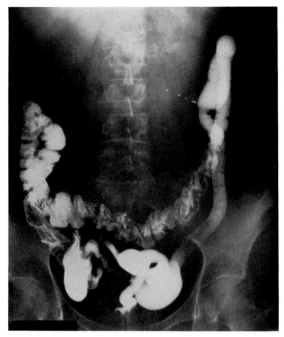

Fig. 16-18. Large intestine (colon)—anterior (P-A) view, postevacuation. (Courtesy Dr. E. I. L. Cilley, Dr. T. W. Crowell, Dr. R. E. Waud, and Dr. G. H. Hoffman.)

Examination

The examination proceeds in the same manner as the barium enema study (p. 376), except that after the patient has eliminated approximately 50% of the barium sulfate mixture, air is injected by means of an air insufflator attached to the Bardex catheter. Fluoroscopy procedures are resumed, and appropriate preevacuation radiographs (see Fig. 16-19) are made.

Note:

Modern disposable barium enema containers will eliminate the need for the patient to evacuate intestinal contents in the lavatory.

Cholecystography

Cholecystography is a functional radiographic examination of the gallbladder by means of an orally ingested contrast medium.

Patient preparation

1. The patient's noon meal on the day before the examination should include two pats of butter or a fried egg.
2. The evening meal should be light and free of fatty foods, as directed on the package of contrast medium tablets.
3. The patient must take the contrast medium tablets with plenty of water approximately *12* hours prior to the examination:

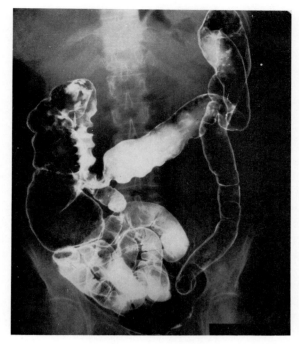

Fig. 16-19. Large intestine (colon)—anterior (P-A) view, air contrast, postevacuation. (Courtesy Dr. E. I. L. Cilley, Dr. T. W. Crowell, Dr. R. E. Waud, and Dr. G. H. Hoffman.)

  a. Sthenic (average build) patients require six tablets (example: Telepaque).
  b. Asthenic (thin, slender) patients require four tablets.
  c. Hypersthenic (large, obese) patients require eight to ten tablets.
 4. On the morning of the examination, the patient must omit breakfast except for water, black coffee, or clear tea.
 5. He must take an enema consisting of warm tap water, using an amount sufficient to produce a clear return.
 6. When the patient is admitted, remove all garments except shoes and socks. Provide a gown and instruct the patient to tie the open ends together in the back.

Note: Recent commercial preparations that are prescribed by some departments and that are taken orally 15 to 18 hours prior to the examination eliminate the necessity for Step 5 (warm water enema).

Contrast media

Various commercial preparations (Telepaque, Oragrafin, or the like) may be purchased from local pharmacies by the patient or provided by the radiology department. (See Step 3 above.)

Note: Inform the patient that varying degrees of diarrhea may result from the ingestion of this type of contrast media, so that it may become necessary for him to control this reaction with some type of paregoric elixir.

Complications

Gas shadows may exist in the intestinal tract; they may be overcome by one of the following:

1. Breathing technique; inspiration or expiration
2. Rotation of the patient
3. Angulation (direction) of the central ray
4. Erect positions; gallbladder will drop approximately 2½ inches in the average size patient
5. Trendelenburg position (anterior, P-A); gallbladder will move slightly cephalad; gas shadows will rise caudad
6. Right lateral decubitus position; gallbladder will drop toward the right midaxillary region; gas shadows will rise toward medial plane
7. Use of Pitressin, carminative (a medium to relieve flatulence, gas) (Use 0.5 ml intradermal injection. **Caution: permission must** be obtained from the referring physician.)

Contrast medium may be absent in the gallbladder; this may be caused by one of the following:

1. Functional disturbance of the patient
2. Gallbladder previously removed
3. Patient vomited contrast medium or had diarrhea
4. Contrast medium ingested too late
5. Improper patient preparation.

ROUTINE RADIOGRAPHIC POSITIONS

Cholecystography (oral)—posterior (A-P) scout (survey) view

> *Functional examination*
> *Film size (scout)—14″ × 17″* *Bucky (or grid)*
> *(regular)—8″ × 10″* *Cone to cover*
> *Cassette*
> *Lengthwise*

Technique

Factors	Screen film cassette (par)
Ma	300
Time	0.3
Mas	90
Thickness in cm	20
Kvp	68
Distance	40

Palpation points

Spinous processes; lateral ribs.

Procedure

Place the patient in the prone position with the median plane of the body over the center line of the table. Rotate the patient's head toward the right side. Extend

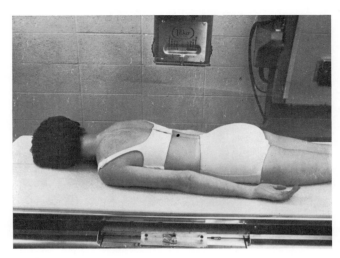

Fig. 16-20. Gallbladder—anterior (P-A) scout position.

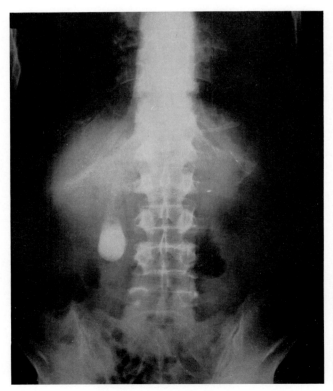

Fig. 16-21. Gallbladder—anterior (P-A) scout view. (Courtesy Dr. E. I. L. Cilley, Dr. T. W. Crowell, Dr. R. E. Waud, and Dr. G. H. Hoffman.)

the arms down the sides. Palpate the second lumbar spinous process and mark this point with a skin pencil. Center the cassette, with right marker, to the selected point.

Central ray
Direct the central ray perpendicular to the center of the film holder. (See Fig. 16-20.)

Immobilization
Employ suspended expiration. A compression band should be used to compress the viscera in obese patients.

Right-left markers
Place a right marker on the right lateral center border of the film holder.

Technical tips
For large or obese patients, center 2 to 3 inches higher than normal. For slender patients, center 2 to 3 inches lower than normal.

Structures demonstrated
Anterior (P-A) scout (survey) view of the abdomen demonstrating the degree of function and the location of the gallbladder by means of an orally ingested contrast medium. (See Fig. 16-21.)

Note:
Locate the gallbladder on the radiograph by measuring from the center of the film, which is in line with the right marker and skin pencil mark on the patient.

Cholecystography (oral)—left anterior oblique (L.A.O.) view

Functional examination
Film size—8″ × 10″   *Bucky (or grid)*
Cassette   *Cone to cover*
Lengthwise

Technique

Factors	Screen film cassette (par)
Ma	300
Time	0.3
Mas	90
Thickness in cm	23
Kvp	74
Distance	40

Palpation points
Spinous processes; lateral ribs.

Procedure
Place the patient in the prone position. Flex the right elbow and knee, rotating the patient into a 20- to 30-degree L.A.O. position. Center a point (transversely)

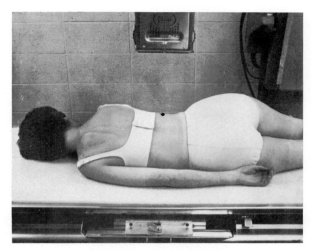

Fig. 16-22. Gallbladder—left anterior oblique (L.A.O.) position.

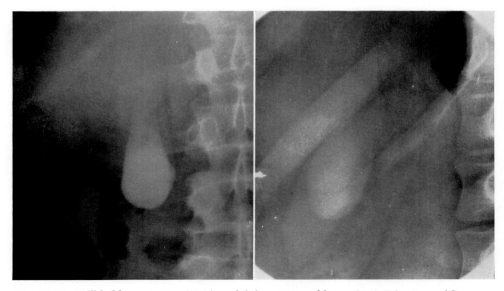

Fig. 16-23. Gallbladder—anterior (P-A) and left anterior oblique (L.A.O.) views. (Courtesy Dr. E. I. L. Cilley, Dr. T. W. Crowell, Dr. R. E. Waud, and Dr. G. H. Hoffman.)

halfway between the spinous processes and the right lateral rib margin over the center line of the table. Center the cassette (longitudinally) in line with the gallbladder (located from the scout film).

Central ray

Direct the central ray perpendicular to the center of the film. (See preceding note.) (See Fig. 16-22.)

Immobilization

Employ suspended expiration.

Right-left markers

Markers are not necessary on this view.

Technical tips

1. Deep suspended *inspiration* may be used to move the gallbladder lower.
2. In large or obese patients, the gallbladder will usually move to the outer third of the lateral abdomen.
3. In slender patients, the gallbladder will usually remain closed to the original anterior (P-A) location.

Structures demonstrated

Left anterior oblique (L.A.O.) view of the abdomen demonstrating the degree of function and the location of the gallbladder (free from superimposed gas shadows) by means of an orally ingested contrast medium. (See Fig. 16-23.)

Note:

For a variation of this view, direct the central ray 15 degrees caudad through the level of the gallbladder to the center of the film holder. When satisfactory preevacuation radiographs (free of superimposed gas shadows) have been completed, provide the patient with a commercial *fatty meal* (Neo-Cholex) preparation per instructions and repeat the radiographic film series (postevacuation) in 20 to 30 minutes.

Cholecystography (oral)—right lateral decubitus view

Functional examination
Film size—8″ × 10″   *Bucky (or grid)*
Grid-cassette   *Cone to cover*
Lengthwise

Technique

Factors	Screen film cassette (*par*)
Ma	300
Time	0.3
Mas	90
Thickness in cm	20
Kvp	68
Distance	40

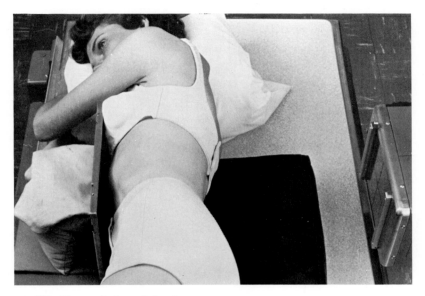

Fig. 16-24. Gallbladder—right lateral decubitus position.

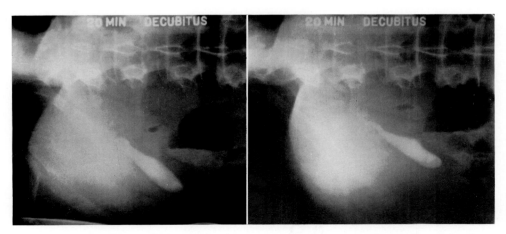

Fig. 16-25. Gallbladder—right lateral decubitus view with expiration and right lateral decubitus view with inspiration. (Courtesy Dr. E. I. L. Cilley, Dr. T. W. Crowell, Dr. R. E. Waud, and Dr. G. H. Hoffman.)

Palpation points

Spinous processes; lateral ribs.

Procedure

Place the patient with his right side on the table. Place a fine-line grid-cassette on edge and against the abdomen with the film center in line with the gall-bladder (located from scout film). The gallbladder tends to drop near the mid-axillary line in this position, so consider this condition when centering.

Central ray

Direct the central ray perpendicular to the center of the film holder. (See Fig. 16-24.)

Immobilization

Employ suspended expiration for one view and suspended inspiration for the second view.

Right-left markers

Place a *decubitus* marker on upper center border of film holder. *R* and *L* markers are not necessary on this view.

Technical tips

In large or obese patients, the gallbladder will usually move slightly superior. In slender patients, the gallbladder will move very close to the midaxillary line and slightly inferior.

Structures demonstrated

Right lateral decubitus (anterior, P-A) view of the right lateral abdomen, demonstrating the degree of function and the layering or stratification of small stones that may concentrate in the fundus of the gallbladder. (See Fig. 16-25.)

Note:

When satisfactory preevacuation radiographs (free of superimposed gas shadows) have been completed, give the patient a *fatty meal* (commercial) preparation per instructions and repeat the film series (postevacuation) in 20 minutes.

The cystic duct may be demonstrated on some patients 10 minutes after the *fatty meal* (commercial) preparation has been ingested.

Cholangiography

Cholangiography is the term used to describe the radiographic examination of the biliary tract. This examination is obtained by three methods: surgical cholangiography, postoperative cholangiography (T tube), and intravenous cholangiography. The purpose of the examination is to detect the presence of small stones or calculi in the bile ducts and, indirectly, to determine the patency of the cystic and common ducts and the condition of the choledochal sphincter.

Surgical cholangiography

Surgical cholangiography is a nonfunctional radiographic examination of the biliary ducts performed in surgery by means of a contrast medium injected directly into these ducts.

Patient preparation

Routine surgical preparation of the patient is performed by surgical personnel.

Contrast media

A sterile 20 cc syringe filled with Diodrast, Renografin, or another selected water-soluble urographic medium is prepared and provided by the surgical department.

Equipment preparation

Provide a mobile radiographic unit, extension cords, and a minimum of two 10″ × 12″ cassettes.

Examination

The cassette is positioned in the surgical table and the radiographic equipment is prepared before the patient arrives in surgery. The patient is positioned on the table in a posterior (A-P) or slight right posterior oblique (R.P.O.) position under aseptic conditions by surgical personnel. After surgically exposing the biliary system, the surgeon aspirates existing bile and probes the biliary ducts for existing stones. The contrast medium is then injected and the sterile field is covered.

Surgical cholangiography—right posterior oblique (R.P.O.) view

> *Nonfunctional Examination*
> *Film size—10″ × 12″*   *Bucky or film tunnel*
> *Grid-cassette*   *Cone to cover*
> *Lengthwise*   *Mobile radiographic unit*

Technique

Factors	Screen film cassette (par)
Ma	300
Time	0.3
Mas	90
Thickness in cm	20
Kvp	68
Distance	40

Palpation point

The center of the biliary system is located by the surgeon.

Procedure

Move the preset mobile radiographic unit into position and make the exposure during the injection.

Central ray

Direct the central ray perpendicular to the center of the film holder.

Immobilization

Employ suspended expiration if the patient is under spinal anesthesia; otherwise, a rapid exposure time is required.

Right-left markers

Preevacuation or Postevacuation markers are placed on the right lateral center border of the film holder.

Structures demonstrated

Right posterior oblique (R.P.O.) view of the right abdominal cavity with the use of a contrast medium to detect the presence of small stones or calculi in the bile ducts, and, indirectly, to determine the patency of the cystic and common ducts, and the condition of the choledochal sphincter.

Note:

Additional postevacuation radiographs may be required.

Postoperative cholangiography (choledochogram, T tube)

A nonfunctional, postoperative (10 days) radiographic examination of the bile ducts by means of a contrast medium injected, through a surgically implanted T tube, directly into the biliary system.

Patient preparation

1. The patient is usually instructed to follow a special regimen prescribed by the referring physician.
2. The evening meal should be light and free of fatty foods.
3. On the morning of the examination, the patient must omit breakfast except for water, black coffee, or clear tea.
4. On the morning of the examination he must take an enema consisting of warm tap water, using an amount sufficient to produce a clear return.
5. When the patient is admitted, remove all garments except shoes and socks. Provide a gown and instruct the patient to tie the open ends together in the front.
6. Make a 14" × 17" posterior (A-P) abdominal scout (survey) radiograph of the patient, centering at the iliac crest. (See p. 397.)

Contrast medium

Fill a sterile 20 cc syringe with Diodrast or other selected contrast medium. (See Table 16-1.)

Equipment preparation

Place a radiolucent sponge mat on the tabletop for the patient's comfort. Provide the following items:

1. Sterile 20 cc syringe with contrast medium (see above)
2. Cannula (tapered)
3. Hemostat (clamp)
4. Emesis basin
5. Cotton sponges

Examination

1. After the scout (survey) radiograph has been completed, the following steps must be carried out:
   a. Expose the T tube (remove the tube tip from the bile receptacle) and insert the cannula into the opening of the T tube.
   b. Allow the bile to drain into the emesis basin. (Repeated deep respiration will aid in this.)
   c. Remove air bubbles from the tube by directing the tube in the vertical position; then clamp the tube with hemostat.
   d. Insert the 20 cc syringe with contrast medium into the cannula orifice.
2. Inform the radiologist that you are prepared, and introduce the radiologist to the patient.
3. Assist the radiologist with lead gloves and lead apron.
4. The radiologist will release the clamp and inject the contrast medium (usually 10 ml).
5. The hemostat is applied and the first exposure is made as rapidly as possible.

Note: Additional injections and exposures may be necessary.

ROUTINE RADIOGRAPHIC POSITION
Postoperative cholangiography (choledochogram, T tube)—right posterior oblique (R. P. O.) view

Nonfunctional examination
Film size—10″ × 12″ (two)   *Bucky*
Cassette   *Cone to cover*
Lengthwise

Technique

Factors	*Screen film cassette (par)* *Regular kvp—12:1 grid*	*Screen film cassette (par)* *High kvp—16:1 grid*
Ma	300	200
Time	0.3	0.1
Mas	90	20
Thickness in cm	21	25
Kvp	76	120
Distance	40	40

Palpation point

Xiphoid process of sternum.

Procedure

Place the patient in the supine position with the left side elevated approximately 35 degrees. Center a point midway between the xiphoid process and the right lateral ribs over the center line of the table. Center the cassette to a point in line with the tip of the xiphoid process.

Central ray

Direct the central ray perpendicular to the center of the film holder.

Immobilization

Place a wedge-shaped positioning sponge (or sponges) beneath the elevated side. Employ suspended expiration for one exposure and suspended inspiration for the second exposure.

Right-left markers

Place numerical sequence markers on the right lateral center border of the film holder.

Structures demonstrated

Right posterior oblique (R.P.O.) view of the right abdominal cavity with the use of a contrast medium to detect the presence of small stones or calculi in the bile ducts (usually ten days to two weeks after surgical removal of the gallbladder). (See Figs. 16-26 and 16-27.)

Note:

A subsequent radiograph (postevacuation) is made after the contrast medium has been aspirated into the syringe by the radiologist.

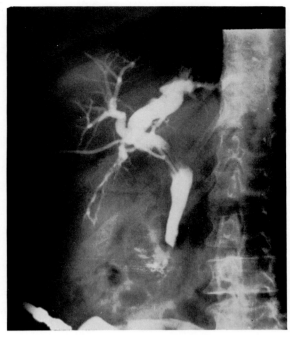

Fig. 16-26. Cholangiogram—postoperative posterior (A-P) view. (Courtesy Dr. E. I. L. Cilley, Dr. T. W. Crowell, Dr. R. E. Waud, and Dr. G. H. Hoffman.)

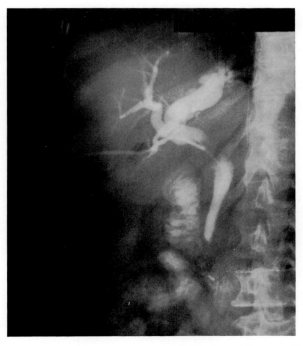

Fig. 16-27. Cholangiogram—postoperative posterior (A-P) view. (Courtesy Dr. E. I. L. Cilley, Dr. T. W. Crowell, Dr. R. E. Waud, and Dr. G. H. Hoffman.)

Intravenous cholangiography

Intravenous cholangiography is a functional radiographic examination of the gallbladder by means of an intravenously injected contrast medium.

Patient preparation

1. The patient's noon meal on the day prior to the examination should include two pats of butter or a fried egg.
2. Between 3 and 5 P.M. on the day prior to the examination, the patient must take 2 ounces of castor oil. *This may be disguised with root beer or orange juice.*
3. The patient must have clear liquids only for the evening meal.
4. On the morning of the examination the patient must take an enema consisting of 1½ to 2 pints of warm soapsuds, followed by a warm water enema until the return is clear.
5. The patient must omit breakfast and all liquids on the morning of the examination.
6. When the patient is admitted, remove all garments except shoes and socks. Provide a short-sleeved gown, and instruct the patient to tie the open ends together in the back.
7. Make a 14″ × 17″ posterior (A-P) abdominal scout (survey) radiograph of the patient, centering at the iliac crest. (See p. 397.)

Contrast media

Fill a sterile 20 cc syringe with Cholografin sodium or another selected contrast medium. Fill a sterile 2 cc syringe with 1 ml of Cholografin sodium (test dose) or another selected contrast medium. (See Table 16-1.)

Equipment preparation

Place a radiolucent sponge mat on the tabletop for the patient's comfort. Provide the following items:

1. A sterile 20 cc syringe with contrast medium
2. A sterile 2 cc syringe with contrast medium (*test dose*)
3. A sterile 21-gauge × 1½-inch needle
4. A sterile 25-gauge × 1-inch needle
5. A sterile towel
6. A tourniquet and sandbag or sponge for support of the arm
7. Alcohol sponges
8. An emesis basin
9. An emergency kit (*consisting in part of* oxygen, Adrenalin° [injectable], and Chlor-trimeton [injectable])

Examination

1. After the scout (survey) radiograph has been completed and checked, make the following preparations:
   a. Place a tourniquet around the upper right arm.
   b. Place a sandbag or sponge under the right extended elbow for support.

°There are some objections to having Adrenalin on an emergency tray.

    c. Place an alcohol-dampened sponge on the antecubital space (anterior elbow surface).

    d. Place the 25-gauge needle on the sterile 2 cc syringe.

2. Inform the radiologist that you are prepared, and introduce the radiologist to the patient.

3. The radiologist will inject the test dose (1 ml); then approximately 10 minutes later he will inject the full dose from the loaded 20 cc syringe.

    Note: Contrast medium instructions caution that injection of the full dose should be made very slowly, over a 10-minute period. Rapid injection will produce nausea and/or vomiting.

4. For visualization of the ducts, serial 10-minute radiographs should be started 10 minutes after the injection.

5. Gallbladder studies may be started 2 hours after the injection.

ROUTINE RADIOGRAPHIC POSITION

Intravenous cholangiography—posterior (A-P) view

Film size—10″ × 12″ (two) *Bucky*
Cassette *Cone to cover*
Lengthwise

Technique

Factors	Screen film, cassette (par) Regular kvp—12:1 grid	Screen film, cassette (par) High kvp—16:1 grid
Ma	300	200
Time	0.3	0.1
Mas	90	20
Thickness in cm	21	25
Kvp	76	120
Distance	40	40

Palpation point

Xiphoid process of the sternum.

Procedure

Place the patient in the supine position with the left side elevated approximately 35 degrees. Center a point midway between the xiphoid process and the right lateral ribs over the center line of the table. Center the cassette to a point in line with the tip of the xiphoid process.

Central ray

Direct the central ray perpendicular to the center of the film holder.

Immobilization

Place wedge-shaped positioning sponges beneath the elevated side. Employ suspended expiration.

Right-left markers

Place time-sequence markers on the right lateral center border of the film holder.

Structures demonstrated

Right posterior oblique (R.P.O.) view of the right abdominal cavity with the use of a contrast medium to detect the presence of small stones or calculi and/or other pathology in the bile ducts or gallbladder.

Note:

For a variation of this view, direct the central ray 20 degrees cephalad through the level of the gallbladder to the center of the film holder.

If the patient has a nonfunctioning gallbladder, this method of administration of the contrast medium will not demonstrate the gallbladder or any defect causing the nonfunction.

Abdomen

The abdomen radiograph is a view of abdominal viscera that includes the gastrointestinal tract, pancreas, spleen, aorta, suprarenal glands, liver, and diaphragm. The abdomen radiographic exposure may be made with the patient in the horizontal, erect or decubitus positions as a scout (survey) film for numerous radiographic series, acute abdominal conditions or foreign bodies.

Abdomen—flat—posterior (A-P) or anterior (P-A) view

Film size—14″ × 17″   *Bucky*
Cassette   *Cone to cover*
Lengthwise

Technique

Factors	Screen film cassette (par)
Ma	300
Time	0.3
Mas	90
Thickness in cm	20
Kvp	68
Distance	40

Patient preparation

Remove all garments except shoes and socks. Provide a gown and instruct the patient to tie the open ends together in the back.

Palpation point

Crest of the ilium.

Procedure

Place the patient in either the supine or prone position, with the median line of the body over the center line of the table. Center the film holder to the crest of the ilium.

Central ray

Direct the central ray perpendicular to the center of the film holder. (See Fig. 16-14.)

Immobilization

For the supine position, elevate the knees with sponges for comfort. For the prone position, elevate the ankles with sponges for comfort. Use a compression band for obese patients. Employ suspended expiration.

Right-left markers

Place a right marker on the right lateral center border of the film holder.

Technical tips

Excellence in longitudinal positioning exists when the symphysis pubis is demonstrated as being transversely bisected by the lower film border.

Structures demonstrated

A posterior (A-P) or anterior (P-A) view of the abdominal viscera demonstrating conformation, size, and shape of the pancreas, spleen, aorta, suprarenal glands, liver, and diaphragm. It serves as an excellent scout (survey) view for intestinal obstructions, numerous tumor masses, calcifications, and foreign bodies.

Abdomen—erect—anterior (P-A) view

> *Film size—14" × 17"*   *Erect bucky*
> *Cassette*   *Cone to cover*
> *Lengthwise*

Technique

Factors	Screen film cassette (par)
Ma	300
Time	0.3
Mas	90
Thickness in cm	20
Kvp	74
Distance	40

Patient preparation

Remove all garments except shoes and socks. Provide a gown and instruct the patient to tie the open ends together in the back.

Palpation point

Crest of the ilium.

Procedure

Place the table in the erect (vertical) position and instruct the patient to stand facing the table with the median line of the body over the center line of the table. Extend the arms along the sides with the hands grasping the edge of the table. Center the film holder 1 inch above the crest of the ilium.

Central ray

Direct the central ray horizontal and perpendicular to the center of the film holder.

Immobilization

Use a compression band. Employ suspended expiration.

Right-left markers

Place a right-erect marker on the right lateral center border of the film holder.

Technical tips

It is necessary to include the *diaphragm* in the radiograph since the free air will rise to and be under it, so adjust the film holder centering to accommodate the size of the patient.

Structures demonstrated

Anterior (P-A) erect view of the abdominal viscera to include the diaphragm for the demonstration of free air under the diaphragm, and for visualization of fluid levels.

Note:

Many routines call for both the erect (upright) and the horizontal flat-plate abdomen radiographs.

Abdomen—lateral decubitus—right or left view

A decubitus position refers to a situation wherein the skin of a given surface of the body is in contact with the tabletop. The patient is horizontal and the central ray is horizontal. Thus, a left anterior decubitus position has the left side down and the anterior surface of the body next to the film; the central ray passes from dorsal to ventral (posterior to anterior) to the film.

> *Film size—14″ × 17″*   *Erect bucky*
> *Cassette*   *Cone to cover*
> *Lengthwise*

Technique

Factors	Screen film cassette (par)
Ma	300
Time	0.3
Mas	90
Thickness in cm	20
Kvp	72
Distance	40

Patient preparation

Remove all garments except shoes and socks. Provide a gown and instruct the patient to tie the open ends together in the back.

Palpation point

Crest of the ilium.

Procedure

Place the table in an erect (vertical) position. Place the patient in the desired lateral position on a stretcher or gurney, which may be rolled to the table. Flex lower elbow beneath pillow. Position the stretcher or gurney so that the crest of the ilium is aligned over the center line of the table, then secure the wheel locks.

Central ray

Direct the central ray horizontal and perpendicular through the median line of the body to the center of the film holder.

Immobilization

Instruct the patient to grasp the edge of the table with his upper hand. Employ suspended expiration.

Right-left markers

Place the correct decubitus marker on the upper lateral center border of the film holder.

Structures demonstrated

Anterior (P-A) or posterior (A-P) lateral decubitus view of the abdominal viscera for demonstration of free air and for visualization of fluid levels.

Urinary excretory system

Radiographic examinations of the urinary excretory system include views of the kidneys, ureters, urinary bladder, and urethra. The examinations are the K.U.B., intravenous pyelogram, retrograde pyelogram, and retrograde urethrogram.

K.U.B.

A K.U.B. is a two-film, radiographic scout (survey) examination of the kidneys, ureters, and urinary bladder without the use of contrast media.

ROUTINE RADIOGRAPHIC POSITION
K.U.B.—posterior (A-P) view

> *Film size—14″ × 17″ (two)*   *Bucky*
> *Cassette*   *Cone to cover*
> *Lengthwise*

Technique

Factors	Screen film cassette (par)
Ma	300
Time	0.3
Mas	90
Thickness in cm	20
Kvp	68
Distance	40

Patient preparation

Remove all garments except shoes and socks. Provide a gown and instruct the patient to tie the open ends together in the back.

Note:

If the examination is prescheduled, instruct patient to follow *Patient Preparation instructions* per Intravenous Pyelography (see p. 401).

Palpation point

Crest of the ilium.

Procedure

Place the patient in the supine position with the median line of the body over the center line of the table. For the first view, center the first film holder to the crest of the ilium. For the second view, center the second film holder 3 inches above the crest of the ilium.

Central ray

Direct the central ray perpendicular to the center of the film holder for each view.

Immobilization

Elevate the knees with sponges for patient comfort. A compression band may be used across large or obese patients. Employ suspended expiration for each view.

Right-left markers

Place a right marker on the right lateral center border of the film holder.

Structures demonstrated

A posterior (A-P) view (two-film scout-survey series) of the abdomen demonstrating stones, calcifications, and certain tumor masses associated with kidneys, ureters, and urinary bladder without the aid of a contrast medium.

Intravenous pyelography (I.V.P.)

Intravenous pyelography is a functional radiographic examination of the kidneys, ureters, and urinary bladder with the use of an intravenously injected contrast medium.

Patient preparation

1. Between 3 and 5 P.M. on the afternoon before the examination the patient must take 2 ounces of castor oil. *This may be disguised with root beer or orange juice.*
2. He may have clear liquids only for the evening meal preceding the day of the examination.
3. On the morning of the examination the patient must take an enema consisting of 1½ to 2 pints of warm soapsuds, followed by a warm water enema until the return is clear.
4. On the morning of the examination, the patient must restrict breakfast to a slice of toast and a half-cup of liquid. He may *not* drink any other liquids that morning.
5. When the patient is admitted, remove all garments except shoes and socks. Provide a short-sleeved gown and instruct the patient to tie the open ends together in the back.
6. Make a 14″ × 17″ posterior (A-P) abdominal scout (survey) radiograph of the patient, centering at the iliac crest. (See p. 397.)

Contrast media

Fill a sterile 2 cc syringe with 1 ml (test dose) of Renografin, Hypaque sodium, or another selected water soluble urographic medium. (See Table 16-1.) Fill a sterile 20 cc or 30 cc syringe with the identical type of contrast medium as used for the test dose.

Equipment preparation

Place a radiolucent sponge mat on the tabletop for the patient's comfort. Provide the following items:

1. A sterile 2 cc syringe with contrast medium (test dose)
2. A sterile 20 cc or 30 cc syringe with contrast medium
3. A sterile 25-gauge × 1-inch needle (test dose)
4. A sterile 21-gauge × 1½-inch needle (main dose)
5. A sterile 18-gauge × 1½-inch needle (filler)
6. A sterile towel
7. A tourniquet and sandbag or sponge for support of the arm
8. Alcohol sponges
9. An emesis basin
10. A compression band and I.V.P. block
11. An emergency kit (*consisting in part of* oxygen, Adrenalin [injectable], and Chlor-trimeton [injectable])

Examination

1. After scout (survey) radiograph has been completed and checked, make the following preparations:
   a. Place a tourniquet around the upper right arm.
   b. Place sandbags or sponges under the right extended elbow for support.
   c. Place alcohol-dampened sponge on antecubital space (anterior elbow surface.
   d. Position the I.V.P. compression block between the anterior superior iliac spines and hold in place with compression band. *Do not tighten compression band.*
   e. Place the 25-gauge needle on the sterile 2 cc syringe and the 21-gauge needle on the sterile 20 cc or 30 cc syringe.
2. Inform the radiologist that you are prepared, and introduce the radiologist to the patient.
3. The radiologist will inject the test dose (1 ml), then approximately 10 minutes later he will inject the full dose from the loaded 20 cc or 30 cc syringe.
4. Immediately after the main injection, apply firm pressure to the I.V.P. block with the compression band and position the table 10 degrees Trendelenburg.
   Note: Some radiologists prefer not to use compression or Trendelenburg positioning.
5. An acceptable radiographic routine series is as follows:
   a. 5 minutes after injection (with pressure)
   b. 15 minutes after injection (with pressure)
   c. 25 minutes after injection (with pressure released)
   d. 35 minutes after injection (erect postvoiding without pressure)
   Note: For hypertensive patients, the radiographic routine series should be 1, 2, and 3 minutes.

ROUTINE RADIOGRAPHIC POSITION
Intravenous pyelography (I.V.P.)—posterior (A-P) view

Film size—14″ × 17″   *Bucky*
Cassette   *Cone to cover*
Lengthwise

Technique

Factors	Screen film cassette (par)
Ma	300
Time	0.3
Mas	90
Thickness in cm	21
Kvp	68
Distance	40

Palpation point

Crest of the ilium.

Procedure

With the patient remaining in the supine position and with the median line of the body over the center line of the table, center the film holder to the crest of the ilium.

Central ray

Direct the central ray perpendicular to the center of the film holder. (See Fig. 16-28.)

Immobilization

With the compression band and I.V.P. block in place and firm pressure applied to the abdomen, employ suspended expiration.

Right-left markers

Place the right and correct time-interval markers on the right lateral center border of the film holder.

Structures demonstrated

Posterior (A-P) view (5-film routine series) of the posterior abdomen with the use of an injectable contrast medium to *functionally* demonstrate stones, calcifications, tumor masses, and other pathology associated with the kidneys, ureters, and urinary bladder. (See Figs. 16-29 and 16-30.)

Note:

For female patients within the childbearing age, cover the pelvis with lead protection and use a 10″ × 12″ film holder *crosswise,* aligning the bottom edge of the film holder with the crest of the ilium for the 5- and 15-minute views.

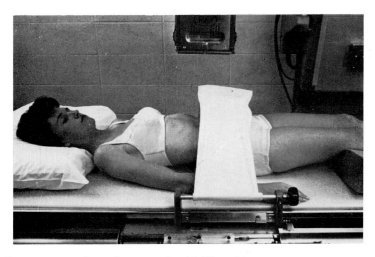

Fig. 16-28. Intravenous pyelography—posterior (A-P) position.

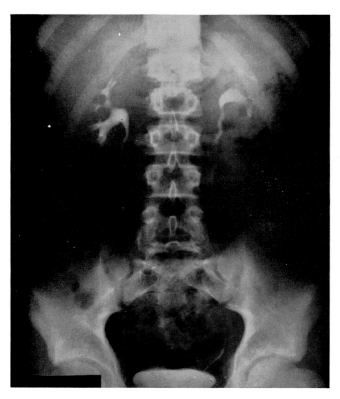

Fig. 16-29. Intravenous pyelogram—posterior (A-P) view. (Courtesy Dr. E. I. L. Cilley, Dr. T. W. Crowell, Dr. R. E. Waud, and Dr. G. H. Hoffman.)

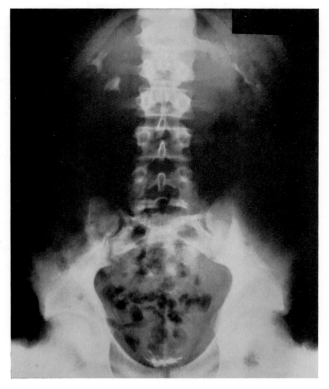

Fig. 16-30. Intravenous pyelogram—erect posterior (A-P) view, postevacuation. (Courtesy Dr. E. I. L. Cilley, Dr. T. W. Crowell, Dr. R. E. Waud, and Dr. G. H. Hoffman.)

Retrograde pyelography—renal pelves and ureters

Retrograde pyelography is a nonfunctional radiographic examination of the kidneys, ureters, urinary bladder, and urethra with the use of a contrast medium injected through ureteral catheters.

Patient preparation

1. Between 3 and 5 P.M. on the afternoon before the examination the patient must take 2 ounces of castor oil. *This may be disguised with root beer or orange juice.*
2. He may have clear liquids only for the evening meal.
3. On the morning of the examination the patient must take an enema consisting of 1½ to 2 pints of soapsuds, followed by a warm water enema until the return is clear.
4. The patient must be instructed to omit breakfast and to drink copious amounts of water a few hours prior to the examination (for urine specimens).
5. Routine surgical preparation of the genitourinary region is performed by surgical personnel.
6. Make a 14″ × 17″ posterior (A-P) abdominal scout (survey) radiograph of the patient, centering at the iliac crest. (See p. 397.)

Contrast medium

Diodrast, Renografin, or another selected water-soluble urographic medium along with a sterilized urographic-retrograde instrument kit is provided by the surgical department.

Equipment preparation

Provide a cystoscopic-radiographic unit or suitable table with leg stirrups, and a minimum of four loaded 14″ × 17″ cassettes.

Examination

The patient is placed in a posterior (A-P) position on the cystoscopy table with the thighs abducted, knees flexed and resting in leg stirrups. A sterile field is prepared around the genitourinary region by the doctor or assistants. A urethral catheter is inserted and a urine specimen collected. A cystoscopic examination is performed, and ureteral catheters inserted, usually as far as the ureteropelvic junction. A scout radiograph is made to demonstrate catheter placement. The contrast medium is then injected. An acceptable radiographic routine series is as follows:

1. A scout (survey) radiograph of the abdomen
2. A radiograph demonstrating the catheters in position
3. A radiograph demonstrating the ureters
4. A radiograph after the contrast medium has been injected and the catheters removed

ROUTINE RADIOGRAPHIC POSITION
Retrograde pyelography—renal pelves and ureters, posterior (A-P) view

Film size—14″ × 17″   *Bucky*
Cassette   *Cone to cover*
Lengthwise

Technique

Factors	Screen film cassette (par)
Ma	300
Time	0.3
Mas	90
Thickness in cm	21
Kvp	68
Distance	40

Palpation point

Crest of the ilium.

Procedure

The patient remains in the supine position with the median line of the body over the center line of the table. The crest of the ilium is precentered over the center line of the fixed Bucky.

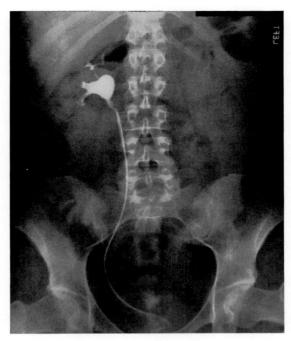

Fig. 16-31. Retrograde pyelogram—posterior (A-P) view. (Courtesy Dr. E. I. L. Cilley, Dr. T. W. Crowell, Dr. R. E. Waud, and Dr. G. H. Hoffman.)

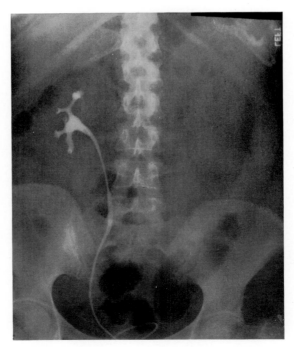

Fig. 16-32. Retrograde pyelogram—posterior (A-P) view. (Courtesy Dr. E. I. L. Cilley, Dr. T. W. Crowell, Dr. R. E. Waud, and Dr. G. H. Hoffman.)

Central ray

The central ray is automatically precentered to the fixed Bucky.

Immobilization

Knees are secured in the leg stirrups. Use a compression band if necessary. Employ suspended expiration.

Right-left markers

Place the right marker on the right lateral center border of the film holder.

Structures demonstrated

Posterior (A-P) views (four-film routine series) of the posterior abdomen with the use of a contrast medium injected through ureteral catheters to demonstrate stones, calcifications, tumor masses, and other pathology associated with the kidneys, ureters, urinary bladder, and urethra. (See Figs. 16-31 and 16-32.)

Retrograde urography—urinary bladder (cystogram)

A retrograde cystogram is a nonfunctional radiographic examination of the urinary bladder with the use of a contrast medium injected through a urethral catheter. This examination may be performed on any regular radiographic table.

Patient preparation

1. In some cases the preparation may be as extensive as that for the intravenous pyelogram (see p. 401); in most cases, however, a routine warm water enema prior to the examination is sufficient.
2. When the patient is admitted, remove all garments except shoes and socks. Provide a gown and instruct the patient to tie the open ends together in the front.
3. Instruct the patient that the bladder must be voided prior to the examination.
4. Make a 10″ × 12″ posterior (A-P) pelvic scout (survey) radiograph, centering the film holder (lengthwise), with the central ray 1 inch above the greater trochanter.

Contrast media

Dilute approximately 75 ml of Renografin, Hypaque sodium, or another selected water-soluble urographic medium (see Table 16-1) with an equal volume of sterile water.

Equipment preparation

Provide the following items:
1. A sterile 50 cc syringe
2. A sterile urethral catheter
3. A sterile two-way stopcock
4. A hemostat (clamp)
5. A sterile kidney basin
6. Adhesive tape
7. Bandage shears

Examination

After the scout (survey) radiograph has been completed and checked, the doctor will introduce a urethral catheter. The bladder will be drained and then irrigated. The contrast medium will be injected through the catheter until the bladder capacity has been reached. The catheter will be clamped and taped to the thigh (usually the left one).

ROUTINE RADIOGRAPHIC POSITIONS

Posterior (A-P), right oblique, and left oblique are the usual routine positions.

Retrograde urography—urinary bladder (cystogram), posterior (A-P) view

Film size—10″ × 12″   *Bucky*
Cassette   *Cone to cover*
Lengthwise

Technique

Factors	Screen film cassette (par)
Ma	300
Time	0.3
Mas	90
Thickness in cm	21
Kvp	68
Distance	40

Palpation point

Greater trochanter of the femur.

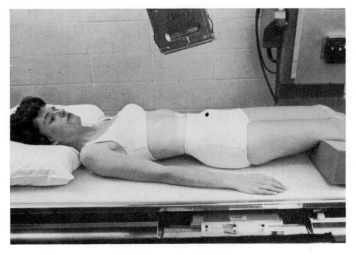

Fig. 16-33. Cystography—posterior (A-P) position.

Procedure

The patient remains in the supine position with the median line of the body over the center line of the table. Center the film holder 1 inch above the greater trochanter.

Central ray

Direct the central ray 15 degrees caudad to the center of the film holder. (See Fig. 16-33.)

Immobilization

Employ suspended expiration.

Right-left markers

Place the right marker on the right lateral center border of the film holder.

Structures demonstrated

Posterior (A-P) view of the pelvic region with the use of a catheter-injected contrast medium to demonstrate stones, calcifications, tumor masses, and other pathology associated with the urinary bladder. (See Fig. 16-34.)

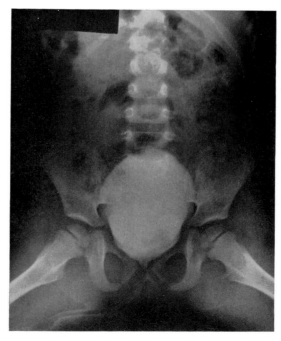

Fig. 16-34. Cystogram—posterior (A-P) view. (Courtesy Dr. E. I. L. Cilley, Dr. T. W. Crowell, Dr. R. E. Waud, and Dr. G. H. Hoffman.)

Retrograde urography—urinary bladder (cystogram), right posterior oblique (R.P.O.) view

Film size—10″ × 12″   *Bucky*
Cassette   *Cone to cover*
Lengthwise

Technique

Factors	Screen film cassette (par)
Ma	300
Time	0.3
Mas	90
Thickness in cm	24
Kvp	74
Distance	40

Palpation points

Greater trochanter of the femur; anterior superior iliac spines.

Procedure

From the supine position, elevate the left side of the body 45 degrees. Flex the right knee, placing the right ankle under the opposite leg. Have the patient grasp the right side of the table with the left hand. Center a point midway between the anterior superior iliac spines over the center line of the table. Center the film holder 1 inch superior to the greater trochanter.

Central ray

Direct the central ray perpendicular to the center of the film holder.

Immobilization

Place wedge-shaped positioning sponges beneath the elevated side. Employ suspended expiration.

Right-left markers

Place an R.P.O. marker on the right lateral center border of the film holder.

Structures demonstrated

Right posterior oblique (R.P.O.) view of the pelvic region with the use of a catheter-injected contrast medium to demonstrate stones, calcifications, tumor masses, and other pathology associated with or contained within the urinary bladder. The prostate gland and urethra may also be demonstrated.

Retrograde urography—urinary bladder (cystogram), left posterior oblique (L.P.O.) view

This view is the reverse of the preceding view.

Retrograde urography—urethra and prostate (urethrography)

A retrograde urethrogram is a nonfunctional radiographic examination of the urethra with the use of a contrast medium injected through a urethral catheter. This examination may be performed on any regular radiographic table.

Patient preparation

1. When the patient is admitted, remove all garments except shoes and socks. Provide a gown and instruct the patient to tie the open ends together in the front.
2. Instruct the patient that the bladder must be voided prior to the examination.
3. Make a 10" × 12" posterior (A-P) pelvic scout (survey) radiograph, centering the film holder (lengthwise), with the central ray in line with the greater trochanter.

Contrast media

Dilute approximately 25 ml of Renografin, Hypaque sodium, or another selected water-soluble urographic medium (see Table 16-1) with an equal volume of sterile water.

Equipment preparation

Provide the following items:
1. A sterile 30 cc or 50 cc syringe
2. A sterile urethral catheter
3. A sterile two-way stopcock
4. A hemostat (clamp)
5. A sterile kidney basin
6. Adhesive tape
7. Bandage shears

Examination

After the scout (survey) radiograph has been completed and checked, the doctor will introduce a urethral catheter. The bladder will be drained and then irrigated. (Radiographic positioning and procedure must now be readied; see the following position.) The doctor next inserts a urethral syringe into the orifice of the urethra and prepares to inject the contrast medium.

ROUTINE RADIOGRAPHIC POSITION
Retrograde urography—urethra and prostate, bicycle view

Film size—10″ × 12″   *Bucky*
Cassette   *Cone to cover*
Crosswise

Technique

Factors	Screen film cassette (par)
Ma	200
Time	0.25
Mas	50
Thickness in cm	16
Kvp	62
Distance	40

Palpation points

Greater trochanter of the femur; symphysis pubis.

Procedure

From the supine position, elevate the left side of the body approximately 35 degrees. Flex the right knee, placing the right ankle under the opposite leg. Have the patient grasp the right side of the table with the left hand. Center the symphysis pubis over the center line of the table. Center the film holder to the greater trochanter.

Central ray

Direct the central ray perpendicular to the center of the film holder. (See Fig. 16-35.)

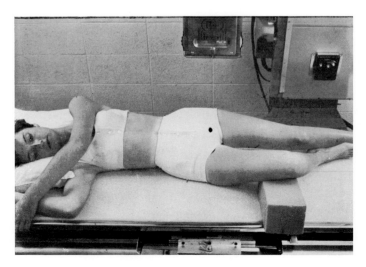

Fig. 16-35. Urethrography—bicycle position.

Immobilization

Place wedge-shaped positioning sponges beneath the elevated side. Employ suspended expiration.

Right-left markers

Place an R.P.O. marker on the right lateral center border of the film holder.

Examination

Extend the penis along the upper thigh. The doctor will inject the contrast medium, and as soon as the urethra distends *fully,* the doctor will signal the technologist. The exposure is then made.

Structures demonstrated

Right posterior oblique (R.P.O.) view of the lower pelvic region with the use of a catheter-injected contrast medium to demonstrate stones or other pathology associated with or contained within the urethra. The prostate gland may also be demonstrated.

Note:

For a variation of this examination, the following is recommended: with the patient in a semisitting position (the arms extended backward for support), abduct the legs and direct the central ray 10 degrees cephalad through the symphysis pubis to the center of the film holder.

Reproductive system
Hysterosalpingography

Hysterosalpingography is a nonfunctional radiographic examination of the uterus, uterine tubes (oviducts), and ovaries with the use of a heavy contrast medium injected through a special uterine catheter.

Patient preparation

1. The patient should be scheduled 7 to 8 days following cessation of menstruation.
2. Instruct the patient to take a warm-water enema (1½ pints) and a cleansing douche prior to the examination.
3. When the patient is admitted, remove all garments except shoes and socks. Provide a gown and instruct the patient to tie the open ends together in the front.
4. Instruct the patient that the bladder must be voided prior to the examination.
5. Make a 10″ × 12″ posterior (A-P) pelvic scout (survey) radiograph of the patient, centering the film holder (lengthwise), with the central ray 2 inches above the greater trochanter.

Contrast medium

Fill a sterile 20 cc syringe with warm Sinografin, Salpix, or another selected contrast medium. (See Table 16-1.)

Equipment preparation

A special, sterilized salpingogram kit is provided by surgical supply or the referring gynecologist.

Examination

After the scout (survey) radiograph has been completed and checked, the patient is placed in the lithotomy* position at the foot-end of the table. The genitourinary region is cleansed by the nurse assistant. The doctor inserts a vaginal speculum and then introduces the special uterine cannula until the tip is engaged in the fallopian orifice. The legs are then extended and the patient is positioned for radiography.

Note:

Some routine series call for fluoroscopy at this stage of progress; if so, follow the equipment preparation procedures per the barium enema studies on pp. 376 and 377, prior to the examination.

---

*Lithotomy position has the patient on her back, the legs flexed on the thighs, the thighs flexed on the belly, and abducted.

ROUTINE RADIOGRAPHIC POSITION

Hysterosalpingography—posterior (A-P) view

Film size—10" × 12"   *Bucky*
Cassette   *Cone to cover*
Lengthwise

Technique

Factors	Screen film cassette (par)
Ma	300
Time	0.3
Mas	90
Thickness in cm	20
Kvp	68
Distance	40

Palpation point

Greater trochanter of the femur.

Procedure

The patient remains in the supine position with the median line of the body over the center line of the table. Center the film holder 2 inches above the greater trochanter.

Central ray

Direct the central ray perpendicular to the center of the film holder.

Immobilization

Employ suspended expiration.

Right-left markers

Place the right marker on the right lateral center border of the film holder.

Examination

The injection of the contrast medium is performed by the doctor. After filling has been completed, the exposure is made.

Note: A 24-hour radiograph may be ordered to determine the presence of stasis.

Structures demonstrated

Posterior (A-P) view of the female pelvic region with the use of a catheter-injected contrast medium to demonstrate absence of patency of one or both uterine tubes, and other pathology associated with the ovaries, uterine tubes, and uterus. (See Fig. 16-36.)

Note:

For oblique views of this region, follow routine procedures for R.P.O. and L.P.O. bicycle positions (see p. 413).

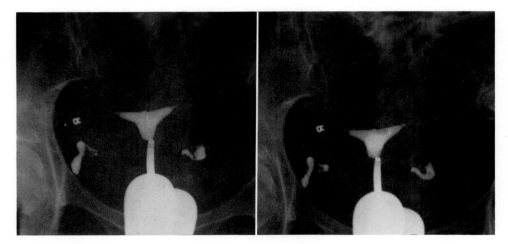

Fig. 16-36. Hysterosalpingogram—immediate posterior (A-P) and 3-minute posterior (A-P) views. (Courtesy Dr. E. I. L. Cilley, Dr. T. W. Crowell, Dr. R. E. Waud, and Dr. G. H. Hoffman.)

Fetography

A fetogram is a routine radiographic examination of the unborn fetus without the use of a contrast medium to determine the following:
1. Position of the fetus for possible placenta previa
2. Question of multiple pregnancy
3. Question of fetal age
4. Question of fetal death

ROUTINE RADIOGRAPHIC POSITION

Fetography—posterior (A-P) view

Film size—14″ × 17″   *Bucky*
Cassette   *Cone to cover*
Lengthwise

Technique

Factors	Screen film, cassette (par) Regular kvp—12:1 grid	Screen film, cassette (par) High kvp—16:1 grid
Ma	200	200
Time	0.5	0.2
Mas	100	40
Thickness in cm	28	28
Kvp	80	125
Distance	40	40

Patient preparation

Remove all garments except shoes and socks. Provide a gown and instruct the patient to tie the open ends together in the back.

Palpation points

Crest of the ilium; symphysis pubis or greater trochanter.

Procedure

Place the patient in the supine position with the median line of the body over the center line of the table. Elevate the knees with a pillow or sponges to relieve strain on the spine. Center the film holder to the crest of the ilium.

Note: It is important that the inferior border of the film holder is aligned 2½ inches below the level of the symphysis pubis (or greater trochanter).

Central ray

Direct the central ray perpendicular to the center of the film holder.

Immobilization

Use a compression band on large abdomens. Rapid, deep respiration prior to the exposure will reduce fetal movement. Employ suspended expiration.

Right-left markers

Place the right marker in the right lateral center border of the film holder.

Structures demonstrated

Posterior (A-P) view of the female abdomen and pelvis to demonstrate relationship, number, age, or pathology associated with the unborn fetus and placenta. (See Fig. 16-37.)

Note:

A lateral view may be requested. However, most radiologists require the posterior (A-P) view only, to reduce radiation exposure to the fetus.

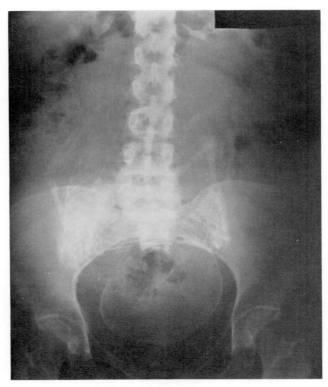

Fig. 16-37. Fetus—posterior (A-P) view. (Courtesy Dr. E. I. L. Cilley, Dr. T. W. Crowell, Dr. R. E. Waud, and Dr. G. H. Hoffman.)

Pelvimetry, Colcher-Sussman method

Pelvimetry is a radiographic examination of the (unborn) fetus with the use of a pelvic measuring device (having a centimeter scale) to determine the size relationship of the fetal head with the pelvic outlet.

ROUTINE RADIOGRAPHIC POSITIONS

Pelvimetry—Colcher-Sussman, posterior (A-P) view

Film size—14″ × 17″   *Bucky*
Cassette   *Cone to cover*
Lengthwise

Technique

Factors	Screen film, cassette (par) Regular kvp—12:1 grid	Screen film, cassette (par) High kvp—16:1 grid
Ma	200	200
Time	0.5	0.2
Mas	100	40
Thickness in cm	28	28
Kvp	80	125
Distance	40	40

Patient preparation

Remove all garments except shoes and socks. Provide a gown and instruct the patient to tie the open ends together in the back.

Palpation points

Symphysis pubis; ischial tuberosities.

Procedure

Place the patient in the supine position with the median line of the body over the center line of the table. Flex the knees, placing the feet flat on the table. Separate the thighs and place the transverse scale of the pelvimeter against the buttocks (see Figs. 16-38 and 16-39) at the level of the ischial tuberosities (10 cm below the upper border of the symphysis pubis). Secure the foot of the pelvimeter with a sandbag. Align the inferior border of the film holder 4 inches below the level of the transverse centimeter scale.

Central ray

Direct the central ray perpendicular to the center of the film holder.

Immobilization

Use a compression band on large abdomens. Rapid, deep respiration prior to the exposure will reduce fetal movement. Employ suspended expiration.

Right-left markers

Place the right marker on the right lateral center border of the film holder.

Structures demonstrated

Posterior (A-P) view of the female pelvis to demonstrate size relationship of the fetal head with the maternal pelvic outlet. (See Fig. 16-40.)

E, Pelvic inlet

T, Pelvic outlet   (ischial tuberosity)

F, Mid-pelvis

G, Top of symphysis pubis

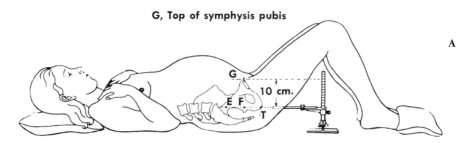

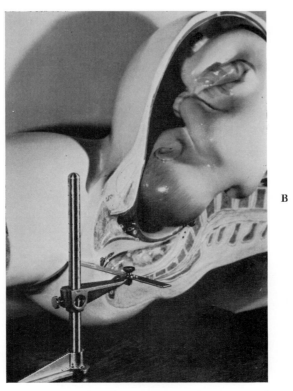

Fig. 16-38. Pelvimetry. **A,** Posterior (A-P) position. **B,** Pelvimeter in place against mannikin. (**A** courtesy X-ray Corporation; **B** courtesy Clay-Adams, Inc.)

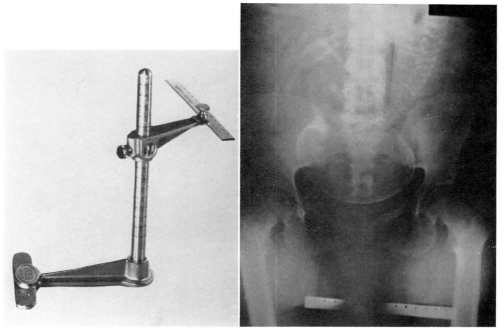

Fig. 16-39   Fig. 16-40

Fig. 16-39. Colcher-Sussman pelvimeter. (Courtesy Picker X-ray Corporation.)

Fig. 16-40. Pelvimetry—posterior (A-P) view. (Courtesy Dr. E. I. L. Cilley, Dr. T. W. Crowell, Dr. R. E. Waud, and Dr. G. H. Hoffman.)

Pelvimetry—Colcher-Sussman, lateral view

    Film size—14″ × 17″   *Bucky*
    Cassette   *Cone to cover*
    Lengthwise

Technique

Factors	Screen film, cassette (par) Regular kvp—12:1 grid	Screen film, cassette (par) High kvp—16:1 grid
Ma	200	200
Time	1.5	0.3
Mas	300	60
Thickness in cm	32	32
Kvp	84	125
Distance	40	40

Patient preparation

Remove all garments except shoes and socks. Provide a gown and instruct the patient to tie the open ends together in the back.

Palpation points

Greater trochanter of the femur; posterior sacrum.

Procedure

Place the patient in a true left lateral position wth the legs together, the knees flexed 90 degrees, and the hips flexed 45 degrees. Place the midaxillary line over the center line of the table. Adjust the height of the pelvimeter to insert the transverse centimeter scale between the gluteal folds. (The transverse centimeter scale should be parallel with the long axis of the femoral shaft. See Fig. 16-41.) Align the inferior border of the film-holder four inches below the center level of the transverse centimeter scale.

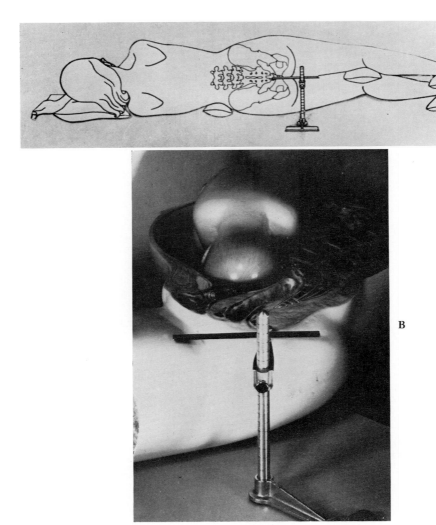

Fig. 16-41. Pelvimetry. **A,** Lateral position. **B,** Lateral position—pelvimeter in place against mannikin. (**A** courtesy Picker X-ray Corporation; **B** courtesy Clay-Adams, Inc.)

Central ray

Direct the central ray perpendicular to the center of the film holder.

Immobilization

Use a compression band. Rapid, deep respiration prior to the exposure will reduce fetal movement. Place sponges between the knees and between and beneath the ankles. Employ suspended expiration.

Right-left markers

Place the left marker on the anterior (patient) side, lateral center border of the film holder.

Structures demonstrated

Left lateral view of the female pelvis to demonstrate size relationship of the fetal head with the maternal pelvic outlet. (See Fig. 16-42.)

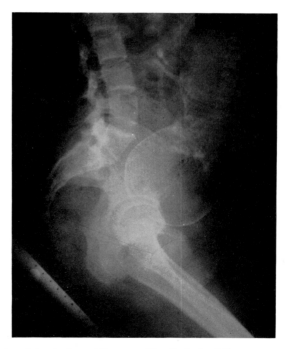

Fig. 16-42. Pelvimetry—lateral view. (Courtesy Dr. E. I. L. Cilley, Dr. T. W. Crowell, Dr. R. E. Waud, and Dr. G. H. Hoffman.)

Bronchography

Bronchography is a nonfunctional fluoroscopic and radiographic examination of the lungs with the use of a directly injected contrast medium.

Patient preparation

When the patient is admitted, remove all garments down to the waist. Provide a gown for female patients and instruct the patient to tie the open ends together in the back.

Make routine anterior (P-A) and lateral radiographs of the lung fields.

Note: The patient may be admitted with nasal catheter preinserted and positioned by the referring physician.

Contrast medium

1. Fill a sterile 20 cc syringe with Lipiodol, Dionosil, or other selected iodized oil that has been warmed to body temperature. (See Table 16-1.)
2. A sterilized bronchogram kit is provided by surgical supply or the referring physician.
3. The contrast medium may be injected by one of the following methods:
    a. Through the nasal pharynx by means of a nasal catheter (the most common method)
    b. Through the oral pharynx by means of a cannula
    c. Through the cricothyroid membrane by means of a needle

Equipment preparation

1. For fluoroscopy preparation, follow the same equipment procedure as for the esophageal examination, p. 363.
2. Provide a sterile 20 cc syringe with contrast medium.
3. Four to six loaded cassettes for spot films must be provided.

Examination

1. Position the patient erect, either sitting or standing, with his back against the fluoroscopy table.
2. Assist the radiologist with lead apron and lead gloves.
3. The assisting doctor or technologist will insert the contrast medium-filled syringe into the external opening of the nasal catheter and inject the iodized oil in small quantities.
4. The radiologist will fluoroscope the patient during this procedure (Step 3) while he is maneuvering (Churchill's maneuvers) the patient into different positions. The Trendelenburg position may also be used.
5. When one side has been filled satisfactorily, radiographs are then made with *essential speed.*
6. Following satisfactory radiography of the region(s) being examined, the catheter is removed and the examination is concluded.

ROUTINE RADIOGRAPHIC POSITIONS

Bronchography—anterior (P-A) view

> *Film size—14″ × 17″*   *Erect film holder*
> *Cassette*   *Cone to cover*
> *Lengthwise*

Technique

Factors	Screen film cassette (par)
Ma	200
Time	1/20
Mas	10
Thickness in cm	20
Kvp	66
Distance	72

Palpation points

Acromion processes, lateral ribs.

Procedure

Place the patient in the erect position with the anterior surface of the chest against the film holder. Center the midline of the body over the center line of the film holder. Align the top of the film holder 3 inches above the acromion processes. Elevate the chin so that it rests on top of the film holder. Place the backs of the hands on the hips. Roll the shoulders anteriorly as far as possible. (See Fig. 12-67.)

Note: *Speed in obtaining this radiograph is essential.*

Central ray

Direct the central ray horizontal and perpendicular to the center of the film holder.

Immobilization

A compression band may be used across the thoracic cage. Employ deep suspended inspiration.

Right-left markers

Place the L marker in the left superior corner of the film holder.

Structures demonstrated

Anterior (P-A) views of the lungs, heart, and the rib structures above the diaphragm. The bronchi and bronchioles are demonstrated with the injected contrast medium. (See Fig. 16-43.)

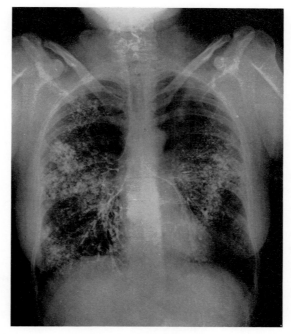

Fig. 16-43. Bronchogram—anterior (P-A) view. (Courtesy Dr. E. I. L. Cilley, Dr. T. W. Crowell, Dr. R. E. Waud, and Dr. G. H. Hoffman.)

Bronchography—lateral view

> *Film size—14″ × 17″*   *Erect film holder*
> *Cassette*   *Cone to cover*
> *Lengthwise*

Technique

Factors	Screen film cassette (par)
Ma	200
Time	0.1
Mas	20
Thickness in cm	30
Kvp	78
Distance	72

Palpation points

Acromion processes; anterior and posterior ribs.

Procedure

Place the patient in the erect position with the lateral surface of the side of the chest being examined against the film holder. Center the midaxillary line of the body over the center line of the film holder. Align the top of the film holder 3 inches above the acromion processes. Cross the arms over the head and rest the forearms on top of the head. Rotate the body into a true lateral position. (See Fig. 12-69.)

Note: *Speed in obtaining this radiograph is essential.*

Central ray

Direct the central ray horizontal and perpendicular to the center of the film holder.

Immobilization

A compression band may be used across the thoracic cage. Employ deep suspended inspiration.

Right-left markers

Place the correct marker in the left superior corner of the film holder.

Structures demonstrated

Lateral views of both lungs superimposed, heart and aorta, and the midthoracic spine. The bronchi and bronchioles are demonstrated with the injected contrast medium. (See Fig. 16-44.)

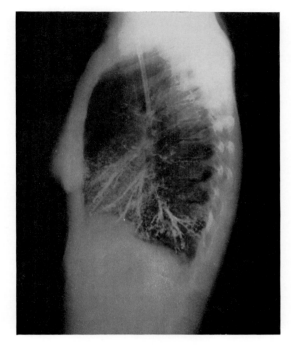

Fig. 16-44. Bronchogram—lateral view. (Courtesy Dr. E. I. L. Cilley, Dr. T. W. Crowell, Dr. R. E. Waud, and Dr. G. H. Hoffman.)

Bronchography—left-right anterior oblique (L.A.O.-R.A.O.) views

Film size—14″ × 17″   *Erect film holder*
Cassette   *Cone to cover*
Lengthwise

Technique

Factors	Screen film cassette (par)
Ma	200
Time	1/15
Mas	13.3
Thickness in cm	24
Kvp	72
Distance	72

Palpation points

Acromion processes; lateral ribs; spinous processes.

Procedure

Place the patient in the erect position with the anterior surface of the chest against the film holder. Align the top of the film holder 3 inches above the acromion processes. Rotate the side of the chest being examined *away* from the film holder 35 degrees. Flex that elbow and place the patient's hand on top of the film holder. Flex the opposite elbow and place the hand on the hip. Align a point midway between the spinous processes and the erect lateral margin of the side being examined over the center line of the film holder. (See Fig. 12-71.)

Central ray

Direct the central ray horizontal and perpendicular to the center of the film holder.

Immobilization

A compression band may be used across the thoracic cage. Employ deep, suspended inspiration.

Right-left markers

Place the correct marker in the left superior corner of the film holder.

Structures demonstrated

Left anterior oblique—maximum view of the right lung field, the trachea, and left bronchial tree. The right bronchi and bronchioles are demonstrated with injected contrast medium.

Right anterior oblique—maximum view of the left lung field, the trachea, the entire right bronchial tree, and left atrium and both ventricles of the heart. The left bronchi and bronchioles are demonstrated with injected contrast medium. (See Fig. 16-45.)

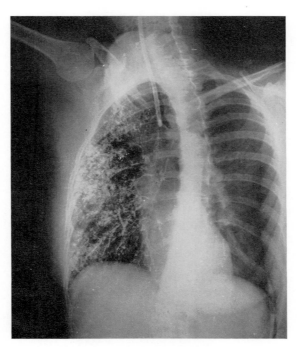

Fig. 16-45. Bronchogram—left anterior oblique (L.A.O.) view. (Courtesy Dr. E. I. L. Cilley, Dr. T. W. Crowell, Dr. R. E. Waud, and Dr. G. H. Hoffman.)

Myelography

Myelography is a nonfunctional fluoroscopic and radiographic examination of the spinal canal (cervical or lumbar injection sites) with the use of a directly injected contrast medium.

Patient preparation

The sterile preparation of the patient is conducted by the doctor or surgical scrub nurse after the patient has been delivered into the radiographic room.

Contrast media

One or more of the following three agents may be used, depending upon the patient's situation and the type of examination:
1. Air or oxygen
2. A water-soluble medium
3. Pantopaque or another selected iodized oil-base contrast medium (See Table 16-1.)

The contrast medium may be furnished by surgical supply or the radiology department.

Equipment preparation

1. For fluoroscopy preparation, follow the same equipment procedure as for the colon examination, pp. 376 and 377.
2. Set the myelogram lock on the fluoroscopy tower.
3. A sterilized myelogram kit is provided by surgical supply.
4. Four to six loaded cassettes for spot films must be provided.

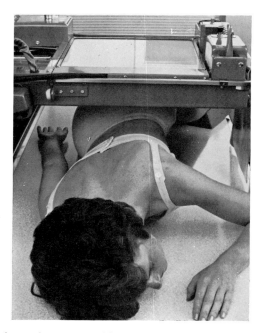

Fig. 16-46. Myelography—right anterior oblique (R.A.O.) position for fluoroscopic spot views.

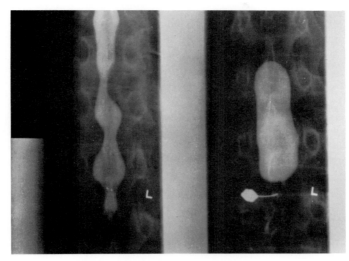

Fig. 16-47. Myelogram—fluoroscopic spot views. (Courtesy Dr. E. I. L. Cilley, Dr. T. W. Crowell, Dr. R. E. Waud, and Dr. G. H. Hoffman.)

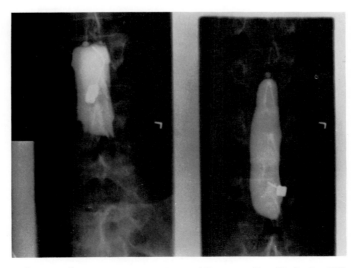

Fig. 16-48. Myelogram—fluoroscopic spot views. (Courtesy Dr. E. I. L. Cilley, Dr. T. W. Crowell, Dr. R. E. Waud, and Dr. G. H. Hoffman.)

Examination

1. The patient is placed in a lateral recumbent or a sitting position (depending upon the region to be examined).
2. The doctor inserts a needle into a predetermined point in the spinal canal and collects spinal fluid for laboratory examination.
3. A similar quantity of the contrast medium is then injected.
4. After repeating this process, the patient is fluoroscoped in the lateral, anterior oblique, and prone positions with varying degrees of the Trendelenburg and semierect table positions. (See Fig. 16-46.)
5. Spot films are made periodically. (See Figs. 16-47 and 16-48.)
6. Upon completion of satisfactory spot films or radiographs, the doctor will aspirate as much of the contrast medium as possible, and the examination is concluded.

Appendix

Meaning of Greek letters often used

α (**alpha**)—A positive particle consisting of two protons and two neutrons (the helium atom nucleus).

β (**beta**)—A negative particle consisting of one electron.

γ (**gamma**)—An electromagnetic wave from radioactive substance.

$\triangle$ (**delta**)—To indicate the change, as in energy.

λ (**lambda**)—Wavelength.

ν (**nu**)—Frequency.

υ (**upsilon**)—Velocity when less than that of light.

ϕ (**phi**)—The work function of a given metal.

Useful constants, laws, definitions, and formulas

Planck's constant—6.62×10^{-27} erg-seconds; simply written as h; a mathematical value that represents the ratio of the energy of any quantum of radiation to its frequency.

c (**the speed of light**)—186,000 miles/second or 3×10^{10} cm/second.

Thermodynamics—

> *Law I:* When mechanical work is transformed into heat or heat into work, the amount of work is always equivalent to the quantity of heat (conservation of energy).

> *Law II:* It is impossible by any continuous self-sustaining process for heat to be transferred from a colder to a hotter body.

Newton's laws—

> *I. Law of inertia:* A body at rest tends to remain at rest, while a body in motion tends to continue in motion in the same straight line unless acted upon by an outside force.

> *II. Law of momentum:* When a force acts upon a body, it changes the momentum of that body. This change of momentum is proportional to the applied force and to the time it acts upon the body.

> *III. Law of reaction:* Every action (force) is accompanied by an equal and opposite reaction (force).

> *IV. Law of gravitation:* Every body in the universe attracts every other body with a force that is directly proportional to the product of the masses (weights) of the two bodies and inversely proportional to the square of the distance between their exact centers.

Density—The ratio of the mass of a homogeneous portion of matter to its volume.

Mass-energy equivalence—The mass of anything increases as its velocity increases, and if the velocity approaches that of light, the mass becomes infinitely large. Mass is constant only when there is no motion. The effect of velocity in mass is significant only when the velocity is near the speed of light. Einstein postulated that the energy of anything is equal to its mass times the square of the speed of light; this is written: $E = mc^2$, where E is the energy, m is the mass at rest, and c is the constant for the speed of light.

Melting point—The temperature, under standard pressure, at which a solid substance begins to melt.

MPD—The maximum permissible dose in rems to the most critical organs is $5(N - 18)$ where N is the age in years and is greater than 18; the MPD in rems to the skin of the whole body is $10(N - 18)$.

Quantum of radiant energy of frequency—$W = h\nu$, where W is the quantum, h is Planck's constant, and ν is the frequency of the energy.

Specific heat—The heat in calories required to raise the temperature of one gram of substance 1 degree centigrade.

Temperature of volatilization—The temperature, under standard pressure, at which a substance begins to vaporize readily.

Thermal conductivity—The quantity of heat that passes in unit time through a unit area of plate whose thickness is unity, when its opposite faces differ in temperature by one degree.

Z number—The atomic number of any element.

Silver stain remover formula:

Water	750 ml
Thiourea	75 grams
Citric acid	75 grams
Water to make	1 liter

Temperature conversion formulas:

$$°C. = °F. - 32 \times 5/9$$
$$°F. = °C. \times 9/5 + 32$$
$$0°K. \text{ (Kelvin or absolute) is } -273.18° C.$$

Sequence of the elements

Element	Symbol	Atomic number	Atomic weight*	K	L	M	N	O	P	Q
				\multicolumn{7}{c}{Orbits with number of electrons contained}
Hydrogen	H	1	1.008	1						
Helium	He	2	4.003	2						
Lithium	Li	3	6.940	2	1					
Beryllium	Be	4	9.013	2	2					
Boron	B	5	10.82	2	3					
Carbon	C	6	12.01	2	4					
Nitrogen	N	7	14.008	2	5					
Oxygen	O	8	16.000	2	6					
Fluorine	F	9	19.000	2	7					
Neon	Ne	10	20.183	2	8					
Sodium	Na	11	22.997	2	8	1				
Magnesium	Mg	12	24.32	2	8	2				
Aluminum	Al	13	26.98	2	8	3				
Silicon	Si	14	28.09	2	8	4				
Phosphorus	P	15	30.975	2	8	5				
Sulfur	S	16	32.006	2	8	6				
Chlorine	Cl	17	35.457	2	8	7				
Argon	A	18	39.994	2	8	8				
Potassium	K	19	39.100	2	8	8	1			
Calcium	Ca	20	40.08	2	8	8	2			
Scandium	Sc	21	44.96	2	8	9	2			
Titanium	Ti	22	47.90	2	8	10	2			
Vanadium	V	23	50.95	2	8	11	2			
Chromium	Cr	24	52.01	2	8	13	1			
Manganese	Mn	25	54.93	2	8	13	2			
Iron	Fe	26	55.85	2	8	14	2			
Cobalt	Co	27	58.94	2	8	15	2			
Nickel	Ni	28	58.69	2	8	16	2			

*A number in parentheses indicates the mass number of the isotope of the longest known half-life.

Sequence of the elements—cont'd

Element	Symbol	Atomic number	Atomic weight	K	L	M	N	O	P	Q
Copper	Cu	29	63.54	2	8	18	1			
Zinc	Zn	30	65.38	2	8	18	2			
Gallium	Ga	31	69.72	2	8	18	3			
Germanium	Ge	32	72.60	2	8	18	4			
Arsenic	As	33	74.91	2	8	18	5			
Selenium	Se	34	78.96	2	8	18	6			
Bromine	Br	35	79.916	2	8	18	7			
Krypton	Kr	36	83.80	2	8	18	8			
Rubidium	Rb	37	85.48	2	8	18	8	1		
Strontium	Sr	38	87.63	2	8	18	8	2		
Yttrium	Y	39	88.92	2	8	18	9	2		
Zirconium	Zr	40	91.22	2	8	18	10	2		
Niobium	Nb	41	92.91	2	8	18	12	1		
Molybdenum	Mo	42	95.95	2	8	18	13	1		
Technetium	Tc	43	99.000	2	8	18	14	1		
Ruthenium	Ru	44	101.7	2	8	18	15	1		
Rhodium	Rh	45	102.91	2	8	18	16	1		
Palladium	Pd	46	106.7	2	8	18	18	0		
Silver	Ag	47	107.880	2	8	18	18	1		
Cadmium	Cd	48	112.41	2	8	18	18	2		
Indium	In	49	114.76	2	8	18	18	3		
Tin	Sn	50	118.70	2	8	18	18	4		
Antimony	Sb	51	121.76	2	8	18	18	5		
Tellurium	Te	52	127.61	2	8	18	18	6		
Iodine	I	53	126.91	2	8	18	18	7		
Xenon	Xe	54	131.3	2	8	18	18	8		
Cesium	Cs	55	132.91	2	8	18	18	8	1	
Barium	Ba	56	137.36	2	8	18	18	8	2	
Lanthanum	La	57	138.92	2	8	18	18	9	2	
Cerium	Ce	58	140.13	2	8	18	20	8	2	
Praseodymium	Pr	59	140.92	2	8	18	21	8	2	
Neodymium	Nd	60	144.27	2	8	18	22	8	2	
Promethium	Pm	61	(145)	2	8	18	23	8	2	
Samarium	Sm	62	150.43	2	8	18	24	8	2	
Europium	Eu	63	152.0	2	8	18	25	8	2	
Gadolinium	Gd	64	156.9	2	8	18	25	9	2	
Terbium	Tb	65	159.2	2	8	18	27	8	2	
Dysprosium	Dy	66	162.46	2	8	18	28	8	2	
Holmium	Ho	67	164.94	2	8	18	29	8	2	
Erbium	Er	68	167.2	2	8	18	30	8	2	
Thulium	Tm	69	169.4	2	8	18	31	8	2	
Ytterbium	Yb	70	173.04	2	8	18	32	8	2	
Lutetium	Lu	71	174.99	2	8	18	32	9	2	
Hafnium	Hf	72	178.6	2	8	18	32	10	2	
Tantalum	Ta	73	180.88	2	8	18	32	11	2	
Tungsten	W	74	183.92	2	8	18	32	12	2	
Rhenium	Re	75	186.31	2	8	18	32	13	2	
Osmium	Os	76	190.2	2	8	18	32	14	2	
Iridium	Ir	77	193.1	2	8	18	32	15	2	
Platinum	Pt	78	195.23	2	8	18	32	17	1	
Gold	Au	79	197.2	2	8	18	32	18	1	
Mercury	Hg	80	200.61	2	8	18	32	18	2	
Thallium	Tl	81	204.39	2	8	18	32	18	3	
Lead	Pb	82	207.21	2	8	18	32	18	4	

Sequence of the elements—cont'd

Element	Symbol	Atomic number	Atomic weight	Orbits with number of electrons contained						
				K	L	M	N	O	P	Q
Bismuth	Bi	83	209.00	2	8	18	32	18	5	
Polonium	Po	84	(210)	2	8	18	32	18	6	
Astatine	At	85	(210)	2	8	18	32	18	7	
Radon	Rn	86	(222)	2	8	18	32	18	8	
Francium	Fr	87	(223)	2	8	18	32	18	8	1
Radium	Ra	88	(226)	2	8	18	32	18	8	2
Actinium	Ac	89	(227)	2	8	18	32	18	9	2
Thorium	Th	90	(232)	2	8	18	32	18	10	2
Protactinium	Pa	91	(231)	2	8	18	32	20	9	2
Uranium	U	92	(238)	2	8	18	32	21	9	2
Neptunium	Np	93	(237)	2	8	18	32	22	9	2
Plutonium	Pu	94	(242)	2	8	18	32	23	9	2
Americium	Am	95	(243)	2	8	18	32	24	9	2
Curium	Cm	96	(247)	2	8	18	32	25	9	2
Berkelium	Bk	97	(249)							
Californium	Cf	98	(251)							
Einsteinium	Es	99	(254)							
Fermium	Fm	100	(253)							
Mendelevium	Md	101	(256)							
Nobelium	No	102	(254)							

Comparison of tungsten with some other elements as a target

Symbol	Z	Density Gm/cm³	Melting point °C.	Temp. of volatilization at 0° C.	Thermal conductivity	Specific heat	Efficiency of anode at 100 kvp
Co	27	8.9	1480			0.09	0.378%
Ni	28	8.9	1450		0.14	0.10	0.392%
Cu	29	8.92	1084		0.92	0.09	0.406%
Mo	42	10.2	2620		0.346	0.07	0.588%
Ag	47	10.5	960.5		0.992	0.05	0.658%
W	**74**	**19.3**	**3370**	**1800**	**0.35**	**0.03**	**1.036%**
Os	76	22.5	2700	2300	0.17	0.03	1.064%
Ir	77	22.4	2350	1400	0.17	0.03	1.078%
Pt	78	21.5	1750	1200	0.17	0.03	1.092%
Pb	82	11.34	327.43		0.082	0.03	1.148%

Useful electrical symbols*

Number	American standard number	Description	Symbol
1	1.	Adjustable	↗
2	6.	Battery	
3	6.3	Battery, multicell	

*Adapted from American standard graphical symbols for electrical diagrams, American Standards Association, Inc., New York. Courtesy Institute of Radio Engineers, Inc., New York.

Useful electrical symbols—cont'd

Number	American standard number	Description	Symbol
4	7.1	Circuit breaker	
5	12.	Coil, operating	
6	14.1	Connector, female contact	
7	14.2	Connector, male contact	
8	14.4	Connectors, separable	
9	15.1.2	Contact, fixed, for switch	
10	15.3.2	Contact, open	
11	15.4	Contact, open, with time closing	
12	15.5	Contact, closed, with time opening	
13	16.2	Contactor, electrically operated with series blowout coil (magnetic contactor)	
14	27.	Fuse	
15	28.	Ground	
16	31.1	Inductor, winding	
17	31.2	Inductor, winding, with magnetic core	
18	31.5	Inductor, adjustable	
19	43.5	Crossed wires, not connected	
20	43.6.2	Crossed wires, connected	
21	50.1	Resistor	
22	50.4	Resistor, variable	
23	56.1	Switch, single throw	
24	56.2	Switch, double throw	
25	56.2.1	Switch, double throw, two-pole	
26	63.	Transformer	
27	63.2	Transformer, magnetic core	
28	63.7.1	Autotransformer, adjustable	
29	64.1.1	Emitting electrode, directly heated	

Useful electrical symbols—cont'd

Number	American standard number	Description	Symbol
30	64.3.1	Anode or plate	⊥
31	64.3.2	Target or x-ray anode	
32	64.6.1	Glass envelope	
33	64.11.6.1	Single unit vacuum tube	
34	64.11.12.1	X-ray tube with filamentary cathode and focusing cup	
35	37.	Meter instrument symbols*	
		Ammeter	A
		Galvanometer	G
		Milliammeter	MA
		Voltmeter	V
		Prereading voltmeter	PV

*The symbols for these instruments are included in the circle located where the meter would be located.

Glossary

Radiographic terminology and definitions

A

a-—A prefix indicating absence of or lacking.

Å—Abbreviation for angstrom unit.

ab-—A prefix indicating off or away from.

abdomen (ab-do'men)—The large inferior cavity of the trunk bounded superiorly by the diaphragm, anteriorly by the ribs and abdominal muscles, bilaterally by the ribs and abdominal muscles, and posteriorly by the vertebral column, psoas and quadratus lumborum muscles.

abduct (ab-dukt')—To move away from the midline of the body, or outwardly.

aberration (ab-er-a'shun)—Deviation from the usual course.

abrasion (ah-bra'zhun)—Excoriation of the cutaneous or mucous surface by mechanical means.

abscess (ab'ses)—A localized collection of pus surrounded by a wall of lymph; an inflammatory exudate.

A.C.—Abbreviation for alternating current.

acanthion (ah-kan'the-on)—A point at the base of the anterior nasal spine.

acetabulum (as-e-tab'u-lum)—The fossa or depression in the lateral and anterior surface of the pelvis for the articulation of the head of the femur.

achlorhydria (ah-klor-hi'dre-ah)—Complete absence of hydrochloric acid in the gastric juice.

acid (as'id)—A compound of an electronegative element with one or more atoms of hydrogen that can be replaced by electropositive atoms when a salt is formed.

acid stopbath—A 28% solution of acetic acid used between the developer and fixer to stop development.

acoustic (ah-koos'tik)—Pertaining to sound or to the sense of hearing.

acromegaly (ak-ro-meg'a-le)—A disease of the pituitary gland in adults that produces overgrowth of bone, especially in the jaws and hands.

acromion (ah-kro'me-on)—Process of the scapula, part of the shoulder girdle.

actinic (ak-tin'ik)—A type of radiation that is capable of producing a chemical change.

ad-—A prefix indicating toward the midline.

adduct (ah-dukt')—To move toward the midline of the body, or inwardly.

adenoma (ad-e-no'mah)—A tumor of glandlike structure.

adipose (ad'e-pōs)—Fatty tissue; obese.

adrenal (ad-re'nal)—A gland of the endocrine system that secretes epinephrine and is located on the proximal poles of each kidney in the human being.

aerated (a'er-a-ted)—Filled with air.

afferent (af'er-ent)—Leading toward the center.

alkali (al'kah-lī)—Opposite of acid; strongly electropositive.

alpha particle (al'fa)—A positively charged particle, consisting of two protons and two neutrons, which is ejected at high speed in certain radioactive disintegrations.

alternating current (A.C.)—This kind of electric current flows for a given length of time in one direction and immediately flows in the opposite direction for the same length of time. It usually consists of 60 complete cycles per second.

441

alveolar (al've-o-lar)—Pertaining to an alveolus. The alveolar process is the process from which the teeth erupt.

ambulatory (am'bu-la-to-re)—Able to walk.

amniography (am"ni-og'rah-fe)—The process of making a radiograph following the replacement of some of the amniotic fluid surrounding the fetus with a contrast medium.

amniotic fluid (am'ni-ot"ic fluid)—The fluid secreted between the amnion and the embryonic disk.

ampere (am'per)—The unit of intensity of an electric current, being the current produced by 1 volt acting through a resistance of 1 ohm.

amphi- (am'fe)—A prefix indicating a bilateral condition, double.

ampulla (am-pul'ah)—A dilatation of a canal or duct.

amputation (am'pu-ta"shun)—The removal (usually surgical) of part or all of an appendage.

AMU—Abbreviation for atomic mass unit.

anabolism (ah-nab'o-lizm)—Any constructive process by which simple substances are converted by living cells into more complex compounds.

anastomosis (a-nas'to-mo"sis)—A communication between two vessels.

anatomy (ah-nat'o-me)—The science of the structure of organs or of organic bodies.

anesthesia (an-es-the'ze-ah)—Loss of feeling or sensation.

anesthesiologist (an-es-the-ze-ol'o-jist)—A specialist in anesthesia.

anesthetic (an-es-thet'ik)—Without the sense of pain or touch; a substance that produces anesthesia.

anesthetist (an-es'the-tist)—An expert in administering anesthetics.

aneurysm (an'ū-rizm)—A circumscribed dilation of the walls of an artery.

angio- (an'je-o)—A prefix pertaining to a vessel, usually a blood vessel.

angiocardiography (an"je-o-kar-de-og'rah-fe)—A radiographic study of the heart and great vessels after being made radiopaque by injection of suitable contrast media.

angiogram (an'je-o-gram)—A radiograph of blood vessels.

angle board—A device used in certain radiographic procedures enabling the technician to place the patient's head in particular angles.

angstrom unit (awng'strem)—One one-hundred millionth of a centimeter, the unit of measure of wavelengths.

anion (an'i-on)—An ion carrying a negative charge.

ankylosis (ang-kil-o'sis)—Stiffness of a joint resulting from either traumatic or intentional union of the joint surfaces.

anode (an'ōd)—The positive part of the x-ray tube in the secondary circuit, made of tungsten imbedded in a copper bar; also called the target.

ante-—A prefix indicating previous or in front of.

antecubital space (an-te-kū'be-tal)—The space in the bend of the elbow on the volar surface of the forearm.

anterior (an-te're-or)—Nearest the head or front.

anti-—A prefix indicating opposition to or against.

antiseptic (an-te-sep'tik)—A substance that will inhibit the growth and development of microorganisms without necessarily destroying them.

antrum (an'trum)—A cavity or chamber; one of the paranasal sinuses in the maxillae. It is also called the maxillary sinus.

anus(ā'nus)—The terminus and outlet of the digestive tract.

aorta (ā-or'tah)—The very large artery arising from the left ventricle of the heart. All of the lesser arteries, except the coronary arteries, arise from it.

A-P—Abbreviation for anteroposterior position or projection.

apex (ā'peks)—The top or summit of any organ; also the pointed end.

aphagia (ah-fa'je-ah)—Loss of the power of swallowing.

aphasia (ah-fa'ze-ah)—Defect or loss of the power of expression by speech, writing, or signs, or of comprehending spoken or written language, due to injury or disease of the brain centers.

apnea (ap-ne'ah)—A partial privation or suspension of breath.

apophyseal joint (ap-o-fiz'e-al)—The true intervertebral joint between the articular processes.

arachnoid (ah-rak′noid)—The delicate membrane of the brain and spinal cord between the dura and pia maters; weblike.

areolar (ah-re′o-lar)—Containing minute interspaces.

arteriography (ar″te-re-og′rah-fe)—The radiographic examination and study of the arteries by injection of a radiopaque solution.

artery (ar′ter-e)—A vessel that conveys blood from the heart.

arthritic (ar-thrit′ik)—Pertaining to or affected with arthritis.

arthritis (ar-thri′tis)—Inflammation of a joint.

arthro-—A prefix indicating relationship with a joint.

arthroclasia (ar-thro-kla′ze-ah)—The breaking down of an ankylosis to secure free movement of the joint.

arthrodesis (ar-throd′e-sis)—The surgical fixation of a joint.

articulate (ar-tik′u-lāt)—To unite so as to form a joint.

articulation (ar-tik-u-la′shun)—Usually indicates motion between two or more bones; any naturally occurring union between two or more bones. The types of articulations are synarthroses—immovable; schindyleses—grooved; gomphoses—sockets; suturae—sutures; diarthroses—movable; arthrodia—gliding; ginglymus—hinge; enarthroses—ball-and-socket; and amphiarthroses—mixed or combinations.

artifact (ar′te-fakt)—Foreign or artificial marks on x-ray films caused by improper processing or faulty equipment.

asterion (as-te′re-on)—The point of junction on the superior surface of the skull of the lambdoidal, parietomastoid, and occipitomastoid sutures.

ataxia (ah-tak′se-ah)—Failure or irregularity of muscular coordination.

atelectasis (at-e-lek′tah-sis)—Imperfect expansion or collapse of the air vesicles of the lungs.

atlas (at′las)—The first cervical vertebra.

atom (at′om)—The ultimate particle of an element; one of the divisions of a molecule, the smallest quantity of a substance that can exist free or uncombined.

atomic number (ah-tom′ik)—The total number of protons in the nucleus of an atom.

atomic weight—The sum of the protons plus the neutrons in the nucleus of an atom.

atony (at′o-ne)—The lack of normal tone or strength.

atresia (ah-tre′ze-ah)—The absence or closure of a normal opening.

atrium (a′tre-um)—The auricle of the heart, a vessel that receives venous blood.

atrophy (at′ro-fe)—Diminution in size of a tissue, organ, or part due to degeneration or decrease in cell size.

attenuation (a-ten′u-a″shun)—The decrease in dose rate of radiation in passing through a material.

atypical (a-tip′e-kal)—Not conformable to type.

auditory meatus (aw′de-to-re)—The opening of the ear.

auricle (aw′re-kl)—The pinna or flap of the ear; also one of the upper chambers of the heart; it receives the blood from the circulatory system.

autopsy (aw′top-se)—The post-mortem examination of a body.

autotransformer—A transformer with a single wrapping or winding of wire, with both ends of the wire attached to the primary alternating current.

axilla (ak-sil′ah)—The armpit.

axis (ak′sis)—The second cervical vertebra.

B

background radiation—In a given area, the sum total of radioactivity from cosmic rays, natural radioactive materials, and whatever may have been introduced into the area.

back-scatter—A term used to describe the rays that are generated when the x-rays capable of penetrating the object strike the surface upon which the film holder lies.

barium sulfate (ba′re-um sul′fāt)—A radiopaque compound used in gastrointestinal studies.

barn—The unit of cross section of a nuclear reaction; 10^{-24} sq. cm. The term describes the target area or cross section in a nuclear reaction.

B.E.—Abbreviation for barium enema.

benign (be-nīn′)—Not endangering health or life.

beta particle (bā′tah)—An electron.

bi-—A prefix indicating two, twofold, or twice.

bilateral (bi-lat′er-al)—Pertaining to or affecting both sides of the body.

biliary (bil′e-a-re)—Pertaining to the bile or its production.

binary fission (bi′na-re)—Division into two equal parts.

bio-—A prefix indicating life or its processes.

biopsy (bi′op-se)—The removal and examination of tissue from the living body for diagnostic purposes.

blastocyst (blas′to-sist)—The stage of development of the embryo following cleavage in which the cells are arranged in a single layer to form a hollow sphere.

bolus (bo′lus)—A rounded mass. The term used for the food mass in the act of deglutition and digestion.

brachial (bra′ke-al)—Brachium; belonging to the arm.

bronchiectasis (brong-ke-ek′tah-sis)—Dilatation of the walls of the bronchi.

bronchiole (brong′ke-ōl)—One of the finer subdivisions of the branched bronchial tree.

broncho-—A prefix indicating association with the trachea.

bronchography (brong-kog′rah-fe)—The radiographic examination and study of the bronchial tree after injection of suitable radiopaque material.

bronchus (brong′kus)—An air tube; one of the divisions of the trachea.

bursa (bur′sah)—A small sac interposed between parts that move upon one another.

bursitis (bur-si′tis)—Inflammation of a bursa. The inflammation may be the result of a foreign substance.

C

c̄—The symbol indicating with.

Ca-—Abbreviation for cancer and for calcium.

calcaneus (kal-ka′ne-us)—The heel bone, largest bone of the tarsus.

calcareous (kal-ka′re-us)—Pertaining to or containing calcium or lime.

calcigerous (kal-sij′er-us)—Producing or carrying calcium salts.

calculus (kal′ku-lus)—A stonelike concretion found in the body.

callus (kal′us)—A new growth of incomplete osseous tissue surrounding the ends of a fractured bone that is in the process of healing.

calvarium (kal-va′re-um)—The cranium.

calyx (ka′liks)—One of the cuplike divisions of the pelvis of the kidney.

canaliculus (kan-al-ik′u-lus)—Any one of a system of minute channels connected with each haversian canal.

cancellous bone (kan′sel-us)—Bone having a reticular, spongy, or latticelike structure.

cancer (kan′ser)—Any type of malignant growth.

cannula (kan′u-lah)—A tube for insertion into the body, its lumen being usually occupied by a trocar during the act of insertion.

canthus (kan′thus)—The angle, either temporal (outer) or nasal (inner), formed by the junction of the eyelids.

cardboard holder—A lightproof holder made of cardboard used for holding certain types of x-ray film. The back side has in it a thin sheet of lead that prevents back-scatter. It is used to produce high contrast and detail in extremity radiographs.

cardio- (kar′de-o)—A prefix pertaining to the heart.

caries (ka′re-ēz)—Decay of bone or of teeth.

carpus (kar′pus)—The bones of the wrist.

cartilage (kar′ti-lij)—Connective tissue containing no vascular network.

cassette (kah-set′)—A device for holding x-ray films during exposure. Cassettes are made in several sizes. The tube side is composed of Bakelite or other radiolucent substance, and the back side contains a thin lead sheet. The back is hinged and fits into the tube side, sealing out all light. Two intensifying screens are mounted inside, one on each side, between which the film is sandwiched.

catabolism (kah-tab′o-lizm)—Destructive metabolism.

catalyst (kat′ah-list)—A substance that alters the velocity of a chemical reaction without undergoing any apparent physical or chemical change itself and without becoming a part of the product formed.

catheter (kath'e-ter)—A tubular surgical instrument for withdrawing fluids from a cavity of the body.

catheterization (kath"e-ter-i-za'shun)—The employment or passage of a catheter.

cathode (kath'ōd)—The negative part of the x-ray tube; the electrons are emitted from it.

cation (kat'i-on)—An ion carrying a positive charge.

caudad (kaw'dad)—Toward the tail or cauda; in man, downward.

caudal (kaw'dal)—Referring to a position near the tail end of the long axis of the body.

cephalad (sef'ah-lad)—Toward the head.

cephalic (se-fal'ik)—Pertaining to the head.

cerebellum (ser-e-bel'um)—That division of the brain behind the cerebrum and above the pons and fourth ventricle concerned with coordination of movements.

cerebrum (ser'ē-brum)—The main portion of the brain.

characteristic fluorescent rays—Rays that are generated in an absorbing material (fluoresce from) as a result of primary x-ray photon bombardment.

characteristic x-rays—X-rays of definite wavelengths, characteristic of a pure substance and emitted by it under proper excitation.

choana (ko'a-nah)—Funnel; opening of the posterior nares into the pharynx.

cholangiogram, operative (ko-lan'je-o-gram)—Radiography of the gallbladder and associated ducts during surgery.

chole- (ko'le)—A combining form denoting relationship to the bile.

cholecystitis (ko"le-sis-ti'tis)—Inflammation of the gallbladder.

cholecystography (ko"le-sis-tog'rah-fe)—Radiography of the gallbladder after opacification.

cholelithiasis (ko"le-li-thi'ah-sis)—The presence of, or a condition associated with, calculi in the gallbladder or bile duct.

chromosome (kro'mo-sōm)—One of several small, dark-staining bodies that appear in the nucleus of a cell especially during mitosis.

chyle (kīl)—The milk-white fluid absorbed by the lacteals during digestion; lymph containing absorbed fat.

chyme (kīm)—Food having undergone gastric digestion only.

cicatrix (sik-a'triks)—A scar; connective tissue that replaces a localized loss of substance.

circumduction (ser-kum-duk'shun)—The movement of a limb in such a manner that its distal part describes a circle, the proximal end being fixed.

circumflex (ser'kum-fleks)—Winding around.

coarctation (ko-ark-ta'shun)—A straightening or pressing together; a condition of stricture or contracture.

coccyx (kok'siks)—The caudal and vestigial terminus of the spinal column.

colloid (kol'oid)—A mixture of microscopic particles so small that the energy of the molecules of the liquid portion is great enough to keep the particles from settling out.

colon (ko'lon)—The large part of the intestine, beginning with the cecum and terminating at the end of the sigmoid flexure.

compact bone—Bone having very dense structure; true bone.

Compton effect—A change in the wavelength of scattered rays and emission of recoil electrons in deep radiation.

condyle (kon'dīl)—Rounded eminence of bone, usually articular.

cone—A funnel-shaped attachment on the x-ray tube housing aperture. Used to control the scattering of x-rays in the air and to limit the x-rays in any given area.

congenital (kon-gen'i-tal)—Existing at or before birth.

contrast (kon'trast)—Defined radiographically, the visible difference between adjacent densities resulting from subject and film characteristics. Generally, contrast is the property of a photographic material that determines the magnitude of the density difference resulting from a given exposure difference.

contusion (kon-tu'zhun)—A bruise; an injury attended with more or less disorganization of the subcutaneous tissue and effusion of blood beneath the skin, but without breaking of the skin.

coracoid (kor'ah-koid)—Shaped like a crow's beak; a process of the scapula.

coronal plane (ko-ro'nal)—A vertical plane extending from left to right and separating anterior from posterior.

coronoid (kor'o-noid)—Crown-shaped; processes found on the mandible and ulna.

cortex (kor'teks)—The outer layer of an organ as distinguished from its inner substance.

costal (kos'tal)—Pertaining to the ribs.

costophrenic angle (kos'to-fren'ik)—The angle formed by the lateral junction of the ribs with the diaphragm.

coulomb (koo'lom)—The unit of quantity in current electricity. The quantity afforded by 1 ampere of current in 1 second flowing against 1 ohm of resistance with a force of 1 volt.

crepitus, bony (krep'i-tus)—The crackling sound produced by the rubbing together of fragments of fractured bone.

cretinism (krē'tin-izm)—A chronic condition due to a congenital lack of thyroid secretion.

cribriform plate (krib're-form)—The sievelike upper plate of the ethmoid.

crista galli (kris'tah gal'le)—A ridge on the ethmoid bone to which the falx cerebri is attached.

cuboid (kū'boid)—The lateral bone of the tarsus between the calcaneus and fourth and fifth metatarsals.

cuneiform (ku-ne'e-form)—Wedge-shaped; bones of the tarsus.

cyanosis (sī-ah-no'sis)—Bluish discoloration of the skin resulting from insufficient quantity of oxygen in the blood.

cyst, dermoid (sist)—A pouch or sac of developmental origin, consisting of a fibrous wall lined with stratified epithelium and containing hair follicles, sweat glands, and sebaceous glands.

cysto- (sis'to)—A prefix pertaining to the urinary bladder. Abbreviation for bladder examination.

D

dactyl (dak'til)—A digit, either finger or toe.

D.C.—Abbreviation for direct current.

decubitus (de-ku'be-tus)—Recumbent or horizontal position.

definition (detail, sharpness)—A term referring to the distinctness with which images of anatomic structures are recorded.

deglutition (deg-loo-tish'un)—The act of swallowing, consummated in three steps: the larynx is elevated; the pharyngeal space is briefly closed while the food bolus is shot back over the tongue; the pharyngeal space then opens to receive the bolus, which is rapidly forced into the upper one third of the esophagus where peristaltic action begins. True peristalsis does not begin in the esophagus. The first step in deglutition is voluntary; the next two steps are involuntary. The entire elapsed time when no respiration occurs is from 5 to 6 seconds.

density, radiographic—The degree of gradation of blackness in a radiograph; the amount of film blackening.

dermis (der'mis)—The corium or true skin.

dermo- (der'mo)—A prefix pertaining to the skin or integument.

desquamation (des-kwah-ma'shun)—The shedding of epithelial elements, chiefly of the skin, in scales or sheets.

detail—The quantity of visibility of the fine structures and marginal sharpness that is demonstrated radiographically.

developer (de-vel'op-er)—The solution in which the films are developed. It brings out the latent image.

di-—A prefix indicating twice or double.

diaphragm (di'ah-fram)—The wall that separates the thorax from the abdomen. It is muscular at the circumference and tendinous in the center.

diaphysis (di-af'is-is)—The shaft of a long bone.

diastole (di-as'to-le)—The heart at rest; the period of dilation of one of the heart chambers.

digestion (di-jest'yun)—The process of converting food into materials for absorption and assimilation.

digit (dij'it)—A finger or toe.

discography (disk-og'rah-fe)—The roentgen examination, by use of contrast media, of the intervertebral discs.

distal (dis'tal)—Farthest from the body or origin; opposite to proximal.

distortion (dis-tor'shun)—The perversion of shape in a radiographic image.

diverticulum (di-ver-tik′u-lum)—A small pouch or blind sac arising from a main structure.

dorsal (dor′sal)—Posterior or rear.

D.U.—Abbreviation for duodenal ulcer.

duodenum (du-o-dē′num)—The first part of the small intestine between the pylorus and jejunum.

dura mater (du′rah ma′ter)—Durable or hard mother. The fibrous outer membrane covering of the brain and spinal cord.

dyspnea (disp-ne′ah)—Difficult breathing.

E

ecchymosis (ek-e-mo′sis)—An extravasation of blood; also a discoloration of the skin caused by the extravasation of blood.

ec-, ecto-—Prefixes indicating outside or away from.

-ectomy (ek′to-me)—A suffix indicating removal of or excision.

edema (e-dē′mah)—Infiltration of serum in a part.

efferent (ef′er-ent)—Carrying away from.

effusion (ef-u′zhun)—A pouring out.

electricity (e-lek-tris′i-te)—One of the forces of nature developed by chemism, magnetism, or friction; also said to be electrons in motion.

electrolyte (e-lek′tro-līt)—A substance capable of conducting an electric current and being decomposed by it.

electromagnetic wave—A wave produced by the oscillation of an electric charge.

electron (e-lek′tron)—The ultimate particle of negative electricity.

electron-volt—An energy unit; the amount of energy acquired when a particle having a charge equal to the fundamental or electronic unit falls through a potential difference of 1 volt.

em-, en-—Prefixes indicating inside of or within.

embolism (em′bo-lizm)—Clot formation causing a stoppage of the flow of blood in a blood vessel.

embryo (em′brē-o)—The product of conception in its earlier stages of development during the first trimester.

emesis (em′e-sis)—Vomitus; the act of vomiting.

emetic (e-met′ik)—Having the power to cause vomiting.

emphysema (em-fi-sē′mah)—Air or gas in a normally airless tissue or an excess of air in normally aerated tissues.

empyema (em-pī-ē′mah)—Pus in a cavity.

emulsion (e-mul′shun)—A liquid, usually water, containing an insoluble substance in suspension; it may be used in a dehydrated form.

encephalography (en-sef-ah-log′rah-fe)—Radiographic examination of the head after a given quantity of spinal fluid has been withdrawn and replaced by an equal quantity of radiopaque or contrast media.

encephalon (en-sef′ah-lon)—That portion of the central nervous system contained within the cranium.

endocrine gland (en′do-krīn)—A gland that secretes a substance or substances directly into the bloodstream. The gland has no common ducts.

endosteum (en-dos′te-um)—The vascular membranous layer of connective tissue lining the medullary cavity of bones.

energy (en′er-jē)—The capacity for doing work. There are two kinds of energy: kinetic, the power of a body in motion; and latent or potential, the power possessed by a body at rest. Radiant energy is a form of kinetic energy that is emitted by all bodies in proportion to their temperature and is propagated by undulations in the luminiferous ether.

enteric (en-ter′ik)—Pertaining to the intestinal tract.

enzyme (en′zīm)—An organic compound produced by living cells, which acts as a catalyst in chemical reactions.

epi-—A prefix indicating the position upon or above.

epicondyle (ep-e-kon′dīl)—An eminence upon a bone above its condyle. It is usually roughened for attachment with muscles or tendons.

epidermis (ep-e-der′mis)—The outer and nonvascular layer of the skin. It is protective and composed of four layers. From inside out the layers are stratum germinativum, stratum granulosum, stratum lucidum, and stratum corneum.

epigastrium (ep-e-gas′tre-um)—Upper and midparts of the abdomen relating to the position of the stomach.

epiphyseal line (ep-e-fiz′e-al)—The line of junction between the epiphysis and the body of the bone; often confusing in the determination of hairline fractures in this region.

epiphysis (e-pif′is-is)—A process of bone that is attached for a time to the body of the bone by cartilage but that later completely ossifies to the body of the bone. The growth in length of the long bones occurs at this cartilaginous joint before maturity of the individual is reached.

epipteric bone (e-pip-ter′ik)—A wormian (supernumerary) bone in the region of the pterion.

epithelium (ep-e-thē′lē-um)—The type of tissue forming the epidermis.

erg—A unit of work. The work done in moving a body 1 cm against a force of 1 dyne.

erythema (er-e-thē′mah)—A redness of the skin following exposure to certain irritants. It is due to congestion of the capillaries.

erythema dose—The minimum quantity of x- or gamma radiation that will produce the appearance of erythema to a particular part of the integument. The quantity of the dose will vary from part to part on the same individual and among different individuals.

E.S.D.—The abbreviation for the radiographic examination of the esophagus, stomach, and duodenum.

esophagus (e-sof′ah-gus)—That portion of the digestive tract between the pharynx and the stomach.

esu—Abbreviation for electrostatic units.

ethmoid (eth′moid)—One of the bones of the cranial section of the skull; sievelike, perforated.

eversion (e-ver′zhun)—Of the foot, turning the foot outwardly or laterally.

exacerbation (eg-sas-er-ba′shun)—An increase in the severity of any symptoms or disease.

excise (ek-sīz′)—To cut out or off.

excrete (eks-krēt′)—To eliminate by means of a duct, tube, tract, or into a common opening.

excretion pyelography or **urography** (eks-krē′shun)—The radiographic examination of the urinary system following intravenous injection of the radiopaque solution. The solution is eliminated by normal processes.

exhale (eks′hāl)—To breathe out.

exostosis (ek-sos-to′sis)—An abnormal bony or osseous outgrowth from a bone surface.

expiration (eks-pira′shun)—Expelling air from the lungs.

extension (eks-ten′shun)—Straightening out, stretching.

external rotation (eks-ter′nal)—Of the humerus; to rotate the hand laterally with the palm forward in the true—posterior (A-P) position.

extirpate (ek-ster′pāt)—To remove a part completely from the body.

exudate (eks′ū-dāt)—A collection of material that has filtered through the walls of vessels into the surrounding tissues.

F

facet (fas′et)—A small plane surface.

femur (fe′mur)—The largest bone of the body, the thigh bone.

fetus (fe′tus)—The unborn offspring of any viviparous animal; in man, the term applies after the second month.

fibrosis (fi-bro′sis)—Development of fibrous tissue.

film emulsion—A dehydrated emulsion of the silver salts of three of the halogens, bromine, chlorine, and iodine, on a suitable base. The base is composed of either cellulose acetate or one of the newer synthetics, each of which is *safe,* i.e., it generates no poisonous gases when burned.

filter—Usually a 1- or 2-mm-thick sheet of aluminum (Al), placed in the tube housing aperture. It is used to filter out the softer rays and reduce the amount of radiation to the patient's skin.

fission (fish′un)—The act of splitting.

fistula (fis′tu-lah)—A narrow canal or tube left by incomplete healing of a wound, incision, or abscess.

fixer—The solution, commonly called hypo, in which the manifest image is fixed and hardened.

flexion (flek'shun)—The act of bending or contracting.

fluorescence (floo-o-res'ens)—The ability of a chemical (calcium tungstate) to give off light in the presence of an activating source.

fluoroscopy (floo-or-os'ko-pe)—The process of examining the tissues by means of a fluorescent screen.

focal-film distance (ffd)—Distance in inches between the focal spot (target) and the film holder and in line with central ray (C.R.).

focal spot—Commonly called the spot, meaning the area on the anode from which the x-rays radiate.

fog—A general or local deposit of silver or silver compound, formed as the result of exposure to extraneous radiation or by chemical action; it is in addition to the legitimate image. Defined radiographically, fog is undesirable cloudiness of a radiographic image.

foramen fo-rā'men)—Perforation or opening (usually in a bone) through which nerves or blood vessels pass.

fornix (for'niks)—Vaultlike space.

fossa (fos'ah)—A pit or depression.

fracture (frak'tūr)—A breaking; a break in continuity of the margin of a bone.

fracture types:

    bumper—In pedestrians, approximately 2 inches distal to the knee.

    buttonhole—Caused by a flying object knocking an actual hole in a bone.

    Colles'—Of the radius, from ½ to 1 inch above the distal end, with posterior and lateral displacement of the hand.

    comminuted—The bone broken into more than two pieces at one site.

    compound—Puncture of the skin at the fracture site.

    compression—Occurring in the vertebrae, smashing part or all of the bone to a lesser thickness.

    contrecoup—Away from the point of trauma, generally opposite, as on the opposite side of the skull from the point of trauma.

    dentate—The fracture presents a serrated surface.

    double—Two fractures at two locations, one each, in any one bone.

    greenstick—In young persons, one side of the bone remains whole, but the other side is fractured.

    impacted—Usually at one end of a long bone, the end being driven into the adjacent end or surface of another bone.

    incomplete—Similar to greenstick fracture; also a hairline not extending through the entire bone.

    oblique—At an angle other than horizontal or vertical.

    Pott's—In the fibula approximately 3 inches above the distal end, with splitting of the internal malleolus.

    reverse Pott's—In the tibia approximately 3 inches above the distal end, with splitting of the external malleolus.

    simple—A noncomplicated fracture.

    Smith's—Same as Colles' fracture except about 5 cm above the distal end.

    spiral—One complete fracture in a spiral shape around the shaft of the bone.

    spontaneous—Occurring spontaneously, as in bones having pathology.

    ununited—In which there has been no union.

frequency (fre'kwen-se)—In harmonic motions, the number of vibrations or cycles in a unit of time.

fundus (fun'dus)—Base; often located at the top of the organ.

fusion (fū'zhun)—The union or blending of things as if melted together.

G

gamete (gam'ēt)—The mature ovum or spermatozoon.

gamma ray (gam'a)—A type of ray (similar to an x-ray but of shorter wavelength) emitted by certain radioactive substances.

gastro-—A prefix pertaining to the gastric region, especially the stomach.

G.B.—Abbreviation for gallbladder.

gene—One of the hereditary units having a specific location on a chromosome.

genetics (je-net′iks)—The laws of generation and heredity; the branch of biology that deals with heredity and variation among related organisms largely in their evolutionary aspects.

G.I.—Abbreviation for gastrointestinal.

glabella (glah-bel′ah)—A point midway between the supraorbital ridges.

gland—An organ that secretes or excretes a substance that may be beneficial or detrimental to life.

glenoid (gle′noid)—Having the shape of a shallow cavity.

glomerulus (glo-mer′u-lus)—Minute mass of coiled capillaries contained within a Bowman's capsule of the kidney.

glottis (glot′is)—Upper opening of the larynx; the epiglottis is the fibrocartilaginous structure that aids in the prevention of solids and liquids entering the larynx and trachea. The glottis is situated upon the upper border of the larynx and is leaf-shaped.

gluteal (gloo′te-al)—The region of the buttocks.

graininess (grān′i-nes)—A mottling of the radiographic image.

-graphy—A suffix pertaining to a graphic record.

grid—A stationary arrangement of thin lead strips. Grids may be an integral part of the Potter-Bucky diaphragm, in which they move across the table; they may be used as stationary devices between the tube and film holder in situations where a Bucky could not be employed.

H

half-value layer—That thickness of a given metal that reduces the intensity of the x-ray beam, in passing through the metal, to exactly one half.

haustra (haws′trah)—Sacculations of the colon.

haversian system (ha-ver′zhan)—From the English anatomist, Havers; system of small canals in the bones.

heel effect—The cathode end of the x-ray tube has a slightly more visible tendency to make a sharper image than has the anode end.

hema-, hemo-—Prefixes pertaining to the blood.

hemangioma (he-man″je-o′mah)—An angioma consisting of blood vessels.

hematoma (hem-ah-to′mah)—A tumor or swelling containing blood.

hepat-—A prefix pertaining to the liver.

hernia (her′nē-ah)—A protrusion of a part of an organ through an opening.

heterogeneous (het-er-o-je′ne-us)—Composed of different substances.

heterogeneous radiation—Beam of x-rays consisting of many x-rays of different wavelengths.

heterozygous (het″er-o-zī′gus)—Containing both genes of an allelomorphic pair. A mixture of the dominant and recessive factors of any characteristic in one individual with the dominant being in evidence.

hiatus (hi-ā′tus)—Normal perforation through the diaphragm.

hiatus hernia—The protrusion of any structure through the esophageal hiatus of the diaphragm.

hilum (hi′lum)—Point of entrance and exit, into and from the lung and kidney, of the nerves and blood vessels.

homeostasis (ho-me-os′tah-sis)—Maintenance of a steady state, or state of equilibrium, in the internal environment.

homogeneous (ho-mo-je′ne-us)—Of uniform character in all parts.

homozygous (ho-mo-zī′gus)—An organism of like germ cells.

htt, HTT—Abbreviations for high-tension transformer.

hydrolysis (hi-drol′is-is)—The decomposition of water.

hyoid (hi-oid′)—The bone between the root of the tongue and the larynx. The hyoid supports the tongue and gives attachment to its muscles. The hyoid is U shaped.

hyper- (hi′per)—A prefix pertaining to an excess.

hypermotility (hi′per-mo-til′i-te)—Excessive motility.

hypersthenic (hi-per-sthen′ik)—Marked by exalted strength or tonicity.

hypertrophy (hi-per′tro-fe)—Excessive growth or overgrowth.

hypo—*see* Fixer.

hypo-—A prefix pertaining to deficient or beneath.

hypochondrium (hi-po-kon′dre-um)—The region below either costal arch.

hypogastrium (hi-po-gas'tre-um)—The lower region of the abdomen, located anteriorly in the median area.

hypophysis (hi-pof'is-is)—The pituitary gland located in the sella turcica under the hypothalamus.

hyposthenic (hi-po-sthen'ik)—Not well developed; feeble, weak.

hypothenar (hi-poth'e-nar)—The ridge on the palm along the bases of the fingers and the ulnar margin.

I

ileo- (il'e-o)—A prefix pertaining to the ileum.

ileum (il'e-um)—The third part of the small intestine between the jejunum and cecum.

ileus (il'e-us)—An obstruction of the intestine producing severe colic.

ilio- (il'e-o)—A prefix pertaining to the ilium.

ilium (il'e-um)—The proximal part of the innominate bone, one of the bones of the pelvis.

incisura angularis (in-si-su'rah ang-gu-lar'is)—The notch formed in the lesser curvature of the stomach at the angle of the junction of the body and the pyloric third. Peristaltic waves on the lesser curvature become quite pronounced as they pass through the incisura.

induration (in-du-ra'shun)—Hardening of a tissue or part.

infarct (in'farkt)—A wedge-shaped area of either hemorrhage or necrosis into an organ caused by loss of blood supply or obstruction of a terminal vessel.

inferior (in-fe're-or)—Lower or below.

inguinal (ing'gwi-nal)—Pertaining to the thigh or inguinal region.

inhale (in-hāl')—To breathe in.

inherent filter—The filtering effect built into modern, shockproof x-ray tubes. The quantity of filtration must be equivalent to a minimum of 0.5 mm of aluminum.

inion (in'e-on)—The external occipital protuberance.

innominate (in-om'i-nāt)—The so-called unnamed bone of the pelvis, composed of the ilium, ischium, and pubis. Also the name applied to the two veins forming the superior vena cava and to one of the arteries branching off the aortic arch; the brachiocephalic trunk.

inspiration (in-spi-ra'shun)—The drawing in of the breath.

insufflation (in-suf-fla'shun)—The blowing of air into a cavity.

intensification factor—The quantity of intensification, expressed numerically as light energy, of the applied source of energy when it passes through the screen emulsion. To find the factor of intensification of an unknown screen: expose a plain film in cardboard with the regular factors; expose an identical film in the cassette containing the unknown screens and using the same factors and object. When the films are dry, place them on an illuminator and check the over-all density, or light transmission, with a light meter or intensimeter. Give a value of 1.0 to the quantity of light transmitted through the plain film that was exposed in the cardboard holder.

intensifying screen—A dehydrated emulsion of certain chemicals (usually calcium tungstate) which fluoresce in the presence of x-rays. The emulsion of calcium tungstate is coated upon a suitable base (usually cardboard). Barium platinocyanide and zinc sulfate are also used.

intermediate—The term applied to tissues that are between radiopaque and radiolucent in regard to x-ray penetration.

internal rotation (in-ter'nal)—Of the humerus; to rotate the hand medially with the palm facing laterally.

intima (in'te-mah)—The lining of blood vessels.

intussusception (in"tus-sus-sep'shun)—The invagination or indigitation of a portion of the intestine into an adjacent portion.

inversion (in-ver'zhun)—Of the foot, turning of the foot inwardly or medially.

ion (i'on)—An atom or group of atoms carrying an electric charge, formed by the dissociation of a dissolved molecule by the action of a solvent.

ionization (i-on-i-za'shun)—Electrolytic dissociation; the production of ions. An atom is said to be ionized when an electron is either gained or lost.

ischium (is'ke-um)—The inferior and posterior part of the innominate bone.

isobar (i'so-bar)—One of two or more chemical elements that have identical atomic weights but different atomic numbers.

isotope (i'so-tōp)—Of a collection of atoms of a given element (having the same number of protons), those atoms possessing a different number of neutrons are the different isotopes of the element.

-itis—A suffix pertaining to inflammation or irritation of some specific tissue, gland, or organ.

I.V.P.—Abbreviation for intravenous pyelography, the injection of a radiopaque solution into one of the antecubital veins. The opacifying medium enters the kidneys via normal circulation, and the calyces, pelves, ureters, and bladder of the urinary system are visualized.

J

jaundice (jawn′dis)—Yellow discoloration of the skin, mucous membranes, and excretions as a result of bile pigments in the blood.

jejunum (je-joo′num)—The second part of the small intestine beginning at the terminal end of the duodenum and terminating at the junction with the ileum.

K

karyokinesis (kar″e-o-ki-ne′sis)—Mitosis.

keloid (ke′loid)—A new growth or tumor of the skin, consisting of whitish ridges, nodules, and plates of dense tissue.

kilovolt (kv) (kil′o-volt)—1,000 volts.

K.U.B.—Abbreviation for radiograph of the kidneys, ureters, and bladder.

kv—Abbreviation for kilovolt or kilovoltage.

kvp—Abbreviation for peak kilovolt or kilovoltage; the peak kilovoltage used in making any x-ray exposure.

kyphosis (ki-fo′sis)—The condition called humpback; convexity turned dorsally.

L

L—Abbreviation for left or left side.

labium (la′be-um)—A lip.

laceration (las-er-a′shun)—A tear, a jagged wound.

lacrimal (lak′re-mal)—One of the bones of the facial section of the skull. Pertaining to tears.

lacteal (lak′te-al)—Lymph vessels that carry the milky-appearing chyle.

lacuna (lah-koo′nah)—A minute cavity of bone or cartilage.

lambdoid (lam′doid)—A suture between the occiput, parietal, and temporal bones; similar in shape to the Greek letter lambda.

lamella (lah-mel′ah)—A small plate or thin layer.

L.A.O.—Abbreviation for left anterior oblique.

larynx (lar′inks)—The voice box. The cartilaginous portion of the air passages extending from the base of the tongue to the trachea.

latent image (la′tent)—The invisible image in the x-ray film emulsion of the radiographed object caused by the remnant rays.

lateral—Outside surface, i.e., outside of the leg, away from the midsagittal plane.

latitude (lat′i-tūd)—The range in exposure factors that will produce a diagnostic radiographic image; the extent of variation between maximum and minimum density in a radiograph consistent with the diagnostic quality of the radiograph. Radiographic latitude increases with *long-scale* contrast.

lobe (lōb)—A division of the lungs, liver, and brain.

lordosis (lor-do′sis)—Curvature of the spine with the convexity forward.

L.P.O.—Abbreviation for left posterior oblique.

lumen (loo′men)—The cavity or hollow space in an organ or tube.

luxation (luks-a′shun)—The displacement of any part, especially of a bone.

lymph (limf)—The clear fluid of the lymphatic system.

-lysis (li′sis)—A suffix meaning gradual decline of a fever; splitting or destruction of a substance or cell.

M

ma—Abbreviation for milliampere or milliamperage.

magnification (mag′ni-fi-ka″shun)—The symmetrical enlargement of the image on the radiograph.

malar (ma′lar)—The malar bone, same as the zygoma.

malignant (mah-lig′nant)—Virulent, compromising or threatening life.

malingerer (mah-ling′ger-er)—One who feigns illness.

mammary gland (mam′a-re)—One of the two or more large compound glands, characteristic of the Mammalia, which, in the female, secrete milk for the nourishment ,of the young.

mandible (man′di-bl)—The bone of the lower jaw.

manifest image (man′i-fest)—Visible image in the film emulsion after the reducing action of the developer.

manubrium (man-oo′bre-um)—The first part of the sternum; a handle.

mas, Ma.S.—Abbreviation for milliampere-seconds. The result of multiplying milliamperes by the time in seconds.

mastectomy (mas-tek′to-me)—Excision of the breast. A *simple mastectomy* is a surgical procedure in which only the mammary gland is removed; a *radical mastectomy* is a surgical procedure in which all of the related lymph glands, nodes, and ducts are removed in addition to the mammary gland.

mastoid (mas′toid)—Part of the temporal bone; shaped like a breast.

maxilla (mak-sil′ah)—The bone of the upper jaw.

maximum tissue differentiation—The ultimate in diagnostic quality of any film, present only when each of the controlling factors is present in its utmost degree. The two major factors are sharpness (definition) and visibility of detail.

meatus (me-a′tus)—An opening or passage.

Meckel's diverticulum—The proximal vestigial portion of the vitelline duct; a small pouch averaging 5 cm in length and located at varying distances—from a few cm to as much as 4 feet—proximal to the ileocecal valve in the lower part of the ileum. It is found in about 2% of all subjects examined.

medial (me′de-al)—Middle side as opposed to lateral, i.e., inside of leg; toward the midsagittal plane.

mediastinum (me′de-as-tī″num)—Midspace of the thoracic cavity, containing the following viscera: bronchi, ascending aorta, aortic arch, upper part of the descending aorta, inferior vena cava, esophagus, thoracic duct, lymphatic duct, and azygos veins.

medulla (me-dul′ah)—The central part of a gland or organ.

medullary canal (med′u-lar-e)—The central canal of the shaft of any long bone; carries the nutritive and nervous supplies; the marrow.

meiosis (mi-o′sis)—The reduction division preceding the formation of gametes, in which the chromosome pairs separate and the chromosome number is reduced to half the somatic number.

meninges (me-nin′jēz)—The membranes of the brain and spinal cord.

mesial (me′se-al)—Medial.

metabolism (me-tab′o-lizm)—Life processes; the chemical changes associated with the assimilation of energy materials into cell protoplasm and the elimination of the waste products of cellular activity. A combination of the processes of anabolism and catabolism.

metacarpus (met-ah-kar′pus)—The bones of the hand.

metaphysis (me-taf′is-is)—The line of junction of the epiphysis with the diaphysis of a long bone; the epiphyseal line.

metastasis (me-tas′tah-sis)—The translocation of disease from its primary site to a secondary site via the blood or lymph. From the Greek word meaning "to transpose."

metatarsus (met-ah-tar′sus)—The bones of the foot.

micturate (mik′tu-rāt)—To urinate.

midaxillary line (mid-ak′sil-ar-e)—An imaginary line drawn or extending from the axilla to the crest of the ilium.

milliampere (ma) (mil″e-am-pēr′)—1/1,000 part of an ampere.

mitosis (mi-to′sis)—Indirect cell division.

mitral valve (mi′tral)—The left atrioventricular valve of the heart, shaped like a miter.

molecule (mol′e-kūl)—The smallest quantity into which a substance can be divided and retain its characteristics and characteristic properties.

moribund (mor′e-bund)—In a dying state.

morula (mor′u-lah)—The segmented ovum in the mulberry stage.

M.P.D.—Abbreviation for the maximum permissible dose.

multipara (mul-tip'ah-rah)—A woman who has given birth to two or more children.

mutant (mu'tant)—An individual showing a permanent transmitted change in its characteristics from those of its parents.

mutation (mu-ta'shun)—A variation from the parent stock that breeds true in future generations.

myelo- (mi'el-o)—A prefix indicating relationship with the spinal cord or bone marrow.

myelogram (mi'el-o-gram)—A radiograph of the spinal cord or a part of it after opacification.

myo-—A prefix pertaining to muscle.

myxedema (mik-se-de'mah)—A condition resulting from hypothyroidism.

N

naris (na'ris)—The nostril.

nasal (na'zal)—The bone of the nose; also pertaining to the nose.

nasion (na'ze-on)—The median point of the nasofrontal suture.

navicular (na-vik'u-lar)—A bone of the tarsus; boat shaped.

necropsy (nek'rop-se)—A post-mortem examination.

necrosis (ne-kro'sis)—The death of a portion of tissue.

neoplasm (ne'o-plazm)—Any new and abnormal growth, such as a tumor.

nephro- (nef'ro)—The prefix pertaining to the kidney.

neural (nū'ral)—Pertaining to the nerves.

neuro- (nū'ro)—A prefix pertaining to the nerves.

neutron (nū'tron)—An atomic particle having the same weight as a proton of the same atom but having no electric charge.

node (nōd)—A knob or protuberance.

no-screen film—An x-ray film with a different and faster speed emulsion than the emulsion of plain film. It is used in cardboard holders for radiographing thin parts (less than 13 cm) where great detail and contrast are desired.

nucha (nu'kah)—The nape of the neck.

nucleus (nu'kle-us)—The essential part or positive particle (atomic) of any atom carrying a positive charge. It may consist of a single proton, or protons, or protons and neutrons.

O

obese (o-bēs')—Extremely fat, corpulent.

ofd, OFD—Abbreviation for object-film distance.

oblique (ob-līk', ob-lēk')—Angular view of a surface or object, not a true posterior (A-P) or lateral position; toward the midsagittal plane.

occiput (ok'si-put)—A bone of the cranial section of the skull; forms the posterior portion and base of the skull.

occlusal plane (ok-klu'sal)—The plane of the masticating surfaces of the molar and bicuspid teeth of the upper and lower jaws when the jaws are closed.

occlusion (ok-klu'shun)—Complete meeting or meshing of the teeth of the upper and lower jaws.

occult (ok-kult')—Hidden or concealed.

odonto- (o-don'to)—A prefix pertaining to a tooth, or meaning like a tooth.

odontoid process (o-don'toid)—Process of the second cervical vertebral body, which extends superiorly through the bony ring of the atlas.

O.G.C.—Abbreviation for oral Graham-Cole.

ohm (ōm)—The unit of electric resistance.

olecranon process (o-lek'rah-non)—The large bony process located proximally on the ulna.

omentum (o-men'tum)—The fold of the peritoneum connected with the stomach.

oocyte (o'o-sīt)—An immature ovum.

oral Graham Cole—A method of administration of gallbladder contrast medium.

organ (or'gan)—Any part of the body having a definite function to perform.

orifice (or'i-fis)—An opening or aperture.

orthodiagraphy (or"tho-di-ag'rah-fe)—The radiographic examination and study of the internal organs to record and measure the size and location.

os—Bone; mouth.

-osis (o-sis)—A suffix indicating condition caused by, or presence of.

osmosis (os-mo'sis)—The movement of substances of different concentrations in solution through a semipermeable membrane.

osseous (os'e-us)—Bony.

ossification (os″e-fi-ka'shun)—Bone formation, growth.

osteo- (os'te-o)—A prefix pertaining to a bone.

osteoblast (os'te-o-blast)—Any one of the cells of mesoblastic origin concerned in the formation of bony tissue.

osteoclast (os'te-o-klast)—A large multinuclear cell found against the surface of bone in small eroded depressions concerned in the removal of bone.

osteocyte (os'te-o-sīt)—A mature bone cell.

osteogenesis (os″te-o-jen'e-sis)—The development of bony tissue.

osteolith (os'te-o-lith)—Petrified bone.

osteology (oste-ol'o-je)—The science of anatomy and the structure of bones.

osteomyelitis (os″te-o-mi-e-li'tis)—Inflammation or infection of bone marrow.

osteoporosis (os″te-o-po-ro'sis)—Abnormal porosity or rarefaction of bone by the enlargement of its canals or the formation of abnormal spaces.

-ostomy (os'to-me)—A suffix pertaining to the surgical removal of a diseased tissue.

oto-—A prefix denoting relationship to the ear.

ovum (o'vum)—The female germ cell.

P

P-A—Abbreviation for posteroanterior (anterior) position or projection.

palatine (pal'ah-tīn)—One of the bones of the facial section of the skull; also a process of the maxilla.

palliate (pal'ē-āt)—To reduce the severity of; to relieve.

palliative therapy (pal'e-a-tiv)—To afford relief but not to cure.

palmar (pah'mar)—Palm surface of the hand.

para-—A prefix pertaining to a place beyond.

paracentesis (par″ah-sen-te'sis)—The puncture of the wall of a cavity of the body.

paralysis (pah-ral'is-is)—Loss or impairment of motor function in a part due to lesion of the neural or muscular mechanism.

paraplasm (par'ah-plazm)—The more fluid, finely granular substance of the cytoplasm of cells.

patella (pah-tel'ah)—Kneecap; largest sesamoid bone in the body, the only sesamoid necessary for normal function.

patent (pā'tent)—Open or exposed.

path—Abbreviation for the pathology.

pathology (pah-thol'o-je)—The branch of medical science dealing with the modifications of functions and changes in structure caused by disease.

P.E., PE, or pe—Abbreviation for photographic effect.

peak kilovoltage—The peak kilovoltage used in making any x-ray exposure.

pelvic straits (pel'vik strates)

    inferior—The plane of the pelvic outlet. The anteroposterior diameter extends from the tip of the coccyx to the subpubic ligament and is 9.5 cm. The transverse diameter extends between the ischial tuberosities and is 11 cm.

    superior—The plane of the pelvic inlet. The anteroposterior, or conjugate, diameter extends from the superior border of the first sacral vertebra to a point ⅛ inch inferior to the superior border of the symphysis pubis and is 11 cm. The transverse diameter at the widest point is 13.5 cm.

pelvimetry (pel-vim'e-tre)—A method of measurement of the size of the bony pelvis.

peri-—A prefix meaning surrounding or around.

pericardium (per-e-kar'de-um)—The closed membranous sac enveloping the heart.

perineum (per-i-ne'um)—The area of the body bounded anteriorly by the pubic arch, posteriorly by the coccyx, and bilaterally by the ischial tuberosities.

periosteum (per-e-os'te-um)—The fibrous membrane covering bone surfaces except at points of tendinous and ligamentous attachment and articular surfaces.

peristalsis (per-e-stal'sis)—The peculiar wavelike contractions of tubular structures as in the digestive tract.

peritoneum (per"i-to-ne"um)—The serous membrane lining the abdomen and surrounding the viscera.

pH—A shortened term introduced by Sörenson to avoid confusion; refers to a total dissociation of ions always totaling 14. As the hydrogen ions increase, the hydroxyl ions decrease in inverse ratio. pH is based on the hydrogen ion concentration. A pH of 7.0 is neutral, the ions of both hydrogen and hydroxyl radicals being even. Any value above 7.0 is alkaline or base, and any value below 7.0 is acidic.

phalanx (fa'lanks)—One of the bones of the fingers or toes.

pharynx (far'inks)—The throat. The musculomembranous pouch situated posteriorly to the nose, mouth, and larynx.

phleboliths (fleb'o-liths)—Small rounded calcium deposits in the walls of veins.

phosphorescence (fos-fo-res'ens)—The ability of a chemical (zinc sulfate) to continue to give off light after the activating source has ceased.

photographic effect (**P.E., PE, pe**)—The ability of a source of energy to cause a latent image formation in the film emulsion in the shape or image of the object through which or from which the energy rays pass to the film.

photon (fo'ton)—A quantum of gamma radiation or light; also used in reference to x-ray.

phrenic (fren'ik)—Pertaining to the diaphragm.

physics (fiz'iks)—The science of matter and forces.

pia mater (pi'ah ma'ter)—The innermost membrane of the meninges containing the blood supply; tender mother.

pkv—Abbreviation for peak kilovoltage.

placenta previa (plah-sen'tah pre've-a)—A placenta that develops in the lower uterine segment, in the zone of dilatation, so that it covers or adjoins the internal os.

placentography (plas-en-tog'rah-fe)—Radiologic visualization of the placenta after the injection of a contrast medium.

plain film—The term denoting the type film most commonly used in cassettes having intensifying screens.

planigram (pla'ne-gram)—A roentgenogram of a selected layer of the body made by planigraphy.

plantar (plan'tar)—The sole surface of the foot.

pleura (ploor'ah)—The serous membrane surrounding the lungs.

pneumoperitoneum (nu"mo-per-i-to-ne'um)—The presence of air or gas in the peritoneal cavity.

pneumothorax (nū-mo-tho'raks)—The presence of air or gas in the pleural cavity.

P-O—Abbreviation for postoperative.

polyp (pol'ip)—A smooth, pedunculated growth from a mucous surface, as of the nose, bladder, rectum, etc. Polyps are the result of hypertrophy of the mucous membrane, or are true tumors.

positron (pos'i-tron)—An atomic particle having the same mass as an electron but having a positive electric charge.

post-—A prefix meaning behind or following.

posterior (pōs-te're-or)—Nearest the back or rear.

pre-—A prefix meaning in front of or preceding.

primipara (pri-mip'ah-rah)—A woman who has given birth to her first child.

proc-, procto-—Prefixes pertaining to the rectum.

pronate (pro'nāt)—Lying prone or face down.

pronation (pro-na'shun)—The act of being in the prone position; of the hand, with the palm down.

prone (prōn)—Lying with the anterior or ventral surface of the face down.

prosthesis (pros'the-sis)—Replacement of a missing part by an artificial substitute.

proteolysis (pro-te-ol'is-is)—Ferments which change proteins into diffusible bodies.

proton (pro'ton)—The nuclear positive corpuscle of electricity.

protoplasm (pro'to-plazm)—The viscid material that constitutes the essential substance of living cells upon which all the vital functions of nutrition, secretion, growth, reproduction, irritability, and motility depend.

proximal (prok'si-mal)—Nearest the body or origin.

ptosis (tŏ'sis)—Dropping, prolapse, or abnormal depression.

pubis (pu'bis)—One of the innominate bones.

pyelography (pi-el-og'rah-fe)—The radiographic examination of the renal pelves, ureters, and bladder after opacification with a suitable radiopaque solution.

pyknic (pik'nik)—Having a short, thick, stocky build.

pylorus (pi-lo'rus)—The muscular and circular opening of the stomach into the duodenum.

pyo-—A prefix pertaining to pus.

pyogenic (pi-o-jen'ik)—Producing pus.

Q

Q.S.—Quantity sufficient to fill to volume.

quadrate (kwod'rāt)—Four-sided.

quantum (kwon'tum)—An elemental unit of energy according to the quantum theory. Its value is $h\nu$, where h is Planck's constant (6.62×10^{-27}), and ν is the frequency of the vibrations or waves with which the energy is associated.

R

R—Abbreviation for right or right side.

r—Abbreviation for roentgen unit.

rad—The unit of absorbed x-ray dose; its quantity is 100 ergs per gram.

radiation (ra-de-a'shun)—The act of radiating or diverging from a central point, such as light rays radiate from a source of light.

radioactive fallout (ra″de-o-ak'tiv)—The dust and other debris rendered radioactive by nuclear fission or neutron bombardment that settles out of the atmosphere while the material is still highly active.

radiograph (ra'de-o-graf)—A permanent photographic record of the structures through which a beam of ionizing radiation has passed.

radiographer (ra″de-og'rah-fer)—A person who is skilled in the art of producing radiographs.

radiographic quality—The characteristic summation of the various factors that combine to produce a radiograph.

radiography (ra″de-og'rah-fe)—The science and art of producing radiographs and skiagraphs.

radiologist (ra-de-ol'o-jist)—A physician who has had specialized training in the use of radiant energy for treatment and diagnosis; this includes x-rays, radium, etc.

radiology (ra-de-ol'o-je)—The science of radiant energy.

radiolucent (ra-de-o-lu'sent)—Permitting the passage of radiant energy or waves.

radiopaque (ra-de-o-pak')—Not permitting the passage of radiant energy or waves.

radius (ra'de-us)—The lateral bone of the forearm.

ramus (ra'mus)—A branch; slender process of bone projecting from the main part.

R.A.O.—Abbreviation for right anterior oblique.

Reid's base line—A line from the infraorbital ridge to the external auditory meatus and the middle line of the occiput.

rem—The abbreviation for roentgen-equivalent-man.

remnant radiation (rem'nant)—That ionizing radiation that produces the radiographic image.

renal (re'nal)—Pertaining to the kidney.

rep—The abbreviation for roentgen-equivalent-physical.

replenisher (re-plen'ish-er)—Solutions for replenishing and strengthening and prolonging the life of the developer and fixer. There is a specific replenisher for each of the two solutions.

retro-—A prefix indicating back or backward.

retrograde pyelography (ret'ro-grād)—Radiography of the renal calyces, pelves, ureters, and bladder after opacification has been accomplished by injection via the urethra.

retrograde urography (ū-rog'rah-fe)—Radiography of the urinary bladder after injection of opacifying material via the urethra.

rickets (rik'ets)—Malformation of bone and cartilage as a result of vitamin D deficiency in the diet.

rigor mortis (rig'or mor'tis)—The muscular rigidity that occurs following death.

roentgen unit—The unit of measure of x-ray; the amount of conductivity of 1 ml of atmospheric air (at saturation) at 0° C. and 760 mm of mercury pressure, exclusive of the wall effect of the chamber.

roentgen-meter—A device that incorporates the principle of a gold-leaf galvanometer to measure a given amount of radiation or r. Radiation causes ionization. Ionization causes an increase in conductivity or electric charges in air.

roentgenologist (rent-gen-ol'o-jist)—A physician who has had specialized training in the use of x-rays.

R.P.O.—Abbreviation meaning right posterior oblique.

ruga (roo'gah)—A fold of the mucosa in the stomach, visible radiographically after barium ingestion.

S

s—The symbol indicating without.

sacrum (sā'krum)—A curved triangular bone composed of five united segments situated between the fifth lumbar vertebra above and the coccyx below and the innominates on each side, and forming the posterior boundary of the pelvis.

sagittal plane (saj'i-tal)—A vertical plane extending from anterior to posterior direction and separating right from left.

sandbags—Bags of sand (or rice) of various sizes and shapes used for immobilization of the part to be x-rayed.

scapula (skap'ū-lah)—The large, flat, triangular bone forming the back of the shoulder.

scattered radiation—Secondary rays. They may be of the same wavelength, or longer, than the primary. They may be characteristic fluorescent rays.

Schmorl's nodule (schmorlz)—A nodule seen in roentgenograms of the spine, due to prolapse of a nucleus pulposus into an adjoining vertebra.

sclerosis (skle-ro'sis)—Hardening.

scoliosis (sko-le-o'sis)—Morbid lateral curvature of the spine.

screen speed—A term used to describe the speed of intensification of the applied energy as it passes through the screen emulsion.

secondary rays—The rays that are generated in the patient as the x-rays pass through the patient.

secrete (se-krēt')—To manufacture a substance and discharge it directly into the bloodstream.

sella turcica (sel'ah tur'si-kah)—The saddle-shaped fossa in the sphenoid wherein is located the pituitary gland.

semilunar (sem-e-loo'nar)—Half-moon shaped.

sepsis (sep'sis)—Poisoning caused by the products of a putrefactive process.

septum (sep'tum)—A partition or division wall.

sequela (se-kwe'lah)—Any lesion or affection following or caused by an attack of disease.

sequestrum (se-kwes'trum)—A detached or dead piece of bone within a cavity, abscess, or wound.

serrate (ser'āt)—Shaped like a sawtooth.

sesamoid (ses'ah-moid)—A small bone shaped like a grain; auxiliary bones found at articular surfaces, especially in the manus or pedis. The patella is the largest of these.

sfd, SFD—Abbreviation for skin-film distance.

Sharpey's fibers (shar'pēz)—The collagenous fibers forming the lamellae that constitute the walls of the haversian canals in bone; same as osteogenic fibers.

sigmoid (sig'moid)—S shaped.

sinus (sī'nus)—A normal cavity in a bone or organ; pathologically in tissues and normally containing pus.

solarization (so'ler-i-za"shun)—A process of transferring the manifest image from a radiograph as either a negative or a positive image to another film by employing either sun or artificial light. A reversal of gradation sequence in the image (usually very dense) obtained on the normal development of films, plates, and papers after giving a very intense or long-continued exposure. A greater exposure than this appears to restore the original sequence of gradation, and a still greater one has been stated to bring about a second reversal.

somatic (so-mat'ik)—Body cells exclusive of germ cells.

sp.gr.—Abbreviation for specific gravity; the weight of a substance judged in comparison with that of a specific standard, usually distilled water at 20° C. and 760 mm of mercury pressure.

spermatocyte (sper′mah-to-sīt)—The parent cell of a spermatid.

spermatozoon (sper″mah-to-zo′on)—A mature male germ cell.

sphenoid (sfen′oid)—Wedge shaped; one of the bones of the cranial section of the skull.

sphincter (sfingk′ter)—A muscle that closes an orifice.

sphygmomanometer (sfig″mo-mah-nom′e-ter)—An instrument for measuring blood pressure.

spina bifida occulta (spi′nah bif′i-da o-kul′ta)—A congenital cleft in the neural arch that is hidden or that has no visible protrusion of the spinal membranes.

splenic (splen′ik)—Pertaining to the spleen.

spondylolisthesis (spon″di-lo-lis-the′sis)—Forward displacement of one vertebra over another, especially pertaining to a separation of the fifth lumbar vertebra from and a slipping forward on the first sacral vertebra.

squamous (skwa′mus)—Flat, or scale shaped.

stasis (sta′sis)—A standing still or stoppage of movement or flow.

stenosis (ste-no′sis)—The narrowing or constriction of a passage.

sterile (ster′il)—Not fertile, infertile, barren; not producing young. Aseptic; not producing microorganisms; free from microorganisms.

sternum (ster′num)—The breastbone. There are three parts: manubrium, handle or first part; body or gladiolus, midportion; xiphoid (xyphoid) process, distal portion.

sthenic (sthen′ik)—Active, strong.

styloid (sti′loid)—Pointed like a stylus.

sub-—A prefix meaning beneath.

subarachnoid space (sub-ah-rak′noid)—The space beneath the arachnoid membrane, which is filled with cerebrospinal fluid.

subluxation (sub-luk-sa′shun)—Incomplete luxation, sprain.

substance (sub′stans)—A solid body; a material object as distinguished from something visionary or shadowy. Any particular kind of matter, whether element, compound, or mixture; any chemical material of which bodies are composed; some authorities restrict a substance to elements and compounds.

sulcus (sul′kus)—A groove or narrow depression.

super-—A prefix meaning above.

superior (su-pe′re-or)—Proximal, upper border or surface.

supination (su-pi-na′shun)—In relation to the hand, the palm turned upward.

supine (su′pīn′)—Lying with the face or ventral surface upward.

suppuration (sup-u-ra′shun)—Pus formation.

supra-—A prefix meaning above.

sustentaculum tali (sus-ten-tak′u-lum ta′li)—A process of the calcaneus that supports the talus.

suture line (su′tūr)—A line of joining or closure.

symphysis (sim′fi-sis)—A line of junction of two bones.

synapsis (si-nap′sis)—The conjugation of homologous chromosomes during meiosis.

syndrome (sin′drom)—A typical set of conditions which characterize a deficiency or disease.

synovia (si-no′ve-ah)—The clear fluid secreted within the synovial membrane.

synovial (si-no′ve-al)—Pertaining to the synovia.

systole (sis′to-le)—The heart at work, or the heart and arteries in a stage of contraction.

T

talus (ta′lus)—The second largest bone of the tarsus, the major weight-supporting bone of the body.

target-film distance (tfd, **TFD**)—The distance in inches between the x-ray tube anode and the film.

target-skin distance (tsd, **TSD**)—The distance in inches between the x-ray tube anode and the skin of the patient. It is used more frequently in x-ray therapy than in radiography.

tarsus (tahr′sus)—The bones of the ankle.

technical (tek′ni-kal)—Of or pertaining to the useful or mechanic arts or to any science, business, profession, sport, or the like; specially appropriate to any art, science, or business.

technique (tek-něk'), **technic** (tek'nik)—*see* technical.

teleroentgenography (tel"e-rent-gen-og'rah-fe)—Radiography at a long target-film distance, usually 6 feet, and of the chest, to avoid magnification.

tenaculum (te-nak'u-lum)—A hooklike instrument for seizing and holding parts.

tetanus (tet'ah-nus)—Sustained contraction of a muscle.

tetany (tet'ah-ne)—A syndrome manifested by sharp flexion of the wrist and ankle joints, cramps, muscle twitchings, and convulsions.

tfd, TFD—Abbreviations for target-film distance.

thalamus (thal'ah-mus)—A mass of gray matter at the base of the brain.

thenar (thē'nar)—The fleshy prominence of the palm of the hand corresponding to the thumb base.

therapeutic dose (ther-ah-pū'tik)—A curative dose.

thermionic emission (ther-me-on'ik e-mish'un)—Release of electrons from the cathode filament by heat.

thoracentesis (tho"rah-sen-te'sis)—Surgical puncture or tapping of the chest wall.

thoracic (tho-ras'ik)—Pertaining to or situated in the chest or thorax.

thoracoplasty (tho-ra'ko-plas-te)—A plastic operation on the thorax.

Thoraeus filter (tho're-us)—A filter used for x-ray therapy. Composition: tin, copper, and aluminum. This kind of filter is used primarily in deep therapy.

thrombus (throm'bus)—A clot of blood formed within the heart or vessels.

thymus (thī'mus)—A ductless glandlike body situated in the anterosuperior part of the mediastinum.

thyroid (thī'roid)—One of the endocrine glands, situated anterior to the trachea.

thyroxin, thyroxine (thi-rok'sin)—The secretion of the thyroid gland; a hormone that is important in iodine metabolism.

tissue (tis'ū)—A group of cells of similar origin, structure, and function.

tomography (to-mog'rah-fe)—A special technique to show in detail images of structures lying in a predetermined plane of tissue, while blurring or eliminating detail in images of structures in other planes.

tonus (tō' nus)—The state of mild contraction exhibited by all healthy muscles.

torsion (tor'shun)—Twisting.

trabecula (trah-bek'u-lah)—A small beam or line visible radiographically in bones. Any one of the fibrous bands extending from the capsule into the interior of an organ.

trachea (tra'ke-ah)—The windpipe.

tragus (tra'gus)—The small prominence of cartilage projecting over the meatus of the external ear.

transformer (trans-for'mer)—An electric device for increasing or decreasing the incoming voltage.

transverse (trans-vers')—At right angles to the longitudinal axis of the body.

trauma (traw'mah)—A wound or injury.

Trendelenburg position (tren-del'en-berg)—A recumbent position of the patient on the table; the patient is usually supine, with the pelvis above the head.

trigone (tri'gōn)—The triangular-shaped area on the floor of the urinary bladder formed by the two ureteral orifices and the urethral orifice.

trochlea (trōk'le-ah)—Grooved convexity at the distal end of the humerus for articulation of the sigmoid of the olecranon process of the ulna.

tsd, TSD—Abbreviations for target-skin distance.

tube target—The target of the anode, usually made of tungsten embedded in a copper block. This is the part of the x-ray tube bombarded by the electron beams to produce x-rays.

tubercle (tu'ber-kl)—A small bony projection; a small nodule.

tuberosity (tu-ber-os'i-te)—A large bony projection.

tuft (tuft)—The terminal end of the terminal phalanx.

U

U.G.I.—The abbreviation for an upper gastrointestinal study.

ulna (ul'nah)—The medial bone of the forearm.

umbilicus (um-bi-li′kus, umbil′i-cus)—The navel; the round, depressed cicatrix in the median line of the abdomen; the former site of attachment of the umbilical cord.

ureter (u-rē′ter)—The tube that conveys the urine from the kidney to the bladder.

urethra (u-rē′thrah)—Canal through which the urine is eliminated from the bladder.

uterus (u′ter-us)—The pear-shaped, muscular organ of the female reproductive system wherein the fetus is developed.

uvula (u′vu-lah)—The median, posterior tip of the soft palate.

V

vagina (vah-ji′nah)—Sheath; passageway from the cervix (neck) of the uterus to the vulva.

varicose vein (var′e-kōs)—An abnormally swollen and tortuous vein.

vascular (vas′ku-lar)—Containing numerous blood vessels.

vein (vān)—A blood vessel carrying blood from the tissues to the heart.

velocity (ve-los′i-te)—The ration of displacement to the time required for this displacement. Time rate of motion in a given direction and sense. Average velocity equals the total distance passed over, divided by the whole time taken.

vena cava (ve′nah ca′vah)—A very large hollow vein.

ventral (ven′tral)—Anterior or front.

ventricle (ven′tre-k′l)—A small cavity or pouch.

ventriculography (ven-trik-u-log′rah-fe)—The radiographic examination of the skull after replacement of a specific quantity of spinal fluid with air or gas.

vertebra (ver′te-brah)—Any one of the bones that comprise the spinal column.

vertebra prominens (prom′i-nens)—The seventh cervical vertebra.

vertex (ver′teks)—The crown of the head; a summit or top.

vestigial (ves-tij′e-al)—Rudimentary; a trace remaining.

villus (vil′us)—Vascular, fingerlike projection of the digestive mucosa.

viscera (vis′er-ah)—Plural of viscus.

viscus (vis′kus) (pl. **viscera**)—Any organ that is enclosed within one of the three great cavities.

vitelline duct (vi-tel′in)—The duct of communication between the yolk sac and the primitive digestive tube in the early stages of fetal life.

vitelline membrane—The external envelope of the ovum.

vitreous (vit′re-us)—Hard and glasslike; hyaline.

void (void)—To cast out as waste matter, as in voiding urine.

volar (vo′lar)—The palm surface of the forearm.

volt—The unit of electric pressure or electromotive force; the force necessary to cause 1 ampere of current to flow against 1 ohm of resistance.

vt, VT—Abbreviations for valve tube.

vulva (vul′vah)—The external female genitalia, composed of the labia majora and minora.

W

watt—The unit of electric power, the result of multiplying volts times amperes.

wavelength—The distance between the peaks or troughs of any two adjacent and like waves.

wormian bones (wer′me-an)—Small supernumerary bones in the skull sutures; those found in the region of the pterion are called epipteric bones.

wound (wōōnd)—A rupture of the continuity of an inner or outer surface of the body.

X

X chromosome—One of the sex chromosomes.

xeroradiography (ze-ro-ra″de-og′rah-fe)—From the Greek word xeros meaning "dry"; physical, rather than chemical, production of a permanent radiograph; production of radiographs without the use of water and other solutions.

xiphoid (zif′oid)—Sword shaped; the distal portion of the sternum.

x-ray—The rays discovered by Dr. Roentgen on Nov. 8, 1895. The roentgen (r) is the unit of measurement. The quantity of roentgen radiation (x-rays) which, when the secondary electrons are fully utilized and the wall effect of the chamber is avoided, produces in 1 ml of atmospheric air at 0° C. and 760 mm of mercury pressure such a degree of conductivity that one electrostatic unit is measured at saturation point. (Actually, it amounts to the degree of ionization produced in 1 ml of air by exposing the chamber to x-rays.)

x-rays—One form of energy released from an x-ray tube as a result of the sudden deceleration, or sudden deceleration and stoppage, of high-speed electrons by a suitable target.

xrt, XRT—Abbreviations for x-ray tube.

Y

Y chromosome—Male sex chromosome in human beings.

Z

zoology (zo-ol′o-je)—The science of animal life.

zygoma (zī-go′mah)—One of the bones of the facial section of the skull.

zygote (zī′gōt)—The fertilized ovum before cleavage.

Index

Asterisk (*) following term indicates location in Glossary (pp. 441-462)